American Cancer Society
Atlas of
Clinical Oncology

Series Volumes

American Cancer Society
Atlas of
Clinical Oncology

Editors

GLENN D. STEELE JR, MD
University of Chicago

THEODORE L. PHILLIPS, MD
University of California

BRUCE A. CHABNER, MD
Harvard Medical School

Managing Editor

TED S. GANSLER, MD, MBA
Director of Health Content, American Cancer Society

American Cancer Society

Atlas of
Clinical Oncology

Cancer of the Lower Gastrointestinal Tract

Christopher G. Willett, MD

Department of Radiation Oncology
Massachusetts General Hospital
Professor
Harvard Medical School
Boston, Massachusetts

2001
B.C. Decker Inc.
Hamilton • London

B.C. Decker Inc.
20 Hughson Street South
P.O. Box 620, L.C.D. 1
Hamilton, Ontario L8N 3K7
Tel: 905-522-7017; 1-800-568-7281
Fax: 905-522-7839
E-mail: info@bcdecker.com
Website: www.bcdecker.com

ISBN 1–55009–110–7
Printed in Canada

Sales and Distribution

United States
B.C. Decker Inc
P.O. Box 785
Lewiston, NY 14092-0785
Tel: 905-522-7017; 1-800-568-7281
Fax: 905-522-7839
E-mail: info@bcdecker.com
Website: www.bcdecker.com

Canada
B.C. Decker Inc.
20 Hughson Street South
P.O. Box 620, L.C.D. 1
Hamilton, Ontario L8N 3K7
Tel: 905-522-7017; 1-800-568-7281
Fax: 905-522-7839
E-mail: info@bcdecker.com
Website: www.bcdecker.com

Foreign Rights
John Scott & Company
International Publishers' Agency
P.O. Box 878
Kimberton, PA 19442
Tel: 610-827-1640
Fax: 610-827-1671

**U.K., Europe, Scandinavia,
Middle East**
Harcourt Publishers Limited
Customer Service Department
Foots Cray High Street
Sidcup, Kent
DA14 5HP, UK
Tel: 44 (0) 208 308 5760
Fax: 44 (0) 181 308 5702
E-mail: cservice@harcourt_brace.com

Australia, New Zealand
Harcourt Australia Pry. Limited
Customer Service Department
STM Division
Locked Bag 16
St. Peters, New South Wales, 2044
Australia
Tel: (02) 9517-8999
Fax: (02) 9517-2249
E-mail: stmp@harcourt.com.au
Website: www.harcourt.com.au

Japan
Igaku-Shoin Ltd.
Foreign Publications Department
3-24-17 Hongo
Bunkyo-ku,Tokyo, Japan 113-8719
Tel: 3 3817 5680
Fax: 3 3815 6776
E-mail: fd@igaku.shoin.co.jp

**Singapore, Malaysia, Thailand,
Philippines, Indonesia, Vietnam,
Pacific Rim**
Harcourt Asia Pte Limited
583 Orchard Road
#09/01, Forum
Singapore 238884
Tel: 65-737-3593
Fax: 65-753-2145

Notice: The authors and publisher have made every effort to ensure that the patient care recommended herein, including choice of drugs and drug dosages, is in accord with the accepted standard and practice at the time of publication. However, since research and regulation constantly change clinical standards, the reader is urged to check the product information sheet included in the package of each drug, which includes recommended doses, warnings, and contraindications. This is particularly important with new or infrequently used drugs.

Contributors

DAVID S. ALBERTS, MD
Arizona Cancer Center
University of Arizona
Tucson, Arizona
Prevention of Colorectal Cancer:
  Epidemiological Evidence and Chemoprevention

ANTHONY L. BACK, MD
Associate Professor
VA Puget Sound Health Care System
University of Washington
Seattle, Washington
Palliative Care for Patients with
  Lower Gastrointestinal Tract Malignancies

WILLIAM R. BRUGGE, MD
Director, Gastrointestinal Endoscopy
Massachusetts General Hospital
Harvard Medical School
Boston, Massachusetts
Endoscopic Management of Colon
  and Rectal Cancer

JEFF CLARK, MD
Massachusetts General Hospital
Dana Farber Cancer Institute
Assistant Professor in Medicine
Harvard Medical School
Boston, Massachusetts
Systemic Therapy Approaches for
  Colorectal Cancer

CAROLYN C. COMPTON, MD, PhD
Professor and Chair
Department of Pathology
McGill University
Montreal, Quebec
Pathology and Staging

EDWARD GIOVANNUCCI, MD, ScD
Associate Professor of Medicine
Channing Laboratory
Department of Medicine
Brigham and Women's Hospital
  & Harvard Medical School
Associate Professor of Nutrition and of
  Epidemiology
Departments of Nutrition and Epidemiology
Harvard School of Public Health
Boston, Massachusetts
Prevention of Colorectal Cancer:
  Epidemiological Evidence and
  Chemoprevention

TIMOTHY D. JENKINS, MD
Instructor of Medicine
University of Pennsylvania
Philadelphia, Pennsylvania
Genetics of Colorectal Carcinoma

BERNARD LEVIN, MD
Vice President for Cancer Prevention
MD Anderson Cancer Center
The University of Texas
Houston, Texas
Colorectal Cancer Prevention and
  Early Detection

MARÍA ELENA MARTÍNEZ, PhD, RD
Arizona Cancer Center
University of Arizona
Research Assistant Professor
College of Public Health
Tucson, Arizona
Prevention of Colorectal Cancer:
  Epidemiological Evidence and
  Chemoprevention

MARK L. MONTGOMERY, MD
Scott and White Clinic
Texas A & M Health Science Center
Temple, Texas
Diagnostic Radiology of Colon and Rectal Cancer

PETER R. MUELLER, MD
Professor of Radiology
Harvard Medical School
Massachusetts General Hospital
Boston, Massachusetts
Diagnostic Radiology of Colon and Rectal Cancer

MARK J. OTT, MD
Massachusetts General Hospital
Division of Surgical Oncology
Assistant Professor of Surgery
Harvard Medical School
Boston, Massachusetts
Surgery of Primary Colon and Rectal Cancer

JEAN-PIERRE E.N. PIERIE, MD, PhD
Chief Resident in Surgery
Department of Surgery
University Medical Center Utrecht
Utrecht, The Netherlands
Surgery of Primary Colon and Rectal Cancer

ANIL K. RUSTGI, MD
T. Grier Miller Associate Professor of
    Medicine & Genetics
Chief of Gastroenterology
University of Pennsylvania
Philadelphia, Pennsylvania
Genetics of Colorectal Carcinoma

DAVID P. RYAN, MD
Instructor in Medicine
Harvard Medical School
Assistant in Medicine
Massachusetts General Hospital
Boston, Massachusetts
Colon and Rectal Carcinoma: An Overview
Anal Cancer

KENNETH K. TANABE, MD
Chief, Division of Surgical Oncology
Massachusetts General Hospital
Associate Professor of Surgery
Harvard Medical School
Boston, Massachusetts
Surgical Management of Metastatic Colon
    and Rectal Cancer

ROGER J. WALTZMAN, MD
Mount Sinai Medical Center
Mount Sinai School of Medicine
Division of Medical Oncology
New York, New York
Palliative Care for Patients with Lower
    Gastrointestinal Tract Malignancies

CHRISTOPHER G. WILLETT, MD
Professor, Harvard Medical School
Clinical Director
Department of Radiation Oncology
Massachusetts General Hospital
Boston, Massachusetts
Colon and Rectal Carcinoma: An Overview
Radiation Therapy in Colon and Rectal Cancer
Anal Cancer

SAM S. YOON, MD
Fellow, Division of Surgical Oncology
Massachusetts General Hospital and
    Harvard Medical School
Boston, Massachusetts
Surgical Management of Metastatic Colon
    and Rectal Cancer

Contents

Preface

Cancer of the Lower Gastrointestinal Tract, An American Cancer Society monograph, is a timely analysis of the biology, diagnosis, and therapy of cancer of the colon, rectum, and anus. This monograph is intended as a useful resource for physicians, scientists, medical students, and allied health personnel in the disciplines of gastroenterology, oncology, and pathology. Renowned contributors from different medical disciplines have written their chapters in a thoughtful, provocative, and visual fashion.

This monograph is divided into 13 chapters. Early chapters (1–2) address the etiology, risk factors, and prevention of colon and rectal cancer followed by chapters (3–5) detailing the revolutionary developments in the genetics and pathology of this malignancy. Chapter 4 comprehensively reviews and outlines the prevention, early detection, and contemporary screening guidelines of colon and rectal cancer. These sections are then followed by chapters (6–7) on endoscopy and diagnostic radiology of colon and rectal cancer. The current multimodality treatment of primary colon and rectal cancer is discussed in three integrative chapters (8–10) from the vantage points of surgery, radiation therapy, and chemotherapy. The challenges and developments in the management of patients with metastatic colon and rectal cancer (surgery, chemotherapy, and innovative and targeted therapies) are presented in two chapters (10–11). Although the focus of this book is colon and rectal cancer, one chapter is dedicated to a comprehensive examination of the epidemiology, biology, and evolving therapy of a unique malignancy, cancer of the anus (12). Finally, the monograph concludes with an excellent discussion of the complex and difficult issues of palliative care for patients with cancer of the lower gastrointestinal tract (13).

I would like to thank Bruce Chabner, MD, and Glenn Steele, Jr, MD, PhD, for their helpful suggestions.

Christopher G. Willett, MD
August, 2000

Dedication

To my friend and colleague, Ira J. Spiro, MD, PhD.

Colon and Rectal Carcinoma: An Overview

DAVID P. RYAN, MD
CHRISTOPHER G. WILLETT, MD

Disease Epidemiology

The incidence of colorectal cancer in the United States has been declining over the last several decades. In 1999, in the United States, there were 129,400 new cases and 56,600 deaths expected.[1] As many as 15 percent of patients with colorectal cancer have a strong family history of the disease, and the relative risk for developing colorectal cancer if at least one first-degree relative has had colorectal cancer is 1.7.[2] The two hereditary syndromes most often identified are familial adenomatous polyposis (FAP) and hereditary nonpolyposis colorectal cancer (HNPCC). FAP is an autosomal dominant condition associated with germline mutations of chromosome 5q21 (adenomatous polyposis coli [APC] gene). In FAP, thousands of adenomatous polyps develop by age 20 and lead to cancer. In the United States, 1 in 5,000 to 10,000 people are affected with FAP, but it accounts for 1 percent of colorectal cancers due to the routine use of prophylactic colectomies when it is found. Total colectomy with mucosal proctectomy, followed by ileoanal anastomosis at a time when polyposis is appreciated, is the treatment of choice. When it is associated with desmoid tumors, osteomas, epidermoid, sebaceous cysts, and periampullary cancers, it is referred to as Gardner's syndrome. When FAP is associated with brain tumors, it is called Turcot's syndrome.

HNPCC is believed to account for 5 to 15 percent of colorectal cancers.[3] It is an autosomal dominant condition associated with germline mutations of mismatch repair genes that lead to errors in DNA replication and DNA instability. The bowel mucosa can appear histologically normal or polypoid or flat adenomas may be present, albeit far fewer than in FAP. The median age for the appearance of cancer is less than 50 years. In women, it can be associated with endometrial and/or ovarian carcinomas. Patients with ulcerative colitis are also at an increased risk of developing colorectal cancer.

Pathology

Most colorectal cancers are thought to develop in a stepwise progression from normal epithelium to adenomatous polyps to adenocarcinoma. Each step is presumably the result of one or many genetic mutations leading to altered cell growth and, eventually, the ability to invade adjacent structures and metastasize.

More than 90 percent of colon cancers are adenocarcinomas. Currently, the World Health Organization (WHO) identifies several variants of adenocarcinoma, including signet-ring and adenosquamous.[4] Undifferentiated, or medullary-type, adenocarcinoma is a recently identified distinct clinicopathologic entity that was not listed by the WHO.[5] Signet-ring cell carcinoma and small-cell carcinoma are the only histologic types of colonic carcinoma that consistently have been found to have a stage-independent adverse effect on outcome. Medullary carcinoma, a rare variant of adenocarcinoma, and mucinous carcinoma have a favorable prognosis when associated with microsatellite instability.

Tumor grade is independently reported and subject to observer variability. Nevertheless, many studies have demonstrated that poorly differentiated tumors have an unfavorable prognosis. This finding has produced a two-tiered system: low grade and high grade. The high-grade tumors are poorly differentiated, whereas the low-grade tumors are well or moderately differentiated.

Staging

The AJCC/UICC TNM staging system is the internationally accepted staging system for colorectal cancer and has replaced the Dukes' and Modified Astler-Collier staging systems in North America.[6] The best estimation of prognosis in colorectal cancer is the anatomic extent of disease by the TNM system. It should be noted that pathologic staging and clinical staging are separate exercises, and the prescripts "p" and "c" are used in the TNM staging system to identify which staging modality is in use. Pathologic staging occurs only after resection of the primary tumor. Clinical staging is based on the clinician's best estimate after evaluation of staging studies (usually endoscopy and computed tomography [CT] scans). In the TNM system, the "T" designation refers to the local extent of the primary tumor through the colorectal mucosa at the time of diagnosis. The "N" designation refers to the presence of tumor within adjacent lymph nodes and is further subclassified by the number of involved nodes. The "M" designation refers to the presence of distant metastatic disease.

CLINICAL MANAGEMENT

Management Overview

Colorectal cancer is diagnosed after routine screening or presentation due to symptoms. The recommendations for screening vary among subspecialty groups.[7] Fecal occult blood testing has been the standard screening tool for many years and still is recommended by most groups. Although not yet proven to be more effective than flexible sigmoidoscopy or double-contrast barium enema, screening with colonoscopy is becoming more common. Screening should begin at age 50 for those patients without a family history and, in those patients with a family history, at least 10 years prior to the age of initial diagnosis of colorectal cancer in a primary relative.

Patients with a history of extensive ulcerative colitis should undergo colonoscopy every 1 to 2 years beginning 10 years after the initial diagnosis. Symptoms from colorectal cancer are variable, and patients can present with obstruction, crampy abdominal pain, fatigue, and bright red blood per rectum.

Once a colon or rectal cancer is suspected, a colonoscopy is required to evaluate the extent of the disease, obtain a biopsy, and exclude simultaneous or synchronous lesions throughout the remainder of the large bowel. Staging studies are then performed to evaluate the extent of local disease and assess for the presence of distant metastases.

The only curative therapy for colorectal cancer is surgical resection of all disease. Patients with advanced T stage or the presence of lymph node metastases may require adjuvant chemotherapy and radiation therapy to improve their overall survival. Patients with metastatic disease at the time of diagnosis are generally not considered curable, except in a very few circumstances. The 5-year survival rate for patients with early stage disease is at least 70 percent and depends on the extent of mucosal invasion; the 5-year survival rate for patients with stage 3 disease is 30 to 60 percent; and the 5-year survival rate for patients with stage 4 disease is < 10 percent.[8]

Staging Studies

If a patient presents with colon cancer, the initial evaluation should include a physical examination, laboratory analysis (complete blood count, electrolytes, creatinine, liver function tests, and carcinoembryonic antigen [CEA]), endoscopy of the entire colon, and a chest x-ray. A high CEA level is predictive of future relapse.[9] The role of further staging studies is controversial in the absence of other indications, for example, abnormal liver function tests to suggest liver metastases. Nevertheless, use of abdominal-pelvic CT scans as part of the initial staging evaluation is becoming more widespread. Approximately 30 percent of patients will have metastatic disease at presentation.

Treatment

Since the primary treatment for colorectal cancers is surgical, nearly all patients will undergo a resection. For colonic tumors, a hemicolectomy is the treatment of choice as removing the entire colon is unnecessary. Surgery for rectal tumors can be divided into procedures that require a colostomy and procedures that spare the anal sphincter. Colostomies are openings in the abdominal wall to which the colon is attached. Fecal contents are emptied through this opening into a colostomy bag. The decision to use a certain procedure for the removal of a rectal tumor is based primarily on the location of the tumor. The major procedure for rectal tumors within approximately 6 cm of the anal verge is the abdominoperineal resection (APR). An APR requires removal of the lower third of the rectum along with the structures that comprise the anal sphincter and is required for tumors close to the anal verge in order to completely remove the tumor. After an APR, patients are left with a colostomy. The major sphincter-sparing procedure is the low anterior resection (LAR), which is used for tumors in the middle and upper rectum. Occasionally, patients will undergo a LAR but have a temporary colostomy that gets reversed (or taken down) at a later date. Local excision has gained popularity in recent years as a means of removing tumors in the lower third of the rectum and sparing the anal sphincter. These approaches appear to be safe for early stage tumors but may require more aggressive use of postoperative radiation and chemotherapy.

For patients with stage 1 colon tumors and most patients with stage 2 tumors, adjuvant therapy is not indicated (Figure 1–1). Adjuvant chemotherapy is indicated for those patients with stage 3 colorectal cancers (patients with nodal metastases). Several randomized studies have established that adjuvant chemotherapy can improve overall survival by 25 to 30 percent.[10–12] The standard regimen is 5-fluorouracil (5-FU) and leucovorin. Leucovorin is a B vitamin that augments the inhibitory effect of 5-FU on DNA synthesis. For patients with rectal cancer that has spread through the bowel wall (T3) or to the lymph nodes, radiation therapy in addition to chemotherapy is indicated (Figure 1–2).[13] Low-dose chemotherapy is administered concurrently with radiation therapy by continuous 24-hour infusion by a pump that patients carry with them. Adjuvant therapy for colorectal cancer is administered for 6 to 8 months. There has been interest in the use of preoperative irradiation and more recently preoperative chemoradiation for patients with clinical stage T3 and T4 tumors of the rectum (Figure 1–3).

After adjuvant therapy is complete, patients are followed serially. Guidelines regarding follow-up vary. Of recurrences, 85 percent occur within the first 3 years after diagnosis. Very few recurrences occur after 5 years from initial diagnosis.

Patients with metastatic disease are considered incurable except for several uncommon situations. Patients with isolated liver or lung metastases may be candidates for resection of the metastatic disease.[14,15] The vast majority of patients who develop stage 4 disease, however, have widespread or unresectable metastatic disease. For many years 5-FU was the initial treatment of choice, but recently the addition of irinotecan (Camptosar, Pharmacia & Upjohn, Inc.) to 5-FU has been shown to improve

T1–2, N0, M0 ⟶ No further therapy

T3, N0, M0 ⟶ Consider adjuvant 5-FU/leucovorin for patients presenting with obstruction or perforation

T4, N0, M0 ⟶ Consider adjuvant chemoradiation followed by 5-FU/leucovorin for patients with invasion of adjacent structures

T4, N_{any}, M0 ⟶ Consider adjuvant chemoradiation followed by 5-FU/leucovorin for patients with invasion of adjacent structures

T_{any}, N1–2, M0 ⟶ Adjuvant 5-FU/leucovorin

Figure 1–1. Postoperative treatment of colon cancer.

Pathologic T1, N0, M0 ⟶ No further therapy

Pathologic T2, N0, M0 ⟶ After LAR/APR: no further therapy
⟶ After local excision: chemoradiation

Pathologic T3, N_{any}, M0 ⟶ Chemoradiation followed by 5-FU/leucovorin

Pathologic T4, N_{any}, M0 ⟶ Chemoradiation followed by 5-FU/leucovorin

Figure 1–2. Postoperative assessment of rectal cancer.

outcome (Figure 1–4).[16,17] For patients treated only with 5-FU as a first-line therapy, second-line chemotherapy with irinotecan has been shown to prolong survival for patients who have progressed on 5-FU.[18,19] There are no approved third-line chemotherapy agents in the United States. The median survival for patients with metastatic disease who receive chemotherapy is 12 to 18 months.

Supportive Care

Since patients with metastatic disease are destined to die from their cancer, end-of-life supportive measures are used to a great degree. Narcotics, antibiotics, radiotherapy for pain management, and antiemetics are used frequently. Recently, the use of erythropoietin via subcutaneous injection for cancer or therapy-related anemia has been demonstrated to reduce the need for blood transfusions.

RESEARCH AND DEVELOPMENT

Screening and Prevention

As colonoscopy becomes less expensive and safer, more physicians are screening patients with this method rather than flexible sigmoidoscopy. Scientif-

ically, this procedure is supported as there has been a trend toward more right-sided colon cancers in recent years. Sigmoidoscopy does not reach the right side of the colon. "Virtual colonoscopy" is an exciting new screening technique that uses the spiral CT scanners to reproduce a three-dimensional picture of the colon.[20,21] Preliminary studies indicate that this method may be a very effective screening tool. Virtual colonoscopy offers patients a noninvasive screening technique.

Dietary measures intended to prevent colorectal cancer are undergoing considerable review. Recently, diets high in fiber were not demonstrated to prevent colon cancer.[22] Nevertheless, several dietary supplements may be beneficial in the prevention of colorectal cancer. There is particular interest in the possibility that folic acid supplementation may prevent colorectal cancer,[23,24] and research into folic acid supplementation is ongoing. Calcium supplementation has also been shown to reduce the risk of subsequent colonic polyps in those patients who have had previous colonic polyps.[25] Lastly, studies demonstrate that regular aspirin use decreases the risk of developing colorectal cancer.[26] New generation cyclooxygenase inhibitors such as the COX-2 inhibitors are currently undergoing prevention studies as preclinical studies

Clinical T1, N0, M0 ⟶ Local excision vs. primary resection with APR/LAR

Clinical T2, N0, M0 ⟶ Surgical resection

Clinical T3, N_{any}, M0 ⟶ Consider preoperative chemoradiation followed by postoperative 5-FU/leucovorin

Clinical T4, N_{any}, M0 ⟶ Preoperative chemoradiation followed by postoperative 5-FU/leucovorin

Figure 1–3. Preoperative assessment of rectal cancer.

First-line therapy: 5-FU/leucovorin/irinotecan

Second-line therapy: Consider oxaliplatin-based regimen
5-FU via different schedule, eg, oral fluoropyrimidines
Consider phase I studies

Special Considerations

1. Isolated liver or lung metastases ——→ refer to surgeon

Figure 1–4. Treatment of metastatic disease in colorectal cancer.

suggested that they too might prevent the development of colorectal cancer.[27]

Diagnostic/Prognosis

For rectal tumors, magnetic resonance imaging (MRI) and ultrasonography have been gaining in popularity because of their ability to predict transmural invasion and nodal metastases; however, they are not yet part of standard staging evaluation. Positron emission tomography (PET) scanning may also become a very useful staging tool in the evaluation of patients with colorectal cancer.[28]

Allelic loss of a portion on chromosome 18q called the DCC gene (deleted in colon cancer) may have as much prognostic importance as lymph node status.[29] Studies are underway that are looking at this gene as well as several other important markers that have been identified in preclinical studies such as p53, K-Ras, and microsatellite instability.

Treatment

In addition to irinotecan, the combination of oxaliplatin (Eloxatin, Sanofi) and 5-FU has also recently been shown to improve progression-free survival compared to 5-FU alone as first-line therapy.[30] Recent focus in the treatment of metastatic colon cancer has turned to the integration of irinotecan and oxaliplatin into first-line therapy. A large National Cancer Institute (NCI)-sponsored study was initiated in 1999 in which patients were randomized to one of three arms: 5-FU/irinotecan versus 5-FU/oxaliplatin versus irinotecan/oxaliplatin.

In the treatment of adjuvant disease, cooperative groups are testing in randomized trials combination therapy versus the standard therapy of 5-FU and leucovorin. Oral 5-FU preparations and thymidylate synthase inhibitors are also undergoing trials in the adjuvant setting as they appear equally efficacious with 5-FU in the metastatic setting.[31]

The NCI is also sponsoring an adjuvant study of a monoclonal antibody against 17-1A, a surface glycoprotein. A small study from Germany suggested that this monoclonal antibody might be just as effective as 5-FU for patients with stage 3 colon cancer.[32] This study is being sponsored by the NCI.

REFERENCES

1. Landis SH, Murray T, Bolden S, et al. Cancer statistics, 1999. CA Cancer J Clin 1999;49:8–31.
2. Fuchs CS, Giovannucci EL, Colditz GA, et al. A prospective study of family history and the risk of colorectal cancer. N Engl J Med 1994;331:1669–74.
3. Aaltonen LA, Salovaara R, Kristo P, et al. Incidence of hereditary nonpolyposis colorectal cancer and the feasibility of molecular screening for the disease. N Engl J Med 1998;338:1481–7.
4. Jass JR, Sobin LH. World Health Organization histological typing of intestinal tumours. 2nd ed. New York: Springer-Verlag; 1989.
5. Lanza G, Gafa R, Matteuzzi M, et al. Medullary-type poorly differentiated adenocarcinoma of the large bowel: a distinct clinicopathologic entity characterized by microsatellite instability and improved survival. J Clin Oncol 1999;17:2429.
6. Cancer AJCC. AJCC Cancer staging manual. 5th ed. Philadelphia: Lippincott-Raven; 1997.
7. Bond JH. Screening guidelines for colorectal cancer. Am J Med 1999;106:7S–10S.
8. Cohen AM, Minsky BD, Schilsky RL. Cancer of the colon. In: DeVita VT, Hellman S, Rosenberg SA, editors. Cancer: principles and practice of oncology. 5th ed. Philadelphia: Lippincott-Raven; 1997.
9. Oncology ASoC. 1997 update of recommendations for the use of tumor markers in breast and colorectal cancer. Adopted on November 7, 1997 by the American Society of Clinical Oncology. J Clin Oncol 1998;16:793–5.

10. Investigators I. Efficacy of adjuvant fluorouracil and folinic acid in colon cancer. Lancet 1995;345:939.

11. Moertel CG, Fleming TR, Macdonald JS, et al. Fluorouracil plus levamisole as effective adjuvant therapy after resection of stage III colon carcinoma: a final report. Ann Intern Med 1995;122:321–6.

12. Haller DG, Catalano PJ, Macdonald JS, et al. Fluorouracil, leucovorin, and levamisole adjuvant therapy for colon cancer: five-year survival report of INT-0098. Proceedings ASCO 1998;17:A982.

13. O'Connell MJ, Martenson JA, Wieand HS, et al. Improving adjuvant therapy for rectal cancer by combining protracted-infusion fluorouracil with radiation therapy after curative surgery. N Engl J Med 1994;331:502–7.

14. Fong Y, Cohen AM, Fortner JG, et al. Liver resection for colorectal metastases. J Clin Oncol 1997;15:938–46.

15. Goldberg RM, Fleming TR, Tangen CM, et al. Surgery for recurrent colon cancer: strategies for identifying resectable recurrence and success rates after resection. Eastern Cooperative Oncology Group, the North Central Cancer Treatment Group, and the Southwest Oncology Group. Ann Intern Med 1998;129:27–35.

16. Douillard JY, Cunningham D, Roth AD, et al. Irinotecan combined with fluorouracil compared with fluorouracil alone as first-line treatment for metastatic colorectal cancer: a multicentre randomised trial. Lancet 2000;355:1041–7.

17. Saltz LB, Cox JV, Blanke C, et al. Irinotecan plus fluorouracil and leucovorin for metastatic colorectal cancer. N Eng J Med 2000; in press.

18. Cunningham D, Pyrhonen S, James RD, et al. Randomised trial of irinotecan plus supportive care versus supportive care alone after fluorouracil failure for patients with metastatic colorectal cancer. Lancet 1998;352:1413–8.

19. Rougier P, Van Cutsem E, Bajetta E, et al. Randomised trial of irinotecan versus fluorouracil by continuous infusion after fluorouracil failure in patients with metastatic colorectal cancer. Lancet 1998;352:1407–12.

20. Ahlquist DA, Hara AK, Johnson CD. Computed tomographic colography and virtual colonoscopy. Gastrointest Endosc Clin N Am 1997;7:439–52.

21. Fenlon HM, Nunes DP, Clarke PD, et al. Colorectal neoplasm detection using virtual colonoscopy: a feasibility study. Gut 1998;43:806–11.

22. Fuchs CS, Giovannucci EL, Colditz GA, et al. Dietary fiber and the risk of colorectal cancer and adenoma in women. N Engl J Med 1999;340:169–76.

23. Giovannucci E, Stampfer MJ, Colditz GA, et al. Folate, methionine, and alcohol intake and risk of colorectal adenoma. J Natl Cancer Inst 1993;85:875–84.

24. Baron JA, Sandler RS, Haile RW, et al. Folate intake, alcohol consumption, cigarette smoking, and risk of colorectal adenomas. J Natl Cancer Inst 1998;90:57–62.

25. Baron JA, Beach M, Mandel JS, et al. Calcium supplements for the prevention of colorectal adenomas. Calcium Polyp Prevention Study Group. N Engl J Med 1999;340:101–7.

26. Giovannucci E, Egan KM, Hunter DJ, et al. Aspirin and the risk of colorectal cancer in women. N Engl J Med 1995;333:609–14.

27. Reddy BS, Rao CV, Seibert K. Evaluation of cyclooxygenase-2 inhibitor for potential chemopreventive properties in colon carcinogenesis. Cancer Res 1996;56:4566–9.

28. Flamen P, Stroobants S, Van Cutsem E, et al. Additional value of whole-body positron emission tomography with fluorine-18-2-fluoro-2-deoxy-D-glucose in recurrent colorectal cancer. J Clin Oncol 1999;17:894–901.

29. Shibata D, Reale MA, Lavin P, et al. The DCC protein and prognosis in colorectal cancer. N Engl J Med 1996;335:1727–32.

30. DeGramont A, Figer A, Seymour M, et al. Leucovorin and fluorouracil with of without oxaliplatin as a first-line treatment in advanced colorectal cancer. J Clin Oncol 2000;18:2938–47.

31. Cocconi G, Cunningham D, Van Cutsem E, et al. Open, randomized, multicenter trial of raltitrexed versus fluorouracil plus high-dose leucovorin in patients with advanced colorectal cancer. Tomudex Colorectal Cancer Study Group. J Clin Oncol 1998;16:2943–52.

32. Riethmuller G, Holz E, Schlimok G, et al. Monoclonal antibody therapy for resected Dukes' C colorectal cancer: seven-year outcome of a multicenter randomized trial. J Clin Oncol 1998;16:1788–94.

2

Prevention of Colorectal Cancer: Epidemiologic Evidence and Chemoprevention

MARÍA ELENA MARTÍNEZ, PhD, RD
EDWARD GIOVANNUCCI, MD, ScD
DAVID S. ALBERTS, MD

One of the most important advances in the field of colorectal cancer has been the recognition that colorectal neoplasia occurs through a stepwise disruption of genes that control cellular replication, differentiation, apoptosis, and DNA repair. Many of the genes implicated in colorectal carcinogenesis are now well characterized,[1] but new ones continue to emerge. Disruptions in the genome occur through a variety of mechanisms, including point mutations, deletions, amplification, and DNA methylation abnormalities. In recent years, remarkable progress has also been made in identifying factors that either enhance or reduce risk of colorectal cancer. Early clues that environmental factors are important in colorectal neoplasia were the substantial geographic variation in incidence of colorectal cancer and the striking increases in the incidence of colorectal cancer in groups that migrated from low- to high-incidence areas. These observations formed the basis for various hypotheses of proposed etiologic factors that influence colorectal carcinogenesis. Many of these hypotheses continue to be evaluated in observational and intervention studies. In this chapter, we summarize the descriptive epidemiology, the analytic epidemiology, the study of gene-environment interactions, and chemoprevention studies of colorectal cancer and its precursor lesion, the adenoma.

DESCRIPTIVE EPIDEMIOLOGY OF COLORECTAL CANCER

Colorectal cancer is overall the third leading cause of cancer deaths in each sex and second overall in the United States.[2] Without preventive actions, approximately 6 percent of individuals in the United States will develop colorectal cancer sometime in their lifetime.[3] Approximately half of diagnosed individuals will die of this disease. Rates of this malignancy are high in essentially all countries that have undergone economic development, and the incidence invariably rises as regions undergo economic development.

Colorectal Cancer Incidence and Mortality in the United States

From the US Surveillance, Epidemiology, and End Results Program (SEER), the American Cancer Society estimates that, in 1999, 94,700 colon and 34,700 rectal cancer cases will have been newly diagnosed.[2] The estimated number of deaths in 1999 is 47,900 for colon cancer and 8,700 for rectal cancer. The annual incidence rate for individuals under 65 years of age is 19.2 per 100,000 and it is 33.7 per 100,000 for those 65 and over.[4] By subsite within the colon and rectum, the most frequent locations are the sigmoid, rectum, and cecum.[5] Between 1991 and 1995, the age-standardized incidence rate of colorectal cancer was 54.5 per 100,000 among men and 38.2 per 100,000 among women. As well, the age-standardized mortality rate was higher among men (26.9 per 100,000) than women (14.9 per 100,000) during this time period. Invasive colorectal cancer is rarely diagnosed in those under age 40 but increases dramatically in middle age and elderly years. The lifetime risk of invasive colorectal cancer is 1 in 17 in both men and women.[2] Despite higher age-standardized rates in men, the absolute number of new cases and deaths is approximately equal in men and women because women tend to live longer.

In the United States, annual age-standardized colorectal cancer mortality rates peaked in the 1940s and have steadily fallen since the 1950s through 1995[6]; however, the decline has been more pronounced among women. Although the rate of left-sided colon cancer remains higher; incidence rates of right-sided colon cancer have increased more rapidly than left-sided colon cancer over the 1976 to 1987 period.[5]

Most colorectal cancers arise in adenomas. Because adenomas are usually asymptomatic, they may be detected years after onset; thus, the appropriate measure of their frequency is prevalence (for example, prevalence at the time of endoscopy or autopsy). The prevalence of adenomas increases with age and is greater in men than women.[7] Autopsy studies suggest that one- to three-fifths of individuals have prevalent adenomas and screening studies of average-risk populations have found that one-fourth to two-fifths of individuals have adenomas.[7]

Racial/Ethnic Differences in Incidence, Mortality, and Survival

The highest colorectal cancer incidence and mortality rates among racial/ethnic groups in the United States are found among African Americans.[8] The age-standardized incidence rate for African-American men from 1990 to 1995 was 59.4 per 100,000; for African-American women, the rate was 45.5 per 100,000. For the same time period, the mortality rate in African Americans was 28.0 per 100,000 for men and 20.1 per 100,000 for women. The lowest incidence rates in the United States are found among Native Americans (21.9 per 100,000 for men and 10.5 per 100,000 for women). Data for mortality rates are not available for Native Americans. Among women, the lowest mortality rates were seen among Hispanics (8.5 per 100,000). By subsite within the colon, incidence rates (1976 to 1987) of cancer of the cecum and ascending colon do not vary appreciably by race.[5] African Americans have higher rates for cancers of the transverse and descending colon, while whites have higher rates for the sigmoid, rectosigmoid, and rectal cancers. In addition, data from the New Mexico Tumor Registry[9] show that over the period of 1969 to 1994, colorectal cancer incidence and mortality rates increased among Native American and Hispanic men and women, whereas those among non-Hispanic whites decreased.

Five-year colon cancer survival rates have increased from 50 to 63 percent in whites and 46 to 53 percent in African Americans between the mid-1970s and the late 1980s and early 1990s in the United States.[2] One-half of the poorer survival among African Americans compared to whites can be attributed to diagnosis of colorectal cancer at later stages.[10] Reduced access to and quality of medical care may also contribute to racial differences.[11]

ANALYTIC EPIDEMIOLOGY OF ETIOLOGIC FACTORS

The wide international variation in colorectal cancer incidence and mortality rates and the changing rates among migrants moving from countries that have low rates to those with high rates suggest that lifestyle and environmental factors influence the development of this malignancy. The following is a summary of findings from analytic epidemiologic studies pertaining to dietary factors, obesity and physical activity, postmenopausal hormone (PMH) use, tobacco, alcohol, and nonsteroidal anti-inflammatory drugs (NSAIDs). In addition, the expanding area of gene-environment interactions is reviewed. Specific factors may influence either the colon or rectum, or both, and etiologic differences among the subsites of the colon may exist. In general, less is known about the etiology of rectal cancer.

Diet

The epidemiologic and experimental evidence that dietary pattern is an important causal determinant of colorectal tumors is compelling. In Western cultures, dietary factors may contribute to the causation of approximately 50 percent of colorectal cancer.[12] However, controversy exists regarding the specific nutrients, foods, or combinations of these that are causally related to the development of colorectal cancer. Various study designs have been used to test specific hypotheses. Ecologic studies compare per capita consumption and cancer incidence and mortality rates among different populations, usually based on national data. Case-control studies compare reported past diet as recalled by cancer cases and cancer-free controls, whereas prospective cohort studies assess diet in cancer-free individuals and correlate specific factors to subsequent cancer occurrence.

Energy Intake

The assessment of the relationship between energy intake and colon cancer presents a challenge because total energy is interrelated with other nutrient and non-nutrient factors that themselves may be related to colon cancer risk. Variation in energy intake among individuals within a population is influenced largely by level of physical activity, metabolic efficiency, and body size.[13] Whether an individual gains or loses weight is determined by a balance between energy intake and expenditure, and even small differences between intake and expenditure over time can lead to appreciable differences in body weight. Results based on total energy intake may have a deceptive interpretation because energy intake may only be acting as a surrogate for one or more of the determinants, such as physical activity, that may influence colon cancer risk.

Results of most published case-control studies have shown a positive association between total energy intake and risk of colon cancer.[14–26] Howe[27] conducted a pooled analysis of 13 case-control studies and found that total energy intake was associated with a higher risk of colon cancer regardless of whether the energy source was fat, protein, or carbohydrate. Slattery and colleagues[28] reported similar findings based on three case-control studies and suggested that total energy intake is more important than the specific energy sources (i.e., fat, protein, or carbohydrate). In contrast to the findings of case-

control studies, cohort studies have shown no relationship or even a slight inverse association between total energy intake and risk of colon cancer.[29–34] In one of these studies,[34] a statistically significant relative risk (RR) of 0.62 was reported between high and low quintiles of energy intake. The reason for the discrepancy between findings from cohort and case-control studies regarding energy intake and colon cancer is unclear and may possibly be related to methodologic biases, such as differential recall or reporting of past diet, selective participation, or survival in case-control studies. Regardless of the reason, from a public health perspective, it may be more informative to examine the role of the determinants of energy intake, such as physical activity and body size, which are reviewed later in the chapter.

Fat and Red Meat

Rates of colon cancer are strongly correlated with national per capita disappearance of animal fat and meat, with correlation coefficients ranging between 0.8 and 0.9.[35,36] A sharp increase in colon cancer incidence rates in Japan in the decades following World War II coincided with an increase in fat intake of 2.5 times.[37] Results of analytic epidemiologic studies also support the association between animal fat and colon cancer; most case-control studies have shown a positive association with intake of animal or saturated fat[14–17,19,20,22,24,38] or red meat,[39–45] with some exceptions.[26,46–48] In the pooled analysis of 13 case-control studies,[27] although a significant association between total energy and colon cancer was observed, intake of saturated, monounsaturated, or polyunsaturated fat was not associated with colon cancer risk independently of total energy. Earlier prospective cohort studies of colon cancer have shown inconsistent findings for the association of fat or red meat consumption and colon cancer.[29,30,49–52] Other cohort studies have shown statistically significant or suggestive positive associations for intake of processed meats and risk of colon cancer.[32–34] Data from the prospective Health Professionals Follow-up Study[32] showed a direct association between red meat consumption and risk of colon cancer, but no association was observed with other sources of fat. In the Nurses' Health Study, approximately a two-fold increase in risk of colon cancer was observed for women in the highest compared to the lowest quintile of animal fat intake.[31] However, when red meat and animal fat intakes were included in the same multivariate model, red meat intake remained a statistically significant risk factor, whereas the association with animal fat did not persist.

Why red meat is frequently associated with increased risk of colorectal cancer remains unclear, but it may be related to meat as a source of fat, saturated fat, protein, carcinogens, or iron, which can act as an antioxidant catalyst. Results of some studies suggest that risk of colorectal cancer may be increased among meat eaters who consume meat with a heavily browned surface, but not increased among those who consume meat with a medium or lightly browned surface.[39,45] When meat is fried, grilled, or broiled at high temperatures for substantial periods of time, mutagenic heterocyclic aromatic amines are formed from heating creatinine with amino acids.[53–55] Over the past decade, close to 20 heterocyclic aromatic amines have been isolated from cooked meat.[55] Ongoing and future investigations should substantiate whether levels of heterocyclic amines consumed in a typical diet are carcinogenic in humans.

Fruit, Vegetables, and Fiber

Early epidemiologic studies found that high consumption of fruit and vegetables was associated with a decreased risk of colorectal cancer. The potential mechanisms of action for the apparent protective effect of fruit and vegetables include inhibition of nitrosamine formation, provision of substrate for formation of antineoplastic agents, dilution and binding of carcinogens, alteration of hormone metabolism, antioxidant effects, and the induction of detoxification enzymes by cruciferous vegetables.[56]

The vast majority of published studies have shown an inverse association between intake of vegetables and colon cancer, whereas inverse associations with fruit consumption are less frequently cited.[19,20,24,38,40,42,43,45,46,50,57–62] This evidence, however, is largely based on data from case-control studies. Trock and colleagues[63] conducted a pooled analysis of six case-control studies and found that a high intake of vegetables was associated with an odds

ratio (OR), an estimate of the RR, for colon cancer of 0.48 (95% confidence interval [CI] = 0.41–0.57) and a weaker inverse association with fiber (OR = 0.58 for upper versus lower categories). The more consistent findings for intake of vegetables as compared to those for fiber may possibly result from better measurement of vegetable sources of fiber than nonvegetable sources. Foods high in fiber have also been shown to be inversely associated with colon cancer risk in most[19,21–23,26,38,44,46,59,64] but not all[14,17,24,31,48] studies. A pooled analysis of 13 case-control studies[65] found a lower risk associated with higher fiber intake (OR = 0.53 for upper versus lower quintile). In contrast, large prospective studies have shown weak or nonexistent inverse associations for fiber and risk of colon cancer.[31–34,66] In studies for which sources of fiber were examined separately,[17,18,21,23–26,31,32,39,40,42,44–46,59,67–73] a reduced risk also appears to be stronger for vegetable sources than for other components. In the most recent and comprehensive prospective study examining the role of fiber and its components on risk of colorectal neoplasms, Fuchs and colleagues[66] found no protective effect against colorectal cancer or adenoma. Furthermore, no important associations were observed when analyses were conducted for cereal, fruit, or vegetable fiber. The causes for the apparent inconsistencies between the case-control and cohort studies are not clear.

Micronutrients

Calcium and Vitamin D. Various study designs have been used to investigate the role of calcium and vitamin D in colorectal carcinogenesis, including human intervention studies on the effect of calcium supplementation on cell proliferation,[74–80] in vitro studies on human epithelial cells,[74] and experimental animal models.[81–84] It is hypothesized[83,85] that calcium might reduce colon cancer risk by binding secondary bile acids and ionized fatty acids to form insoluble soaps in the lumen of the colon, thus reducing the proliferative stimulus of these compounds on colon mucosa. Calcium can also directly influence the proliferative activity of the colon mucosa.[75] Despite all the data accumulated thus far, the roles of calcium and vitamin D as colorectal anticarcinogens remain unclear.

Results of analytic epidemiologic studies that have examined the association between calcium as a risk factor for colorectal cancer have been inconsistent.[86] Data from the large cohort studies are consistent in showing weak, nonsignificant inverse associations with no evidence of a dose-response relationship.[86] In a recently published prospective study,[87] for which data from three dietary questionnaires were collected prospectively over 6 years, the results did not support a major inverse association between calcium intake and risk of colorectal cancer over a 6-year period (1986 to 1992). Nonsignificant, inverse associations were observed for dietary calcium and risk of colorectal cancer using the baseline dietary questionnaire (RR = 0.80; 95% CI = 0.60–1.07), the average intake based on the three questionnaires (RR − 0.74; 95% CI = 0.36–1.50), and the consistent intake based on the three questionnaires (RR = 0.70; 95% CI = 0.35–1.39). These results are consistent with a modest effect as also indicated by calcium intervention trials on colorectal adenoma recurrence (see chemoprevention section).

Epidemiologic data on vitamin D and colorectal cancer are sparse.[86] Four[30,87–89] of the five prospective studies have reported inverse associations for dietary vitamin D and colon or colorectal cancer, but this relation was only significant in the Western Electric study.[30] Of the three published case-control studies of vitamin D and colon or colorectal cancer, two[24,62] show inconsistent, nonsignificant findings and one[90] reported a significant inverse association. Of interest, stronger associations were seen when supplemental or total (dietary plus supplemental) vitamin D intake was considered in these studies. In the Nurses' Health Study,[87] overall stronger inverse associations were seen for vitamin D than for calcium. Results based on three questionnaires showed significant inverse associations with colorectal cancer for women who remained in the upper tertile of total vitamin D intake on all three questionnaires as compared to those who were in the lower tertile (RR = 0.33; 95% CI = 0.16–0.70) and for women in the upper versus the lower category of average intake of total vitamin D (RR = 0.42; 95% CI = 0.19–0.91). However, many of the women in the highest tertile were taking multivitamin supplements, a major source of vitamin D

in this population; therefore, other vitamin or mineral components could also be important.

Folate and Methionine. In addition to animal data,[91] an increasing epidemiologic body of evidence shows a potential role for folate in reducing risk for colorectal cancer. Five case-control studies have found a higher risk of colon cancer among individuals with low folate intakes.[26,62,90,92,93] Among four prospective studies that provide information on the relation between folate and colorectal cancer, three[94–96] support an inverse association between higher folate intake and lower cancer risk; another study,[97] which did not have comprehensive dietary data, showed an inverse association between plasma folate level and risk of colon cancer. Some evidence from small studies suggests a similar inverse relationship between folate and large bowel dysplasia or cancer associated with chronic ulcerative colitis.[98,99] In numerous studies that have not directly assessed folate, diets high in vegetables, the major dietary source of folate, have frequently been inversely associated with risk of colon cancer.[100] Folate intake has been consistently associated with lower risk of colon adenomas,[101–103] which typically arise a decade or more before a subsequent malignancy. Recent results indicate that increased consumption of folic acid from supplements, after a period of 15 or more years, may decrease risk of colon cancer by about 75 percent.[96] Additional evidence for a role for folate is that inherited variation in the activity of methylene tetrahydrofolate reductase (MTHFR), a critical enzyme in the production of the form of folate that supplies the methyl group for methionine synthesis,[104] influences risk of colon cancer[97,105] (Figure 2–1). This gene-nutrient interaction is discussed in more detail in a following section in this chapter. In a recently published study, Martínez and colleagues[106] found total folate (dietary plus supplemental) to be inversely related to the frequency of K-ras mutations in adenomatous polyps.

The mechanisms whereby folate may reduce carcinogenesis are unclear. Different endogenous forms of folate, 5-methyl tetrahydrofolate and 5,10-methylene tetrahydrofolate, are essential for DNA methylation and DNA synthesis, respectively (see Figure 2–1). When levels of 5,10-methylene tetrahydrofolate, which is required to convert deoxyuridy-

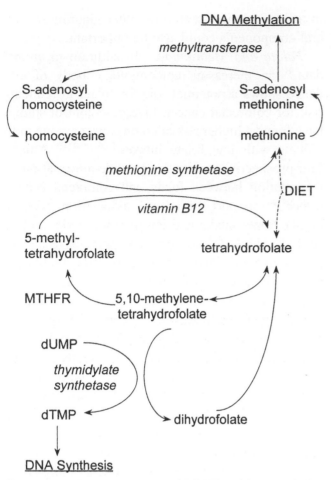

Figure 2–1. The metabolic role of MTHFR in folate metabolism involving DNA methylation and DNA synthesis.

late to thymidylate, are low, misincorporation of uracil for thymidine may occur during DNA synthesis,[107] possibly increasing spontaneous mutation rates,[108] sensitivity to DNA-damaging agents,[109] frequency of chromosomal aberrations,[110,111] and errors in DNA replication.[111–113] Folate deficiency is related to massive incorporation of uracil into human DNA and to increased chromosomal breaks, and these abnormalities are reversed with folic acid supplementation.[114] When methionine intake is low, levels of S-adenosylmethionine decrease, which stimulates the enzyme MTHFR to convert 5,10-methylene tetrahydrofolate into 5-methyl tetrahydrofolate (see Figure 2–1). Homocysteine is methylated by 5-methyl tetrahydrofolate to form methionine. If compensatory production of methionine is hindered by an insufficient folate level, the supply of methyl groups for DNA methylation may be inadequate. DNA hypomethylation is among the earliest events observed in

colon carcinogenesism,[115–120] although whether it directly influences the process remains unproven.

Besides folate, another dietary factor that may affect DNA methylation is methionine, which can be directly converted to S-adenosylmethionine.[121] An inverse association between sources of methionine, such as fish and poultry, and colon cancer or adenoma has been reported.[32–34,51,103,122–126] However, the inverse association between methionine and colorectal adenoma has only been directly examined in one study of two large cohorts.[102] In the Health Professionals Follow-up Study,[95] the increased risk in colon cancer was marked among men with lower intakes of folate and methionine in the presence of high alcohol consumption, whereas among individuals with high folate intake, there appeared to be little association between alcohol intake and cancer risk. The proposed mechanism for these observations relates to dietary factors that influence methyl group availability. The role of folate, methionine, and alcohol in colon carcinogenesis underscores the importance of considering complex dietary interactions when assessing cancer risk.

The consistent findings from diverse study designs and populations, the finding that a genetic polymorphism in a folate-metabolizing gene (MTHFR) is associated with risk of colorectal cancer, animal data, and the critical role for folate in DNA synthesis and methylation indicate an important role for folate.

Obesity and Physical Activity

Evidence for the deleterious effect of obesity, assessed by body mass index (BMI), on risk of colon cancer is derived from prospective[30,34,127–137] and retrospective[19,20,22,138,139] epidemiologic studies. The evidence appears to be stronger for men than for women. In one study,[137] women who had a BMI greater than 29 kg/m^2 had a RR of 1.45 (95% CI = 1.02–2.07) in comparison with women whose BMI was less than 21 kg/m^2. Data on body fat distribution and colon cancer risk are very limited. One study of men[129] reported a strong positive association between waist-to-hip ratio and waist circumference with colon cancer risk. When comparing upper to lower quintiles, the relative risk for waist-to-hip ratio was 3.41 (95%

CI = 1.52–7.66) and for waist circumference it was 2.56 (95% CI = 1.33–4.96). Of interest, the two studies among women[34,137] reported suggestive but not statistically significant positive associations between waist-to-hip ratio and risk of colon cancer. Possibly, these measures of adipose distribution are stronger predictors of colon cancer risk for men than for women because of the male tendency for central adiposity.

Results of prospective[49,72,127,128,137,140–147] and retrospective[21–23,44,123,138,148–163] studies support an inverse association between physical activity and risk of colon but not rectal cancer.[22,128,142–144,154,164,165] The results are consistent whether assessing active versus non-active individuals or sedentary versus active (Figure 2–2). In a prospective study of female nurses,[137] leisure-time physical activity and body size were assessed in relation to the subsequent development of colon cancer. Women who were in the upper quintile of activity were at almost half the risk of developing colon cancer compared to nonactive women (RR = 0.54; 95% CI = 0.33–0.90). These findings are supported by results of other published studies, including those of the Health Professionals Follow-up Study,[129] a large prospective study of men. When physical activity and BMI are assessed jointly, the highest risk of colon cancer occurs among those both physically inactive and with high BMI levels.[28,129]

Although physical activity is often associated with other lifestyle factors that are themselves risk factors for colon cancer (i.e., obesity, diet, cigarette smoking, etc.), the inverse association appears to be independent of these factors. In spite of the wide variation in physical assessment methodology among studies, including type of activity (leisure-time or occupational) and method of assessment, considerable consistency was found. Based on a recent comprehensive review of the literature, Colditz and colleagues[166] reported approximately a 50 percent reduction in incidence of colon cancer among individuals with the highest level of physical activity. Several biologic mechanisms have been proposed for the inverse association between physical activity and colon cancer.[167] Martínez and colleagues[168] recently showed that a higher level of leisure-time activity was significantly inversely related to the concentration of prostaglandin E_2 (PGE$_2$) in the rectal mucosa, suggesting a potential mechanism acting through PGE$_2$ synthesis. Hyperinsulinemia may also be important, as this condition is related to physical inactivity, high body mass, and central deposition of adipose, and insulin is a mitogen for normal and neoplastic colonic epithelial cells.[169]

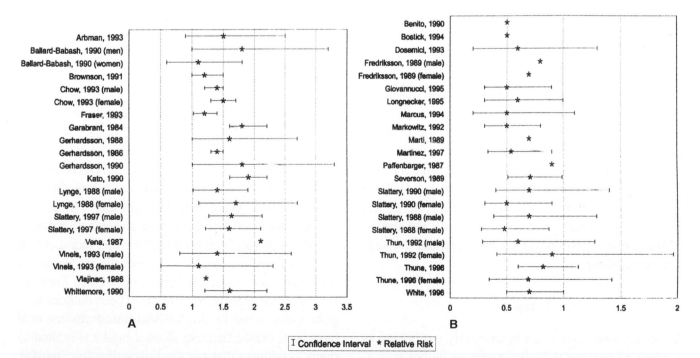

Figure 2–2. Summary of epidemiologic studies of colon (excluding rectum) cancer and physical activity. *A,* Low versus high activity, *B,* high versus low activity.

Supporting a role for insulin are recent studies that have found diabetes mellitus to be a risk factor[170] and a prospective analysis of insulin that found a direct association with colon cancer risk.[171]

Postmenopausal Hormone Use

Excess colorectal cancer mortality among nuns[172] and positive correlations in incidence and mortality rates of colon and breast cancers[173–175] have implicated a hormonal etiology for colorectal cancer. Although studies on reproductive factors and colorectal cancer have provided conflicting results, PMH has been associated with a decreased risk of colon or colorectal cancer in the majority of case-control and cohort studies.[127,136,176–191] In the Nurses' Health Study,[185] current PMH use was associated with a decreased risk of colorectal cancer (RR = 0.65; 95% CI = 0.50–0.83) compared to non-users; the relation for past use was weaker (RR = 0.84; 95% CI = 0.67–1.05) and disappeared 5 years after hormone use was stopped (RR = 0.92; 95% CI = 0.70–1.21). This investigation is one of three large prospective studies[180,190] to report an inverse association between colorectal cancer and estrogen use in postmenopausal women. A large multicenter case-control study[191] also indicated that women who used PMH had a lower colon cancer risk (OR = 0.82; 95% CI = 0.67–0.99), and recent use was associated with approximately a 30 percent reduction in risk (OR = 0.71; 95% CI = 0.56–0.89). Results of another large case-control study[182] also showed an inverse association between PMH and colorectal cancer, particularly among recent users (RR = 0.54; 95% CI = 0.36–0.81). Overall, the results of recent studies show inverse associations ranging from 0.5 to 0.8 for the use of PMH. A causal association would be of important public health significance. Given the relative consistency of results based on the use of PMH, the inconsistency for other reproductive factors is puzzling.

Tobacco

Although tobacco had not been clearly implicated as a cause of colorectal malignancies, a higher risk of adenomatous polyps has been consistently observed among smokers in numerous studies.[192] A very long induction period between smoking and risk of colorectal cancer was hypothesized based on results from two large cohort studies.[193,194] Subsequently, the vast majority of published studies have reported positive associations between cigarette smoking and colorectal cancer,[127,195–204] though several studies did not support an association.[205–208] Of note, three of the nonsupportive studies[205–207] were conducted in Sweden, suggesting that some factor, possibly genetic, in Swedes may counter the impact of smoking. In a review of the published data, Giovannucci and Martínez[192] suggested that the evidence earlier in the decade tended not to support the hypothesis that smoking influenced colorectal carcinogenesis because a sufficient lag period had not elapsed between smoking and colorectal cancer risk. With the assumption that an increased risk emerges only about four decades after one begins smoking, a relatively consistent pattern materializes. The consistent finding of a positive association between smoking and the risk of adenomas probably results from a presumably much shorter induction period for these lesions. One study found that polycyclic aromatic hydrocarbons (PAHs) form DNA adducts in human colon mucosa.[209] The overall evidence supports the hypothesis that tobacco smoke is an initiator of colorectal carcinogenesis and the requirement for a very long induction period, possibly up to four decades.

Alcohol

An association between alcohol intake and colon cancer risk has been observed in many ecologic,[12] cohort,[95,127,133,210–215] and population-based case-control studies.[16,216–222] Further, alcohol has been consistently related to higher risk of colorectal adenoma.[102] In a recent extensive review,[12] Kune and Vitetta concluded that a positive association between alcohol intake and colorectal cancer was found in 5 of 7 correlational studies, in 9 of 10 of the studies using population-based controls, but in only 5 of 17 studies that used hospital-based controls. These authors suggested that some of the hospital-based studies may have been biased because alcohol intake is related to many conditions that require hospitalization, causing an overestimate of intake among controls. Kune and

Vitetta also found that in three of the four cohort studies that did not demonstrate an association, the alcohol data collected were limited.

The mechanism of action whereby alcohol increases risk for colorectal cancer is unknown. An intriguing possibility is the property of alcohol as an antagonist of folate and methionine metabolism.[121,223] The alcohol breakdown product acetaldehyde may inactivate methyltetrahydrofolate, the form of folate required for methionine synthesis.[224] In rodents, the carcinogenicity of methyl-deficient diets is enhanced by ethanol.[225] Based on these considerations, it was postulated that specific combinations of diet might be particularly deleterious.[95] In a cohort study of men,[95] alcohol, folate, and methionine intakes individually were moderately associated with risk of colon cancer, but combinations of high alcohol and low methionine and folate intakes yielded striking relative risks of 3.3 for total colon cancer and 7.4 for distal colon cancer. Further, among men with high intakes of folate or methionine, alcohol levels of greater than two drinks per day were not associated with risk of colon cancer. These findings suggest that the role of alcohol may depend on other dietary factors, particularly those related to methyl group metabolism.

Nonsteroidal Anti-inflammatory Drugs

Evidence in favor of a protective effect of non-steroidal anti-inflammatory drugs (NSAIDs) (e.g., aspirin, indomethacin, ibuprofen, piroxicam, sulindac) on colorectal cancer stems from epidemiologic,[226–230] animal,[231–234] and intervention studies among individuals with familial adenomatous polyposis.[235–237] In addition, patients with rheumatoid arthritis, who generally have higher use of NSAIDs, have lower incidence and mortality rates of gastrointestinal malignancies.[238,239] Supporting evidence is also derived from observational studies of NSAIDs and colorectal adenomas.[229,240–242]

Results of the epidemiologic studies are consistent with an approximate 50 percent reduction in colorectal cancer risk associated with use of aspirin or other NSAIDs, although in one study[243] a positive association was observed. Perhaps the strongest evidence to date for the preventive activity of aspirin has been derived from the Nurses' Health Study.[230] Results of this large cohort study showed a statistically significant reduction of colorectal cancer in women after 20 years of consistent (two or more aspirin tablets per week) aspirin use (RR = 0.56; 95% CI = 0.36–0.90; p = .008), independent of other known risk factors, including diet. Another similar prospective study in male health professionals reported RRs of comparable magnitude.[229]

Unfortunately, standard doses of NSAIDs, such as those used for arthritis treatment, are associated with a significant incidence of erosive mucosal disease in the upper gastrointestinal tract and occasionally lead to ulceration. Thus, NSAID administration at standard doses does not seem to be a feasible strategy for primary prevention of colorectal cancer in average risk persons. The evidence supporting a protective effect of NSAIDs on colon cancer is, nevertheless, provocative, and perhaps use in high-risk individuals is warranted.

Insulin-Like Growth Factors

The insulin-like growth (IGF) factor axis is organized into IGFs, IGF binding proteins (IGFBPs), IGF proteases, and cell membrane-associated receptors. The IGF axis influences cellular proliferation and apoptosis and, for many cell types, IGF-1 is required to progress through the cell cycle.[244] IGF binding proteins can oppose actions to IGF-1; this action may occur in part by binding and thus sequestering IGF-1[245] and possibly by inhibitory effects mediated by specific IGFBP-3 membrane-associated receptors.[246] Since high cellular turnover tends to increase the rate at which genetic alterations accumulate in cells, it is plausible that the IGF axis influences cancer rates for the numerous cell types that express IGF-1 receptors. In addition, IGF-1 has been shown to be important for the survival of transformed cells.[247]

Normal colorectal epithelia and cancer cells express IGF-1 receptors, which stimulate mitogenesis when activated by IGF-1 in vitro.[248–252] Acromegaly, a condition characterized by chronically elevated growth hormone levels resulting from a pituitary adenoma and IGF-1 hypersecretion, is associated with increased epithelial cell proliferation in the sigmoid colon[253] and elevated risk of benign and malignant colon tumors.[254–263] In a recent study of 129 patients with biochemically proven acromegaly, the prevalence of colorectal neoplasia found during a colonoscopic examination was considerably higher than would be expected based on published rates for asymptomatic screened controls; the odds ratio was 13.5 (95% CI = 3.1–75) for colorectal cancer and 4.2 (95% CI = 2.5–6.8) for adenoma.[261]

In a study of U.S. physicians, baseline plasma IGF-1, IGF-2, and IGFBP-3 levels among 193 men diagnosed with colorectal cancer over a 12-year follow-up period were compared with levels from 318 age- and smoking-matched controls.[264] Men in the top quintile of IGF-1 had a RR of 1.36 (95% CI = 0.72–2.55; p = .51), but after further adjustment for IGFBP-3, the RR was 2.51 (95% CI = 1.15–5.46; p = .02). For IGFBP-3, the RR for top versus bottom quintile was 0.47 (95% CI = 0.23–0.95; p = .07); when further adjusted for IGF-1, the RR was 0.28 (95% CI = 0.12–0.66; p = .005). The IGF-2 level was unrelated to risk of colorectal cancer. A preliminary analysis in the Nurses' Health Study[265] found that high IGF-1 and low IGFBP-3 levels increased risk of colorectal adenomas and adenomas $\geq$ 1 cm in diameter or those with a villous component (tubulovillous, villous, in situ cancers), but not of small, tubular adenomas. These results indicate that the IGF axis influences adenoma progression and increases risk of colorectal cancer. Modifiable determinants of IGF levels are poorly understood and a better understanding may lead to preventive approaches.

GENE-ENVIRONMENT INTERACTIONS AND GENETIC SUSCEPTIBILITY

Susceptibility to colorectal cancer may be related in part to interindividual variability in biotransformation of endogenous and exogenous substances. This variability in susceptibility could have important implications for colorectal cancer prevention. At the present time, interventions focus on the notion that all individuals in the population respond uniformly to carcinogenic exposures. It is possible to construct a molecular-based approach to primary and secondary prevention of colorectal cancer based on

the identification of individuals who may be more vulnerable to the effects of certain carcinogens (Figure 2–3). For example, in individuals with the high-risk genotype, an aggressive intervention may include more frequent colonoscopy screenings, chemopreventive agents, and behavior modification involving avoiding the relevant carcinogenic factors. For the individuals with the low-risk genotype, the standard intervention can include screening as per the standard guidelines, with continued focus on the lifestyle factors. The following is a discussion of some examples of potential gene-environment interactions.

Xenobiotic Metabolizing Genes

A current area of research involves the role of genetic variability in susceptibility to the adverse effects of specific risk factors. Differences in human response to carcinogens have been linked to heritable differences in polymorphic metabolism of xenobiotic chemicals. For example, if heterocyclic amines found in cigarette smoke condensate or those formed by cooking meat at high temperatures are involved in colorectal carcinogenesis, genetic polymorphisms in the various enzymes involved in metabolism of these carcinogens are likely to influence the risk of this malignancy. Individuals with this type of susceptibility are at increased risk only if exposed to particular carcinogens. The metabolism of many of these compounds is mediated in part by cytochromes P450 1A1 (CYP1A1) and 1A2 (CYP1A2), which generate reactive metabolites that can produce DNA adducts. Enhanced metabolic activation of polycyclic aromatic hydrocarbons (PAHs) has been observed in homozygotes for an Msp I mutation in the 3'-end of CYP1A1. Some data show that the polymorphism associated with enhanced activation of CYP1A1 is related to higher risk for colorectal carcinoma in situ and cancer.[266] A polymorphism that causes a highly inducible state of CYP1A2 has also been described[267]; however, since the exact locus of genetic variation remains to be identified, CYP1A2 polymorphisms can only be determined by phenotypic assays.

Acetylation polymorphisms resulting from different forms of the N-acetyltransferase gene 1

(NAT1) and 2 (NAT2) lead to either fast or slow acetylation of xenobiotics. Rapid acetylation may only be important among individuals who consume a diet high in meats that are significant sources of heterocyclic amines. In studies that have found that rapid NAT2 increased risk of colon cancer, the association was greatest among those in the higher quartiles of meat consumption.[268,269] It has been suggested that rapid NAT2 acetylation of heterocyclic amines formed in cooking of meat may be related to colon cancer risk.[268] Furthermore, when the role of cooked meat preference and phenotype combinations of NAT2 and CYP1A2 in colorectal neoplasia was assessed,[268] the combination of well-done meat cooking preference and rapid-rapid phenotypes was associated with an odds ratio of 6.45; however, these findings have not been replicated by more recent studies.[270,271] The role of NAT1 has not been adequately studied because, up until recently, it was thought to be monomorphic. In contrast to enzymes that may activate carcinogens, glutathione S-transferases (GSTs) detoxify carcinogens, including smoking-related carcinogens formed by CYP1A1, by conjugating them with glutathione. Cytosolic GSTs are a supergene family, are widely distributed in the mammalian species, and are grouped into five classes on the basis of subunit composition: α (A), μ (M), π (P), τ (T), and σ (Z). The GSTM1-null genotype, which is associated with enzyme inactivity of GSTμ, has been shown to be more frequent among patients with colorectal cancer,[272,273] although this finding has not been universal.[274]

Research involving xenobiotic metabolizing genes is relatively new and will no doubt continue to intensify in the near future. To date, sample sizes for studies attempting to uncover gene-environment interactions have been small, limiting the potential for detecting significant findings.

Methylenetetrahydrofolate Reductase and Folic Acid

Another example of a gene-diet interaction involves the MTHFR gene, folic acid, and colorectal cancer.[105] As noted earlier, diets low in folate and methionine and high in alcohol are associated with a higher risk of colorectal cancer.[95] Such a dietary pat-

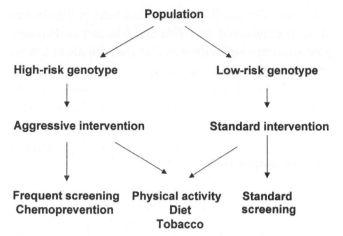
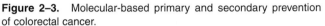

Figure 2–3. Molecular-based primary and secondary prevention of colorectal cancer.

tern results in a methyl-deficient diet, thus enhancing colorectal cancer risk by altering DNA methylation or by influencing the production of thymidine, which is required for DNA synthesis.[275] MTHFR is an enzyme that regulates the metabolism of folate and methionine by converting 5,10-methylene-tetrahydrofolate to 5-methyltetrahydrofolate, the form of folate required for methionine synthesis (see Figure 2–1). In a study of men, Chen and colleagues[105] observed a lower risk of colorectal cancer for individuals with the MTHFR variant homozygous genotype (TT) who consumed more methionine (OR = 0.27; 95% CI = 0.06–1.20) or had a higher folate intake (OR = 0.44; 95% CI = 0.13–1.55) as compared with those with the variant heterozygous (CT) or the wild-type homozygous (CC) with lower intakes of methionine or folate. Furthermore, among men with the variant homozygous genotype, those in the high alcohol category had a 15-fold risk of colorectal cancer compared to those in the low category, indicating that the benefit associated with MTHFR is eliminated with high alcohol consumption. Based on their findings, the authors suggested that the risk of colorectal cancer associated with the MTHFR homozygous variant genotype may differ depending on the folate and methionine content of the diet as well as alcohol intake. Similar findings were also reported by Ma and colleagues[97] in a later publication. A recent case-control study by Slattery and colleagues[276] found a weaker association for the TT genotype in men (OR = 0.8; CI = 0.6–1.1) and women (OR = 0.9; CI = 0.6–1.2).

Although the results were weaker than in the studies in men conducted by Chen and Ma and colleagues, one striking similarity was that individuals at lowest overall risk were those with the TT genotype and low risk based on methyl status (low alcohol/high folate and high methionine); if methyl status was poor (high alcohol/low folate and low methionine status), the subjects with the TT and CC genotypes were at similar risk.

Glutathione S-Transferases and Cruciferous Vegetables

Vegetables contain several compounds that possess a variety of anticarcinogenic properties.[277] Specifically, the anticarcinogenic properties of cruciferous vegetables have been mainly attributed to the degradation products of glucosionolates (e.g., isothiocyanates and indoles), which induce detoxification enzymes.[278] A possible mechanism of action of isothiocyanates is thought to be through the induction of GSTs.[279] These enzymes catalyze the conjugation of glutathione with a large number of compounds bearing an electrophilic center, including carcinogens. There is some support in the literature for the role of GSTs in the metabolism of isothiocyanates in man.[280] In terms of individual isoenzymes, GSTM1 and GSTP1 appear to be the most efficient catalysts that rapidly conjugate isothiocyanates to glutathione, which is then excreted in the urine.[281] GSTM1 is involved in the detoxification of tobacco-related carcinogens, such as epoxides and hydroxylated metabolites of benzo[a]pyrene. While there have been several studies of the impact of GSTM1 deficiencies on susceptibility to a range of cancers, there have been no similar studies of GSTP1. Since these polymorphisms have only recently been identified, the literature regarding their role in carcinogenesis is unclear. The only study reported in the literature that has addressed the interaction between cruciferous vegetables, GSTs polymorphisms, and colorectal neoplasia[282] found a lower prevalence of colorectal adenomas among people with the GSTM1-null genotype when comparing individuals in the highest versus lowest quartile of broccoli intake (OR = 0.36; 95% CI = 0.19–0.68). Nevertheless, the hypothesis that crucif-

erous vegetable consumption might decrease risk of colorectal cancer through their increase in GST activity is plausible and is currently being addressed in several study settings.

CHEMOPREVENTION

In addition to observational and animal studies, chemoprevention trials can provide an additional setting where the cancer-inhibitory effect of specific agents can be tested. A major challenge related to chemoprevention trials is that very large numbers of participants must be enrolled to detect a meaningful effect in a reasonable time frame. Chemoprevention would be extremely attractive for general use if agents with virtually no side effects could be identified. To the degree that potential agents have significant toxicities, they must be confined to use on select populations. To date, NSAIDs, the most clearly active chemopreventive agents, have significant side effects, most notably gastrointestinal bleeding and upper gastrointestinal symptoms. The probability of such side effects is large enough that some NSAIDs are unacceptable for use in individuals who do not have cancer. In those with a high risk of colorectal cancer, however, the use of these agents may be justified. The level of potential toxicity has to be considered in light of the probability that the person faces a high risk of colorectal cancer.

To date, the most common study design for colorectal cancer chemoprevention has been to test the effects of specific agents on adenoma recurrence among individuals with a history of adenomatous polyps. In this setting, individuals who have undergone removal of one or more adenomas are randomized to intervention or placebo (although not all have a true placebo arm). Participants are then followed for a period of approximately 3 years, at which time they undergo a colonoscopy for detection of additional adenomas. Although this design provides a convenient model in which to test these interventions, effects of agents at earlier or later stages in the colorectal carcinogenesis sequence are not tested. Specifically, results of these trials do not provide evidence for the role of agents in the occurrence of new (initial) adenomas. More importantly, since these trials focus on relatively early stages, they do not assess whether the agent in question is related to colorectal cancer development from large dysplastic adenomas. Even the larger trials may not have sufficient statistical power to test the effect of the intervention on the formation of large adenomas, which are more clinically important. Since the follow-up time in these trials generally is not longer than 4 years, it is entirely possible that null findings are the result of an insufficient follow-up period.

Several agents have been tested or are being evaluated for chemopreventive potential of colorectal cancer. They include folic acid, bile acid modifiers (for example, calcium, wheat bran fiber, low fat, high fruit and vegetables and fiber, and ursodeoxycholic acid), and NSAIDs (for example, piroxicam, sulindac, sulindac sulfone, celecoxib [Celebrex®]). The following is a review of agents, to date, that have been investigated or show promise as interventions for colorectal cancer prevention.

Bile Acid Agents: Fiber, Calcium, Ursodeoxycholic Acid

For almost half a century, bile acids have been suspected to be important colorectal carcinogens. The primary bile acids, cholic and chenodeoxycholic acids, are synthesized in the liver and then secreted into the intestines through the bile duct. In the colon, the bile salts that have not been reabsorbed through the small intestine are metabolized by anaerobic bacteria into the secondary bile acids, deoxycholic and lithocholic acids, and small amounts are converted into ursodeoxycholic acid. Of the bile acids, deoxycholic is hypothesized to have an important role in carcinogenesis. Evidence from experimental[283,284] and observational[285,286] studies supports the hypothesis that decreasing the level or concentration of deoxycholic acid lessens the likelihood of neoplastic transformation, although the role in human colorectal cancer remains controversial.

Fiber may have a role in colorectal cancer prevention through various mechanisms involving bile acid metabolism. Fiber increases the water content of stool, which reduces the carcinogenic concentration of secondary bile acids. By altering the pH in the gut, fiber decreases the rate of conversion of primary to secondary bile acids.[287] Previously published small intervention trials have tested the influence of wheat bran fiber on colorectal carcinogenesis (Table 2–1). However, the recently published results of a large chemoprevention trial[288] found that a dietary supplement of wheat bran fiber had no significant reduction in the recurrence of colorectal adenomas. Likewise, in the Polyp Prevention Trial, no effect of a low-fat, high fiber and fruit intervention was shown on adenoma recurrence.

Calcium may alter the pH in the gut and thus influence bile acid balance and colon cancer risk by decreasing cellular proliferation.[85,289] Two studies evaluating the combined effects of calcium and wheat bran fiber have been conducted. In one study,[290] a randomized, double-blinded, placebo-controlled trial design evaluated the effects of wheat bran fiber and calcium on fecal bile acids. The results suggested that fiber and calcium individually and in combination lower the concentrations of total bile acid, as well as each bile acid component. In the other study,[291] rectal mucosal proliferation was not lessened by wheat bran fiber or calcium supplementation or a combination of the two. In addition, the results of an intervention trial of calcium supplementation (1,200 mg of elemental calcium versus placebo) among 913 participants found a moderate but statistically significant reduction in risk of adenoma recurrence.[292] The recurrence rate in the calcium group was 31 percent and that in the placebo group was 38 percent (RR = 0.76; 95% CI = 0.60–0.96). Similar results were observed in the European Calcium Fibre Polyp Prevention trial,[293] although the lower recurrence rate among the calcium group was not statistically significant in the small study.

Ursodeoxycholic acid, generally found in trace amounts in the human colon bile acid pool, is produced by bacterial enzymes from chenodcoxycholic acid.[294] Addition of ursodeoxycholic acid to the diet decreases the concentration of deoxycholic acid and the formation of tumors in rodents.[295] The potential benefit of 600 mg daily ursodeoxycholic acid is currently being tested in a double-blind, placebo-controlled trial on the 3-year adenoma recurrence rates among 1,200 participants with a history of adenomatous polyps (see Table 2–1). Collection of blood and stool samples for analysis of baseline and study endpoint bile acid concentrations is being conducted

Table 2–1. SELECTED DIETARY AND CHEMOPREVENTIVE AGENT TRIALS OF COLORECTAL CANCER INCIDENCE OR ADENOMATOUS POLYP RECURRENCE			
Study	Agent(s) Tested	Follow-up (years)	Relative Risk
Cancer			
NPSC	Selenium, 200 µg	5	0.42
ATBC	β carotene, 20 mg	6	β carotene: 1.05
	Vitamin E, 50 IU		Vitamin E: 0.83
Adenoma Recurrence			
MacLennan	WBF, 25 g	4	WBF: 1.2
	β carotene, 20 mg		β carotene: 1.5
Greenberg	β carotene, 25 mg	4	β carotene: 1.01
	Vitamin E, 400 IU + Vitamin C, I g		Vitamin E + Vitamin C: 1.08
McKeown-Eyssen	WBF, 20 g	2	1.2
McKeown-Eyssen	Vitamin C, 400 mg	2	0.86
	+ Vitamin E, 400 mg		
Roncucci	Vitamin A, 30,000 IU	1.5	Vitamins: 0.11
	+ Vitamin E, 70 mg		Lactulose: 0.31
	+ Vitamin C, 1 g		
Baron	Lactulose Calcium, 1200 mg	4	0.83
Faivre	Calcium, 2 g	3	Calcium: 0.66
	Ispaghula husk fiber, 3.5 g		Fiber: 1.67
PPT	Low fat + High fruit & vegetables + fiber	4	OR: 0.88; RR: 0.99
Alberts	WBF, 13 g	3	1.00
Baron*	Aspirin, 80 mg and 325 mg + Folic acid, 1000 µg	3	Ongoing
Giovannucci*	Folic acid, 1000 µg	3	Ongoing

*Personal communications.
NPSC = nutritional prevention of skin cancer; WBF = wheat bran fiber; ATBC = alpha-tocopherol beta-carotene; PPT = polyp prevention trial.
Data from Clark LC et al.[307]
The ATBC Study Group.[306]
MacLennan R et al.[308]
Greenberg ER et al.[309]
McKeown-Eyssen GE, Bright-See E, Bruce WR, et al. A randomized trial of a low fat high fibre diet in the recurrence of colorectal polyps. J Clin Epidemiol 1994; 47:525–36.
McKeown-Eyssen GE, Holloway C, Jazmaji V, et al. A randomized trial of vitamins C and E in the prevention of recurrence of colorectal polyps. Cancer Res 1988;8:470–5.
Roncucci L, DiDonccto P, Carati L, et al. Antioxidant vitamins or lactulose for the prevention of the recurrence of colorectal adenomas. Dis Colon Rectum 1903;36:227–34.
Baron JA et al.[292]
Faivre J et al.[293]
Schatzkin A, Lanze E, Corle D, et al. Lack of an effect of a low-fat, high-fiber diet on the recurrence of colorectal adenomas. Polyp Prevention Trial I Study Group. N Engl J Med 2000;342:1149–55.
Alberts DS et al.[288]

to evaluate the extent to which the mechanism of ursodeoxycholic acid's effect on the risk of new polyp formation involves alteration of secondary bile acids.

NSAIDs

Interest in NSAIDs as a means of chemoprevention was stimulated by results of animal and observational epidemiologic studies that suggested that aspirin use was associated with substantially decreased colorectal cancer risk.[228,230] Aspirin, piroxicam, sulindac, sulindac sulfone, and celecoxib are the NSAIDs being considered as colorectal cancer chemopreventive agents.

It has become clear that some NSAIDs will not be suitable candidates for chemoprevention because of their significant toxicities, including increased risk of gastrointestinal bleeding, ulcers, and kidney damage.[296] The action of most NSAIDs involves their inhibition of the enzyme cyclooxygenase.[297] There are two cyclooxygenases: the first, and the most abundant, COX-1, is involved in normal maintenance of cellular function; the second, COX-2, is induced by injury or inflammation. The recent focus of research on cyclooxygenase inhibitors has been the identification of agents that block COX-2.

Sulindac decreases the prevalence of colorectal polyps in familial adenomatous polyposis patients, possibly by depression of proliferation, induction of apoptosis,[298] or alteration of bile acid concentration.[299] Although sulindac may operate via inhibition of cyclooxygenase and thus reduce prostaglandin synthesis, the oxidized metabolite of sulindac, sulindac sulfone, was recently shown to inhibit cell growth in vitro and colon tumor formation in vivo, and induce apoptosis without inhibiting either COX-1 or COX-2.[300–302] The sulfone appears as powerful as sulindac in depressing colon tumor formation, suggesting a novel sulfone-induced signal transduction pathway route to enhanced apoptosis in neoplastic colorectal cells.[302]

In the Physicians' Health Study,[303] 22,071 healthy volunteers were randomized to either 325 mg of aspirin every other day or placebo to examine the impact of aspirin on cardiovascular disease risk. After 5 years of follow-up, there was no reduction in risk of colorectal cancer for the aspirin group compared to placebo (RR = 1.15; 95% CI = 0.80–1.65). Given that a protective effect of aspirin was suggested only after 20 years of regular use in the Nurses' Health Study cohort,[230] the null results in the Physicians' Health Study could have been due to short duration in follow-up. Investigators at Dartmouth University are currently conducting a multicenter clinical adenoma recurrence trial of aspirin (325 mg/day vs. 80 mg/day vs. placebo) with or without folic acid in patients with a history of colorectal adenomatous polyps (see Table 2–1). The results of this and other intervention trials will aid in establishing an optimal dose and, more importantly, in determining the benefits and risk of such intervention.

Celecoxib, almost exclusively a COX-2 inhibitor, is presently one of the most promising of the modern-day NSAIDs. In experimental systems, it has been shown to lessen aberrant crypt formation[304] and the incidence, multiplicity, and weight burden of induced tumors.[305] In these studies, celecoxib apparently induced no toxic side effects generally associated with NSAIDs (i.e., weight loss, gastrointestinal ulcers, mucosal damage, or bleeding). Chemoprevention trials of celecoxib are presently in advanced planning stages and should be initiated soon.

Folic Acid

As described previously, increasing epidemiologic, genetic, and experimental evidence support a preventive role of folic acid on colorectal carcinogenesis. The generally nontoxic nature of this agent, a vitamin, makes it an ideal candidate for chemoprevention. Ongoing trials are assessing the role of folic acid on recurrent adenomas (see Table 2–1).

Antioxidants and Other Micronutrients

Chemoprevention trials that tested the anticarcinogenic potential of antioxidant nutrients have shown mixed results for the development of colorectal cancer[306,307] (see Table 2–1) or adenoma recurrence.[308–310] A greater than 50 percent reduction in colorectal cancer incidence was shown for selenium, in the form of braker's yeast intervention, in the Nutritional Prevention of Skin Cancer.[307] Since these results were based on secondary endpoint data among a population of selenium-deficient areas in the United States, additional large trials will be needed to confirm this provocative finding.

CONCLUSION

The past decade has been an exciting and challenging one for progress in the prevention of colorectal cancer. As this century comes to a close, the prospect of colorectal cancer no longer remaining a major source of cancer mortality appears promising. The genetic events underlying this disease continue to be elucidated rapidly; the lesion that leads to colorectal cancer, the adenoma, has been identified, and the basic process by which this lesion becomes more dysplastic and, eventually, invasive is also well described. A critical area for future investigations is the validation of intermediate markers in the carcinogenic process. Until such markers are developed, progress in chemoprevention will be slow since studies that use incidence and survival are lengthy. Additionally, since relatively few adenomatous polyps progress to malignant lesions, the identification of factors that predict the rate of progression more accurately continues to be an important task. As the biology and molecular basis of this disease become better understood, and we continue to discover agents that offer promising means of intervening, there is potential for also understanding important mechanisms by which these agents may influence risk.

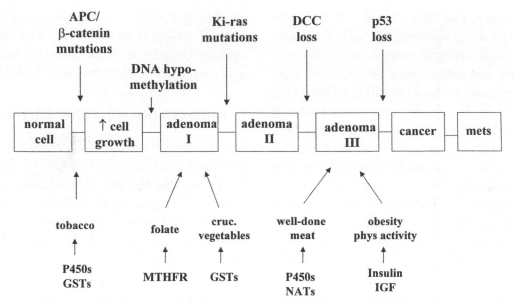

Figure 2–4.   Proposed model of gene-environment interactions in the pathogenesis of colorectal cancer.

As a result of recent epidemiologic studies that have examined various risk factors in relation to adenoma and carcinoma, a hypothetical model for colorectal carcinogenesis that takes into account environmental factors, genetic predisposition, and molecular events is proposed (Figure 2–4). A model such as this can perhaps be helpful in understanding where in the carcinogenesis sequence we can intervene most effectively. Studies are now beginning to examine suspected etiologic factors in relation to mutations in certain genes (e.g., p53 tumor suppressor gene, the K-ras proto-oncogene), including specific types of mutations (e.g., transition mutations at a specific codon). Examples of such studies are just beginning to emerge in the literature.[106,204] By linking certain exposures to specific genetic alterations, we may enhance our ability to reach firm conclusions from epidemiologic investigations.

Although the precise mechanisms remain to be elucidated, several dietary and lifestyle factors are likely to have a major impact on colorectal cancer. Physical inactivity, excess body weight, and a central deposition of adiposity are consistent risk factors for colon cancer. Also, excess alcohol consumption, probably in combination with a diet low in some micronutrients such as folate and methionine, and smoking early in life are likely to increase risk. Diet and nutritional factors are clearly important, but the role of specific dietary factors beyond

general overconsumption of energy remains unresolved. Recent epidemiologic studies have tended not to support a strong impact of fiber; instead, some micronutrients or phytochemicals in fiber-rich foods may be important. Folic acid is one such nutrient that has received attention lately and is being studied in randomized intervention trials. Recent evidence also points to a role of growth factors such as 1GF-1 and 1GFBP-3, but our understanding of modifiable factors that influence levels of these is poor at present. Agents with chemopreventive properties, such as aspirin and postmenopausal estrogens, have potential adverse effects as well as other benefits, so a careful consideration of the risk-benefit ratio is required before general recommendations can be made.

REFERENCES

1. Vogelstein B, Fearon ER, Hamilton SR, et al. Genetic alterations during colorectal-tumor development. N Engl J Med 1988;319:525–32.
2. Landis SH, Murray T, Bolden S, Wingo PA. Cancer statistics, 1999. CA Cancer J Clin 1999;49:8–31.
3. Byers T, Levin B, Rothenberger JD, et al. American Cancer Society guidelines for screening and surveillance for early detection of colorectal polyps and cancer: update 1997. CA Cancer J Clin 1997;47:154–67.
4. Miller BA, Ries LAG, Hankey BF, et al. SEER Cancer Statistics Review 1973–1989. Bethesda (MD): National Cancer Institute, 1992.

5. Devesa SS, Chow WH. Variation in colorectal cancer incidence in the United States by subsite of origin. Cancer 1993;71:3819–26.

6. Ries LAG, Kosary CL, Hankey BF, et al. SEER cancer statistics review, 1973–1995. Bethesda (MD): National Cancer Institute, 1998.

7. Markowitz AJ, Winawer SJ. Management of colorectal polyps. CA Cancer J Clin 1997;47:93–112.

8. American Cancer Society. Cancer facts and figures for African Americans 1998–1999. Atlanta (GA): American Cancer Society, 1998.

9. Chao A, Gilliland FD, Hunt WC, et al. Increasing incidence of colon and rectal cancer among Hispanics and American Indians in New Mexico (United States), 1969–94. Cancer Causes Control 1998;9:137–44.

10. Mayberry RM, Coates RJ, Hill HA, et al. Determinants of black/white differences in colon cancer survival. J Natl Cancer Inst 1995;87:1686–93.

11. Jessup JM, Menck MR, Fremgen A, Winchester DP. Diagnosing colorectal carcinoma: clinical and molecular approaches. CA Cancer J Clin 1997;47:70–92.

12. Kune GA, Vitetta L. Alcohol consumption and the etiology of colorectal cancer: a review of the scientific evidence from 1957 to 1991. Nutr Cancer 1992;18: 97–111.

13. Willett WC, Stampfer MJ. Total energy intake: implications for epidemiologic analyses. Am J Epidemiol 1986;124:17–27.

14. Jain M, Cook GM, Davis FG, et al. A case-control study of diet and colo-rectal cancer. Int J Cancer 1980;26: 757–68.

15. Bristol JB, Emmett PM, Heaton KW, Williamson RC. Sugar, fat, and the risk of colorectal cancer. BMJ 1985;291:1467–70.

16. Potter JD, McMichael AJ. Diet and cancer of the colon and rectum: a case-control study. J Natl Cancer Inst 1986;76:557–69.

17. Lyon JL, Mahoney AW, West DW, et al. Energy intake: its relationship to colon cancer risk. J Natl Cancer Inst 1987;78:853–61.

18. Kune S, Kune GA, Watson LF. Case-control study of dietary etiologic factors: the Melbourne Colorectal Cancer Study. Nutr Cancer 1987;9:21–42.

19. Graham S, Marshall J, Haughey B, et al. Dietary epidemiology of cancer of the colon in western New York. Am J Epidemiol 1988;128:490–503.

20. West DW, Slattery ML, Robison LM, et al. Dietary intake and colon cancer: sex- and anatomic site-specific associations. Am J Epidemiol 1989;130:883–94.

21. Slattery ML, Schumacher MC, Smith KR, et al. Physical activity, diet, and risk of colon cancer in Utah. Am J Epidemiol 1988;128:989–99.

22. Whittemore AS, Wu-Williams AH, Lee M, et al. Diet, physical activity and colorectal cancer among Chinese in North America and China. J Natl Cancer Inst 1990;82:915–26.

23. Gerhardsson de Verdier M, Hagman U, Steineck G, et al. Diet, body mass and colorectal cancer: a case-referent study in Stockholm. Int J Cancer 1990;46:832–8.

24. Peters RK, Pike MC, Garabrandt D, Mack TM. Diet and colon cancer in Los Angeles County, California. Cancer Causes Control 1992;3:457–73.

25. Iscovich JM, L'Abbe KA, Castelleto R, et al. Colon cancer in Argentina. II. Risk from fiber, fat and nutrients. Int J Cancer 1992;51:858–61.

26. Meyer F, White E. Alcohol and nutrients in relation to colon cancer in middle-aged adults. Am J Epidemiol 1993;138:225–36.

27. Howe GR. Advances in the biology and therapy of colorectal cancer. Presentation from M.D. Anderson's Thirty-seventh Annual Clinical Conference; 1993. M.D. Anderson Cancer Center, Houston, Texas. p. 56–8

28. Slattery ML, Potter J, Caan B, et al. Energy balance and colon cancer—beyond physical activity. Cancer Res 1997;57:75–80.

29. Stemmermann GN, Nomura AM, Heilbrun LK. Dietary fat and the risk of colorectal cancer. Cancer Res 1984;44:4633–7.

30. Garland C, Shekelle RB, Barrett-Conner E, et al. Dietary vitamin D and calcium and risk of colorectal cancer: a 19-year prospective study in men. Lancet 1985;1:307–9.

31. Willett WC, Stampfer MJ, Colditz GA, et al. Relation of meat, fat, and fiber intake to the risk of colon cancer in a prospective study among women. N Engl J Med 1990;323:1664–72.

32. Giovannucci E, Rimm EB, Stampfer MJ, et al. Intake of fat, meat, and fiber in relation to risk of colon cancer in men. Cancer Res 1994;54:2390–7.

33. Goldbohm RA, van den Brandt PA, van't Veer P, et al. A prospective cohort study on the relation between meat consumption and the risk of colon cancer. Cancer Res 1994;54:718–23.

34. Bostick RM, Potter JD, Kushi LH, et al. Sugar, meat, and fat intake, and non-dietary risk factors for colon cancer incidence in Iowa women (United States). Cancer Causes Control 1994;5:38–52.

35. Armstrong B, Doll R. Environmental factors and cancer incidence and mortality in different countries, with special reference to dietary practices. Int J Cancer 1975;15:617–31.

36. Rose DP, Boyar AP, Wynder EL. International comparisons of mortality rates for cancer of the breast, ovary, prostate, and colon, and per capita food consumption. Cancer 1986;58:2263–71.

37. Aoki K, Hayakawa N, Kurihara M, Suzuki S. Death rates for malignant neoplasms for selected sites by sex and five-year age group in 33 countries, 1953–57 to 1983–87. International Union Against Cancer. Nagoya, Japan: University of Nagoya Coop Press, 1992.

38. Kune GA, Kune S, Watson LF. The nutritional causes of colorectal cancer: an introduction to the Melbourne Study. Nutr Cancer 1987;9:5–56.

39. Gerhardsson de Verdier M, Hagman U, Peters RK, et al. Meat, cooking methods and colorectal cancer: a case-referent study in Stockholm. Int J Cancer 1991; 49:520–5.

40. Manousos O, Day NE, Trichopoulos D, et al. Diet and colorectal cancer: a case-control study in Greece. Int J Cancer 1983;32:1–5.

41. La Vecchia C, Negri E, Decarli A, et al. A case-control study of diet and colo-rectal cancer in northern Italy. Int J Cancer 1988;41:492–8.

42. Miller AB, Howe GR, Jain M, et al. Food items and food groups as risk factors in a case-control study of diet and colo-rectal cancer. Int J Cancer 1983;32:155–61.

43. Young TB, Wolf DA. Case-control study of proximal and distal colon cancer and diet in Wisconsin. Int J Cancer 1988;42:167–75.

44. Benito E, Obrador A, Stiggelbout A, et al. A population-based case-control study of colorectal cancer in Majorca. I. Dietary factors. Int J Cancer 1990;45: 69–76.

45. Lee HP, Gourley L, Duffy SW, et al. Colorectal cancer and diet in an Asian population—a case-control study among Singapore Chinese. Int J Cancer 1989; 43:1007–16.

46. Macquart-Moulin G, Riboli E, Cornee J, et al. Case-control study on colorectal cancer and diet in Marseilles. Int J Cancer 1986;38:183–91.

47. Berta JL, Coste T, Rautureau J, et al. Diet and recto-colonic cancers. Results of a case-control study. Gastroenterol Clin Biol 1985;9:348–53.

48. Tuyns AJ, Haelterman M, Kaaks R. Colorectal cancer and the intake of nutrients: oligosaccharides are a risk factor, fats are not. A case-control study in Belgium. Nutr Cancer 1987;10:181–96.

49. Gerhardsson M, Floderus B, Norell SE. Physical activity and colon cancer risk. Int J Epidemiol 1988;17: 743–6.

50. Bjelke E. Epidemiology of colorectal cancer, with emphasis on diet. In: Davis W, Harrup KR, Stathopoulous G, eds. Human cancer. Its characterization and treatment. Amsterdam, Exerpta Medica, Int.: Congress Series No. 484. 1980. p. 158–74.

51. Hirayama T. A large-scale study on cancer risks by diet—with special reference to the risk reducing effects of green-yellow vegetable consumption. In Hayashi Y, Magao M, Sugimura T, et al. eds. Diet, nutrition, and cancer. Japan Scientific Societies Press, 1986. p. 41–53.

52. Phillips RL, Snowdon DA. Association of meat and coffee use with cancers of the large bowel, breast, and prostate among Seventh-Day Adventists: preliminary results. Cancer Res 1983;43(suppl):2403S–8S.

53. Sugimura T, Sato S. Mutagens-carcinogens in foods. Cancer Res 1983;43:2415S–21S.

54. Sugimura T. Carcinogenicity of mutagenic heterocyclic amines formed during the cooking process. Mutat Res 1985;150:33–41.

55. Wakabayashi K, Nagao M, Esumi H, Sugimura T. Food-derived mutagens and carcinogens. Cancer Res 1992;52:2092s–8s.

56. Steinmetz KA, Potter JD. Vegetables, fruit and cancer. I. Epidemiology. Cancer Causes Control 1991;2: 325–57.

57. Phillips RL. Role of life-style and dietary habits in risk of cancer among Seventh-Day Adventists. Cancer Res 1975;35:3513–22.

58. Mayne ST, Janerich DT, Greenwald P, et al. Dietary beta carotene and lung cancer risk in U.S. nonsmokers. J Natl Cancer Inst 1994;86:33–8.

59. Modan B, Barell V, Lubin F, et al. Low-fiber intake as an etiologic factor in cancer of the colon. J Natl Cancer Inst 1975;55:15–8.

60. Tuyns AJ, Kaaks R, Haelterman M. Colorectal cancer and the consumption of foods: a case-control study in Belgium. Nutr Cancer 1988;11:189–204.

61. Steinmetz KA, Kushi LH, Bostick RM, et al. Vegetables, fruit, and colon cancer in the Iowa Women's Health Study. Am J Epidemiol 1994;139:1–15.

62. Benito E, Stiggelbout A, Bosch FX, et al. Nutritional factors in colorectal cancer risk: a case-control study in Majorca. Int J Cancer 1991;49:161–7.

63. Trock B, Lanza E, Greenwald P. Dietary fiber, vegetables, and colon cancer: critical review and meta-analyses of the epidemiologic evidence. J Natl Cancer Inst 1990;82:650–61.

64. Zaridze D, Filipchenko V, Kustov V, et al. Diet and colorectal cancer: results of two case-control studies in Russia. Eur J Cancer 1993;29A:112–5.

65. Howe GR, Benito E, Castelleto R, et al. Dietary intake of fiber and decreased risk of cancers of the colon and rectum: evidence from the combined analysis of 13 case-control studies. J Natl Cancer Inst 1992;84: 1887–96.

66. Fuchs CS, Colditz GA, Stampfer MJ, et al. Dietary fiber and the risk of colorectal cancer and adenoma in women. N Engl J Med 1999;340:169–76.

67. Zaridze DG. Environmental etiology of large-bowel cancer. J Natl Cancer Inst 1983;70:389–400.

68. Freudenheim JL, Graham S, Marshall JR, et al. A case-control study of diet and rectal cancer in western New York. Am J Epidemiol 1990;131:612–24.

69. Hu J, Liu Y, Yu Y, et al. Diet and cancer of the colon and rectum: a case-control study in China. Int J Epidemiol 1991;20:362–7.

70. Bidoli E, Franceschi S, Talamini R, et al. Food consumption and cancer of the colon and rectum in north-eastern Italy. Int J Cancer 1992;50:223–9.

71. Dales LG, Friedman GD, Ury HK, et al. A case-control study of relationships of diet and other traits to colorectal cancer in American blacks. Am J Epidemiol 1979;109:132–44.

72. Thun MJ, Calle EE, Namboodiri MM, et al. Risk factors for fatal colon cancer in a large prospective study. J Natl Cancer Inst 1992;84:1491–500.

73. Heilbrun L, Nomura A, Hankin J, Stemmermann G. Diet and colorectal cancer with special reference to fiber intake. Int J Cancer 1989;44:1–6.

74. Buset M, Kipkin M, Winawer S, et al. Inhibition of human colonic epithelial cell proliferation in vivo and in vitro by calcium. Cancer Res 1986;46:5426–30.

75. Lipkin M, Newmark H. Effect of added dietary calcium on colonic epithelial-cell proliferation in subjects at high risk for familial colonic cancer. N Engl J Med 1985;313:1381–4.

76. Gregoire RC, Stern HS, Yeung KS, et al. Effect of calcium supplementation on mucosal cell proliferation in high risk patients for colon cancer. Gut 1989;30:376–82.

77. Rozen P, Fireman Z, Fine N, et al. Oral calcium suppresses increased rectal epithelial proliferation of persons at risk of colorectal cancer. Gut 1989;30:650–5.

78. Stern HS, Gregoire RC, Kashtan H, et al. Long-term effects of dietary calcium on risk markers for colon cancer in patients with familial polyposis. Surgery 1990;108:528–33.

79. Wargovich MJ, Isbel G, Shabot M, et al. Calcium supplementation decreases rectal epithelial cell proliferation in subjects with sporadic adenoma. Gastroenterology 1992;103:92–7.

80. Kleibeuker JH, Welberg JW, Mulder NH, et al. Epithelial cell proliferation in the sigmoid colon of patients with adenomatous polyps increases during oral calcium supplementation. Br J Cancer 1993;67:500–3.

81. Wargovich MJ, Eng VW, Newmark HL, Bruce WR. Calcium ameliorates the toxic effect of deoxycholic acid on colonic epithelium. Carcinogenesis 1983;4:1205–7.

82. Wargovich MJ, Eng VWS, Newmark H. Calcium inhibits the damaging and compensatory proliferative effects of fatty acids on mouse colon epithelium. Cancer Lett 1984;23:253–8.

83. van der Meer R, de Vries HT. Differential binding of glycine- and taurine-conjugated bile acids to insoluble calcium phosphate. Biochem J 1985;229:265–8.

84. Pence BC, Buddingh F. Inhibition of dietary fat-promoted colon carcinogenesis in rats by supplemental calcium or vitamin D_3. Carcinogenesis 1988;9:187–90.

85. Newmark HL, Wargovich MJ, Bruce WR. Colon cancer and dietary fat, phosphate, and calcium: a hypothesis. J Natl Cancer Inst 1984;72:1323–5.

86. Martinez ME, Willett WC. Calcium, vitamin D, and colorectal cancer: a review of the epidemiologic evidence. Cancer Epidemiol Biomarkers Prev 1998;7:163–8.

87. Martínez ME, Giovannucci EL, Colditz GA, et al. Calcium, vitamin D, and the occurrence of colorectal cancer among women. J Natl Cancer Inst 1996;88:1375–82.

88. Bostick RM, Potter JD, Sellers TA, et al. Relation of calcium, vitamin D, and dairy food intake to incidence of colon cancer in older women. Am J Epidemiol 1993;137:1302–17.

89. Kearney J, Giovannucci E, Rimm EB, et al. Calcium, vitamin D and dairy foods and the occurrence of colon cancer in men. Am J Epidemiol 1996;143:907–17.

90. Ferraroni M, La Vecchia C, D'Avanzo B, et al. Selected micronutrient intake and the risk of colorectal cancer. Br J Cancer 1994;70:1150–5.

91. Cravo ML, Mason JB, Dayal Y, et al. Folate deficiency enhances the development of colonic neoplasia in dimethylhydrazine-treated rats. Cancer Res 1992;52:5002–6.

92. Freudenheim JL, Graham S, Marshall JR, et al. Folate intake and carcinogenesis of the colon and rectum. Int J Epidemiol 1991;20:368–74.

93. White E, Shannon JS, Patterson RE. Relationship between vitamin and calcium supplement use and colon cancer. Cancer Epidemiol Biomarkers Prev 1997;6:769–74.

94. Glynn SA, Albanes D, Pietinen P, et al. Colorectal cancer and folate status: a nested case-control study among male smokers. Cancer Epidemiol Biomarkers Prev 1996;5:487–94.

95. Giovannucci E, Rimm EB, Ascherio A, et al. Alcohol, low-methionine-low-folate diets, and risk of colon cancer in men. J Natl Cancer Inst 1995;87:265–73.

96. Giovannucci E, Stampfer MJ, Colditz GA, et al. Multivitamin use, folate, and colon cancer in women in the Nurses' Health Study. Ann Intern Med 1998;129:517–24.

97. Ma J, Stampfer MJ, Giovannucci E, et al. Methylenetetrahydrofolate reductase polymorphism, dietary interactions, and risk of colorectal cancer. Cancer Res 1997;57:1098–102.

98. Lashner BA, Heidenreich PA, Su GL, et al. Effect of folate supplementation on the incidence of dysplasia and cancer in chronic ulcerative colitis: a case-control study. Gastroenterology 1989;97:255–9.

99. Lashner BA. Red blood cell folate is associated with the development of dysplasia and cancer in ulcerative colitis. J Cancer Res Clin Oncol 1993;119:549–54.

100. Giovannucci E, Willett WC. Dietary factors and risk of colon cancer. Ann Med 1994;26:443–52.

101. Bird CL, Swendseid ME, Witte JS, et al. Red cell and plasma folate, folate consumption, and the risk of

colorectal adenomatous polyps. Cancer Epidemiol Biomarkers Prev 1995;4:709–14.

102. Giovannucci E, Stampfer MJ, Colditz GA, et al. Folate, methionine, and alcohol intake and risk of colorectal adenoma. J Natl Cancer Inst 1993;85:875–84.

103. Benito E, Cabeza E, Moreno V, et al. Diet and colorectal adenomas: a case-control study in Majorca. Int J Cancer 1993;55:213–9.

104. Kutzbach C, Stokstad ELR. Mammalian methylenetetrahydrofolate reductase. Partial purification, properties, and inhibition by S-adenosylmethionine. Biochem Biophys Acta 1971;250:459–77.

105. Chen J, Giovannucci E, Kelsey K, et al. A methylenetetrahydrofolate reductase polymorphism and the risk of colorectal cancer. Cancer Res 1996;56:4862–4.

106. Martínez ME, Maltzman T, Marshall JR, et al. Risk factors for Ki-ras protooncogene mutation in sporadic colorectal adenomas. Cancer Res 1999;59:5181–5.

107. Wickramasinghe SN, Fida S. Bone marrow cells from vitamin B_{12}- and folate-deficient patients misincorporate uracil into DNA. Blood 1994;83:1656–61.

108. Weinberg G, Ullman B, Martin DW Jr. Mutator phenotypes in mammalian cell mutants with distinct biochemical defects and abnormal deoxyribonucleoside triphosphate pools. Proc Natl Acad Sci U S A 1981; 78:2447–51.

109. Meuth M. Role of deoxynucleoside triphosphate pools in the cytotoxic and mutagenic effects of DNA alkylating agents. Somat Cell Genet 1981;7:89–102.

110. Sutherland GR. The role of nucleotides in human fragile site expression. Mutat Res 1988;200:207–13.

111. Fencch M, Rinaldi J. The relationship between micronuclei in human lymphocytes and plasma levels of vitamin C, vitamin E, vitamin B12 and folic acid. Carcinogenesis 1994;15:1405–11.

112. Hunting DJ, Dresler SL. Dependence of u.v.-induced DNA excision repair on deoxyribonucleoside triphosphate concentrations in permeable human fibroblasts: a model for the inhibition of repair by hydroxyurea. Carcinogenesis 1985;6:1525–8.

113. James SJ, Basnakian AG, Miller BJ. In vitro folate deficiency induces deoxynucleotide pool imbalance, apoptosis, and mutagenesis in Chinese hamster ovary cells. Cancer Res 1994;54:5075–80.

114. Blount BC, Mack MM, Wehr CM, et al. Folate deficiency causes uracil misincorporation into human DNA and chromosome breakage: implications for cancer and neuronal damage. Proc Natl Acad Sci U S A 1997;94:3290–5.

115. Cravo M, Fidalgo P, Pereira AD, et al. DNA methylation as an intermediate biomarker in colorectal cancer: modulation by folic acid supplementation. Eur J Cancer Prev 1994;3:473–9.

116. Feinberg AP, Vogelstein B. Hypomethylation distinguishes genes of some human cancers from their normal counterparts. Nature 1983;301:89–92.

117. Goelz SE, Vogelstein B, Hamilton SR, Feinberg AP. Hypomethylation of DNA from benign and malignant human colon neoplasms. Science 1985;228:187–90.

118. Feinberg AP, Gehrke CW, Kuo KC, Ehrlich M. Reduced genomic 5-methylcytosine content in human colonic neoplasia. Cancer Res 1988;48:1159–61.

119. Issa J-PJ, Vertino PM, Wu J, et al. Increased cytosine DNA-methyltransferase activity during colon cancer progression. J Natl Cancer Inst 1993;85:1235–40.

120. Makos M, Nelkin BD, Lerman MI, et al. Distinct hypermethylation patterns occur at altered chromosome loci in human lung and colon cancer. Proc Natl Acad Sci U S A 1992;89:1929–33.

121. Finkelstein JD, Cello JP, Kyle WE. Ethanol-induced changes in methionine metabolism in rat liver. Biochem Biophys Res Commun 1974;61:525–31.

122. Willett WC, Stampfer MJ, Colditz GA, et al. Relation of meat, fat and fiber intake to colon cancer risk in a prospective study among women [abstract]. Am J Epidemiol 1989;130:820.

123. Kato I, Tominaga S, Matsuura A, et al. A comparative case-control study of colorectal cancer and adenoma. Jpn J Cancer Res 1990;81:1101–8.

124. Giovannucci E, Stampfer MJ, Colditz GA, et al. Relationship of diet to risk of colorectal adenoma in men. J Natl Cancer Inst 1992;84:91–8.

125. Neugut AI, Garbowski GC, Lee WC, et al. Dietary risk factors for the incidence and recurrence of colorectal adenomatous polyps: a case-control study. Ann Intern Med 1993;118:91–5.

126. Sandler RS, Lyles CM, Peipins LA, et al. Diet and risk of colorectal adenomas: macronutrients, cholesterol and fiber. J Natl Cancer Inst 1993;85:884–91.

127. Wu AH, Paganini-Hill A, Ross RK, Henderson BE. Alcohol, physical activity and other risk factors for colorectal cancer: a prospective study. Br J Cancer 1987;55:687–94.

128. Lee IM, Paffenbarger RS Jr, Hsieh CC. Physical activity and risk of developing colorectal cancer among college alumni. J Natl Cancer Inst 1991;83:1324–9.

129. Giovannucci E, Ascherio A, Rimm EB, et al. Physical activity, obesity, and risk for colon cancer and adenoma in men. Ann Intern Med 1995;122:327–34.

130. Lew EA, Garfinkel L. Variations in mortality by weight among 750,000 men and women. J Chronic Dis 1979;32:563–76.

131. Waaler HT. Height, weight and mortality. The Norwegian experience. Acta Med Scand Suppl 1984;679: 1–56.

132. Phillips RL, Snowdon DA. Dietary relationships with fatal colorectal cancer among Seventh-Day Adventists. J Natl Cancer Inst 1985;74:307–17.

133. Klatsky AL, Armstrong MA, Friedman GD, Hiatt RA. The relations of alcoholic beverage use to colon and rectal cancer. Am J Epidemiol 1988;128:1007–15.

134. Must A, Jacques PF, Dallal GE, et al. Long-term morbidity and mortality of overweight adolescents. A follow-up of the Harvard Growth Study of 1922 to 1935. N Engl J Med 1992;327:1350–5.

135. Le Marchand L, Wilkins LR, Mi MP. Obesity in youth and middle age and risk of colorectal cancer in men. Cancer Causes Control 1992;3:349–54.

136. Chute CG, Willett WC, Colditz GA, et al. A prospective study of reproductive history and exogenous estrogens on the risk of colorectal cancer in women. Epidemiology 1991;2:201–7.

137. Martinez ME, Giovannucci E, Spiegelman D, et al. Leisure-time physical activity, body size, and colon cancer in women. Nurses' Health Study Research Group. J Natl Cancer Inst 1997;89:948–55.

138. Kune G, Kune S, Wason L. Body weight and physical activity as predictors of colorectal cancer risk. Nutr Cancer 1990;13:9–17.

139. Dietz AT, Newcomb PA, Marcus PM, Strer BE. The association of body size and large bowel cancer risk in Wisconsin (United States) women. Cancer Causes Control 1995;6:30–6.

140. Ballard-Barbash R, Schatzkin A, Albanes D, et al. Physical activity and risk of large bowel cancer in the Framingham Study. Cancer Res 1990;50:3610–3.

141. Albanes D, Blair A, Taylor PR. Physical activity and risk of cancer in the NHANES I population. Am J Public Health 1989;79:744–50.

142. Severson RK, Nomura AMY, Grove JS, Stemmermann GN. A prospective analysis of physical activity and cancer. Am J Epidemiol 1989;130:522–9.

143. Lynge E, Thygesen L. Use of surveillance systems for occupational cancer: data from the Danish national system. Int J Epidemiol 1988;17:493–500.

144. Paffenbarger RSJ, Hyde RT, Wing AL. Physical activity and incidence of cancer in diverse populations: a preliminary report. Am J Clin Nutr 1987;45(Suppl):312–7.

145. Gerhardsson M, Norell SE, Kiviranta H, et al. Sedentary jobs and colon cancer. Am J Epidemiol 1986;123:775–80.

146. Marti B, Minder CE. Physische Berufsktivitaatund Kolonkarzinommortalitaat bei Schweizer Mannern 1979–1982. Soz Praventivmed 1989;34:30–7.

147. Thune I, Lung E. Physical activity and risk of colorectal cancer in men and women. Br J Cancer 1996;73:1134–40.

148. Markowitz S, Morabia A, Garibaldi K, Wynder E. Effect of occupational and recreational activity on the risk of colorectal cancer among males: a case-control study. Int J Epidemiol 1992;21:1057–62.

149. Peters RK, Garabrant DH, Yu MC, Mack TM. A case-control study of occupational and dietary factors in colorectal cancer in young men by subsite. Cancer Res 1989;49:5459–68.

150. Brownson RC, Zahm SH, Chang JC, Blair A. Occupational risk of colon cancer. An analysis of anatomic subsite. Am J Epidemiol 1989;130:675–87.

151. Kato I, Tominaga S, Ikari A. A case-control study of male colorectal cancer in Aichi Prefecture, Japan: with special reference to occupational activity level, drinking habits and family history. Jpn J Cancer Res 1990;81:115–21.

152. Fredriksson M, Bengtsson NO, Hardell L, Axelson O. Colon cancer, physical activity, and occupational exposures. A case-control study. Cancer 1989;63:1838–42.

153. Fraser G, Pearce N. Occupational physical activity and risk of cancer of the colon and rectum in New Zealand males. Cancer Causes Control 1993;4:45–50.

154. Longnecker MP, Gerhardsson de Verdier M, Frumkin H, Carpenter C. A case-control study of physical activity in relation to risk of cancer of the right colon and rectum in men. Int J Epidemiol 1995;24:42–50.

155. Slattery ML, Abd-Elghany N, Kerber R, Schumacher MC. Physical activity and colon cancer: a comparison of various indicators of physical activity to evaluate the association. Epidemiology 1990;1:481–5.

156. Chow WH, Dosemeci M, Zheng W, et al. Physical activity and occupational risk of colon cancer in Shanghai, China. Int J Epidemiol 1993;22:23–9.

157. Arbman G, Axelson O, Fredriksson M, et al. Do occupational factors influence the risk of colon and rectal cancer in different ways? Cancer 1993;72:2543–9.

158. Gerhardsson de Verdier M, Steineck G, Hagman U, et al. Physical activity and colon cancer: a case-referent study in Stockholm. Int J Cancer 1990;46:985–99.

159. Vineis P, Ciccone G, Magnino A. Asbestos exposure, physical activity and colon cancer: a case-control study. Tumori 1993;79:301–3.

160. Vlajinac H, Jarebinski M, Adanja B. Relationship of some biosocial factors to colon cancer in Belgrade. Neoplasma 1987;34:503–7.

161. Dosemeci M, Hayes RB, Vetter R, et al. Occupational physical activity, socioeconomic status, and risks of 15 cancer sites in Turkey. Cancer Causes Control 1993;4:313–21.

162. Marcus PM, Newcomb PA, Storer BE. Early adulthood physical activity and colon cancer risk among Wisconsin women. Cancer Epidemiol Biomarkers Prev 1994;3:641–4.

163. White E, Jacobs EJ, Daling JR. Physical activity in relation to colon cancer in middle-aged men and women. Am J Epidemiol 1996;144:42–50.

164. Vena JE, Graham S, Zielezny M, et al. Lifetime occupational exercise and colon cancer. Am J Epidemiol 1985;122:357–65.

165. Garabrant DH, Peters JM, Mack TM, Berstein L. Job activity and colon cancer risk. Am J Epidemiol 1984;119:1005–14.

166. Colditz G, Cannuscio C, Frazier A. Physical activity and reduced risk of colon cancer: implications for prevention. Cancer Causes Control 1997;8:649–67.

167. Bartram HP, Wynder EL. Physical activity and colon cancer risk? Physiological considerations. Am J Gastroenterol 1989;84:109–12.

168. Martinez ME, Heddens D, Earnest DL, et al. Physical activity, body mass index, and prostaglandin E2 levels in rectal mucosa. J Natl Cancer Inst 1999;91:950–3.

169. Giovannucci E. Insulin and colon cancer. Cancer Causes Control 1995;6:164–79.

170. Hu FB, Manson JE, Liu S, et al. Prospective study of adult onset diabetes mellitus (Type 2) and risk of colorectal cancer in women. J Natl Cancer Inst 1999;91:542–7.

171. Schoen RE, Tangen CM, Kuller LH, et al. Increased blood glucose and insulin, body size, and incident colorectal cancer. J Natl Cancer Inst 1999;91:1147–54.

172. Fraumeni JF Jr, Lloyd JW, Smith EM, Wagoner JK. Cancer mortality among nuns: role of marital status in etiology of neoplastic disease in women. J Natl Cancer Inst 1969;42:455–68.

173. Howell MA. The association between colorectal cancer and breast cancer. J Chronic Dis 1976;29:243–61.

174. Boyle P, Robertson C. Breast cancer and colon cancer incidence in females in Scotland, 1960–84. J Natl Cancer Inst 1987;79:1175–9.

175. La Vecchia C, Decarli A. Correlations between cancer mortality rates from various Italian regions. Tumori 1985;71:441–8.

176. Davis FG, Furner SE, Persky V, Koch M. The influence of parity and exogenous female hormones on the risk of colorectal cancer. Int J Cancer 1989;43:587–90.

177. Furner SE, Davis FG, Nelson RL, Haenszel W. A case-control study of large bowel cancer and hormone exposure in women. Cancer Res 1989;49:4936–40.

178. Gerhardsson de Verdier M, London S. Reproductive factors, exogenous female hormones, and colorectal cancer by subsite. Cancer Causes Control 1992;3:355–60.

179. Jacobs EJ, White E, Weiss NS. Exogenous hormones, reproductive history, and colon cancer (Seattle, Washington, USA). Cancer Causes Control 1994;5:359–66.

180. Calle EE, Miracle-McMahill HL, Thun MJ, Heath CW, Jr. Estrogen replacement therapy and risk of fatal colon cancer in a prospective cohort of postmenopausal women. J Natl Cancer Inst 1995;87:517–23.

181. Marcus PM, Newcomb PA, Young T, Storer BE. The association of reproductive and menstrual characteristics and colon and rectal cancer risk in Wisconsin women. Ann Epidemiol 1995;5:303–9.

182. Newcomb PA, Storer BE. Postmenopausal hormone use and risk of large-bowel cancer. J Natl Cancer Inst 1995;87:1067–71.

183. Folsom AR, Mink PJ, Sellers TA, et al. Hormone replacement therapy and morbidity and mortality in a prospective study of postmenopausal women. Am J Public Health 1995;85:1128–32.

184. Fernandez E, La Vecchia C, A'Avanzo B, et al. Oral contraceptives, hormone replacement therapy and the risk of colorectal cancer. Br J Cancer 1996;73:1431–5.

185. Grodstein F, Martinez ME, Platz EA, et al. Postmenopausal hormone use and risk for colorectal cancer and adenoma. Ann Intern Med 1998;128:705–12.

186. Weiss NS, Daling JR, Chow WH. Incidence of cancer of the large bowel in women in relation to reproductive and hormonal factors. J Natl Cancer Inst 1981;67:57–60.

187. Wu-Williams AH, Lee M, Whittemore AS, et al. Reproductive factors and colorectal cancer risk among Chinese females. Cancer Res 1991;51:2307–11.

188. Risch HA, Howe GR. Menopausal hormone use and colorectal cancer in Saskatchewan: a record linkage cohort study. Cancer Epidemiol Biomarkers Prev 1995;4:21–8.

189. Peters RK, Pike MC, Chang WWL, Mack MT. Reproductive factors and colon cancer. Br J Cancer 1990;61:741–8.

190. Troisi R, Schairer C, Chow W-H, et al. A prospective study of menopausal hormones and risk of colorectal cancer. Cancer Causes Control 1997;8:130–8.

191. Kampman E, Potter JD, Slattery ML, et al. Hormone replacement therapy, reproductive history, and colon cancer: a multicenter, case-control study in the United States. Cancer Causes Control 1997;8:146–58.

192. Giovannucci E, Martínez ME. Tobacco, colorectal cancer, and adenomas: a review of the evidence. J Natl Cancer Inst 1996;88:1717–30.

193. Giovannucci E, Rimm EB, Stampfer MJ, et al. A prospective study of cigarette smoking and risk of colorectal adenoma and colorectal cancer in U.S. men. J Natl Cancer Inst 1994;86:183–91.

194. Giovannucci E, Colditz GA, Stampfer MJ, et al. A prospective study of cigarette smoking and risk of colorectal adenoma and colorectal cancer in U.S. women. J Natl Cancer Inst 1994;86:192–9.

195. Slattery ML, West DW, Robison LM, et al. Tobacco, alcohol, coffee, and caffeine as risk factors for colon cancer in a low-risk population. Epidemiology 1990;1:141–5.

196. Heineman EF, Zahm SH, McLaughlin JK, Vaught JB. Increased risk of colorectal cancer among smokers: results of a 26-year follow-up of US veterans and a review. Int J Cancer 1994;59:728–38.

197. Newcomb PA, Storer BE, Marcus PM. Cigarette smoking in relation to risk of large bowel cancer in women. Cancer Res 1995;55:4906–9.

198. Slattery ML, Potter JD, Friedman GD, et al. Tobacco use and colon cancer. Int J Cancer 1997;70:259–64.

199. Hsing AW, McLaughlin JK, Chow W-H, et al. Risk factors for colorectal cancer in a prospective study among U.S. white men. Int J Cancer 1998;77:549–53.

200. Knekt P, Hakama M, Järvinen R, et al. Smoking and risk of colorectal cancer. Br J Cancer 1998;78:136–9.

201. Le Marchand L, Wilkens LR, Kolonel LN, et al. Associations of sedentary lifestyle, obesity, smoking, alcohol use, and diabetes with the risk of colorectal cancer. Cancer Res 1997;57:4787–94.

202. Yamada K, Araki S, Tamura M, et al. Case-control study of colorectal carcinoma in situ and cancer in relation to cigarette smoking and alcohol use (Japan). Cancer Causes Control 1997;8:780–5.

203. Chyou P-H, Nomura AMY, Stemmermann GN. A prospective study of colon and rectal cancer among Hawaii Japanese men. Ann Epidemiol 1996;6:276–82.

204. Freedman AN, Michalek AM, Marshall JR, et al. The relationship between smoking exposure and p53 overexpression in colorectal cancer. Genet Epidemiol 1995;12:333.

205. Baron JA, Gerhardsson de Verdier M, Ekbom A. Coffee, tea, tobacco, and cancer of the large bowel. Cancer Epidemiol Biomarkers Prev 1994;3:565–70.

206. Nordlund LA, Carstensen JM, Pershagen G. Cancer incidence in female smokers: a 26-year follow-up. Int J Cancer 1997;73:625–8.

207. Nyrén O, Bergström R, Nyström L, et al. Smoking and colorectal cancer: a 20-year follow-up study of Swedish construction workers. J Natl Cancer Inst 1996;88:1302–7.

208. Tavani A, Pregnolato A, La Vecchia C, et al. Coffee and tea intake and risk of cancers of the colon and rectum: a study of 3,530 cases and 7,057 controls. Int J Cancer 1997;73:193–7.

209. Alexandrov K, Rojas M, Kadlubar FF, et al. Evidence of anti-benzo[a]pyrene diolepoxide-DNA adduct formation in human colon mucosa. Carcinogenesis 1996;17:2081–3.

210. Hirayama T. Association between alcohol consumption and cancer of the sigmoid colon: observations from a Japanese cohort study. Lancet 1989;725–7.

211. Stemmermann GN, Nomura AMY, Chyou P-H, Yoshizawa C. Prospective study of alcohol intake and large bowel cancer. Dig Dis Sci 1990;35:1414–20.

212. Carstensen JM, Bygren LO, Hatschek T. Cancer incidence among Swedish brewery workers. Int J Cancer 1990;45:393–6.

213. Bjelke E. Epidemiologic studies of cancer of the stomach, colon and rectum; with special emphasis on the role of diet. Scand J Gastroenterol Suppl 1974;31:1–235.

214. Williams RR, Horm JW. Association of cancer sites with tobacco and alcohol consumption and socio-economic status of patients: interview study from the Third National Cancer Survey. J Natl Cancer Inst 1977;58:525–47.

215. Dean G, MacLennan R, McLoughlin H, Shelley E. Causes of death of blue-collar workers at a Dublin brewery 1954–73. Br J Cancer 1979;40:581–9.

216. Freudenheim JL, Graham S, Marshall JR, et al. Lifetime alcohol intake and risk of rectal cancer in Western New York. Nutr Cancer 1990;13:101–9.

217. Longnecker MP. A case-control study of alcoholic beverage consumption in relation to risk of cancer of the right colon and rectum in men. Cancer Causes Control 1990;1:5–14.

218. Kune S, Kune GA, Watson LF. Case-control study of alcoholic beverages as etiological factors: the Melbourne colorectal cancer study. Nutr Cancer 1987;9:43–56.

219. Tuyns AJ, Pequignot G, Gignoux M, Valla A. Cancers of the digestive tract, alcohol and tobacco. Int J Cancer 1982;30:9–11.

220. Ward K, Moriarty KJ, O'Neill S, et al. Alcohol and colorectal cancer [abstract]. Gut 1983;24:A981.

221. Kabat GC, Howson CP, Wynder EL. Beer consumption and rectal cancer. Int J Epidemiol 1986;15:494–501.

222. Newcomb PA, Storer BE, Marcus PM. Cancer of the large bowel in women in relation to alcohol consumption: a case-control study in Wisconsin (United States). Cancer Causes Control 1993;4:405–11.

223. Barak AJ, Beckenhauer HC, Tuma DJ, Badakhsh S. Effects of prolonged ethanol feeding on methionine metabolism in rat liver. Biochem Cell Biol 1987;65:230–3.

224. Shaw S, Jayatilleke E, Herbert V, Colman N. Cleavage of folates during ethanol metabolism: role of acetaldehyde/xanthine oxidase-generated superoxide. Biochem J 1989;257:277–80.

225. Porta EA, Markell N, Dorado RD. Chronic alcoholism enhances hepatocarcinogenicity of diethylnitrosamine in rats fed a marginally methyl-deficient diet. Hepatology 1985;5:1120–5.

226. Kune GA, Kune S, Watson LF. Colorectal cancer risk, chronic illnesses, operations, and medications: case control results from the Melbourne Colorectal Cancer Study. Cancer Res 1988;48:4399–404.

227. Rosenberg L, Palmer J, Zauber A, et al. A hypothesis: nonsteroidal anti-inflammatory drugs reduce the incidence of large-bowel cancer. J Natl Cancer Inst 1991;83:355–8.

228. Thun MJ, Namboodiri MM, Heath CW Jr. Aspirin use and reduced risk of fatal colon cancer. N Engl J Med 1991;325:1593–6.

229. Giovannucci E, Rimm EB, Stampfer MJ, et al. Aspirin use and the risk for colorectal cancer and adenoma in male health professionals. Ann Intern Med 1994;121:241–6.

230. Giovannucci E, Egan KM, Hunter DJ, et al. Aspirin and the risk of colorectal cancer in women. N Engl J Med 1995;333:609–14.

231. Narisawa T, Sato M, Tani M, et al. Inhibition of development of methylnitrosourea-induced rat colon tumors by indomethacin treatment. Cancer Res 1981;41:1954–7.

232. Pollard M, Luckert PH. Effect of piroxicam in primary intestinal tumors induced in rats by N-methylnitrosourea. Cancer Lett 1984;25:117–21.

233. Reddy BS, Maruyama H, Kelloff G. Dose-related inhibition of colon carcinogenesis by dietary piroxicam, a nonsteroidal antiinflammatory drug, during different stages of rat colon tumor development. Cancer Res 1987;47:5340–6.

234. Moorghen M, Ince P, Finney KJ, et al. A protective effect of sulindac against chemically-induced primary colonic tumours in mice. J Pathol 1988;156: 341–7.

235. Rigau J, Pique JM, Rubio E, et al. Effects of long-term sulindac therapy on colonic polyposis. Ann Intern Med 1991;115:952–4.

236. Labayle D, Fischer D, Vielh P, et al. Sulindac causes regression of rectal polyps in familial adenomatous polyposis. Gastroenterology 1991;101:635–9.

237. Giardiello FM, Hamilton SR, Krush AJ, et al. Treatment of colonic and rectal adenomas with sulindac in familial adenomatous polyposis. N Engl J Med 1993;328:1313–6.

238. Laakso M, Mutru O, Isomaki H, Koota K. Cancer mortality in patients with rheumatoid arthritis. J Rheumatol 1986;13:522–6.

239. Gridley G, McLaughlin JK, Ekbom A, et al. Incidence of cancer among patients with rheumatoid arthritis. J Natl Cancer Inst 1993;85:307–11.

240. Suh O, Mettlin C, Petrelli NJ. Aspirin use, cancer, and polyps of the large bowel. Cancer 1993;72:1171–7.

241. Logan RF, Little J, Hawtin PG, Hardcastle JD. Effect of aspirin and non-steroidal anti-inflammatory drugs on colorectal adenomas: case-control study of subjects participating in the Nottingham faecal occult blood screening programme. BMJ 1993;307:285–9.

242. Martinez ME, McPherson RS, Levin B, Annegers JF. Aspirin and other nonsteroidal anti-inflammatory drugs and risk of colorectal adenomatous polyps among endoscoped individuals. Cancer Epidemiol Biomarkers Prev 1995;4:703–7.

243. Paganini-Hill A, Chao A, Ross R, Henderson B. Aspirin use and chronic diseases: a cohort study of the elderly. BMJ 1989;299:1247–50.

244. Aaronson S. Growth factors and cancer. Science 1991; 254:1146–53.

245. Rechler M. Growth inhibition by insulin-like growth factor (IGF) binding protein-3—what's IGF got to do with it? Endocrinology 1997;138:2645–7.

246. Rajah R, Valentinis B, Cohen P. Insulin-like growth factor (IGF)-binding protein-3 induces apoptosis and mediates the effects of transforming growth factor-β1 on programmed cell death through a p53 and IGF-independent mechanism. J Biol Chem 1997; 272:12181–8.

247. Baserga R. The insulin-like growth factor I receptor: a key to tumor growth? Cancer Res 1995;55:249–52.

248. Pollak MN, Perdue JF, Margolese RG, et al. Presence of somatomedin receptors on primary human breast and colon carcinomas. Cancer Lett 1987;38:223–30.

249. Guo YS, Narayan S, Yallampalli C, Singh P. Characterization of insulinlike growth factor I receptors in human colon cancer. Gastroenterology 1992;102: 1101–8.

250. Watkins L, Lewis L, Levine A. Characterization of the synergistic effect of insulin and transferrin and the regulation of their receptors on a human colon carcinoma cell line. Int J Cancer 1990;45:372–5.

251. Koenuma M, Yamori T, Tsuruo T. Insulin and insulin-like growth factor 1 stimulate proliferation of metastatic variants of colon carcinoma 26. Jpn J Cancer Res 1989;80:51–8.

252. Bjork J, Nilsson J, Hultcrantz R, Johansson C. Growth-regulatory effects of sensory neuropeptides, epidermal growth factor, insulin, and somatostatin on the non-transformed intestinal epithelial cell line IEC-6 and the colon cancer cell line HT 29. Scand J Gastroenterol 1993;28:879–84.

253. Cats A, Dullaart R, Kleibeuker J, et al. Increased epithelial cell proliferation in the colon of patients with acromegaly. Cancer Res 1996;56:523–6.

254. Klein I, Parveen G, Gavaler J, Vanthiel D. Colonic polyps in patients with acromegaly. Ann Intern Med 1982;97:27–30.

255. Ituarte E, Petrini J, Hershman J. Acromegaly and colon cancer. Ann Intern Med 1984;101:627–8.

256. Pines A, Rozen P, Ron E, Gilat T. Gastrointestinal tumors in acromegalic patients. Am J Gastroenterol 1985;80:266–9.

257. Ritter M, Richter W, Schwandt P. Acromegaly and colon cancer. Ann Intern Med 1987;106:636–7.

258. Ziel F, Peters A. Acromegaly and gastrointestinal adenocarcinomas. Ann Intern Med 1988;109:514–5.

259. Brunner J, Johnson C, Zafar S, et al. Colon cancer and polyps in acromegaly: increased risk associated with family history of colon cancer. Clin Endocrinol (Oxf) 1990;32:65–71.

260. Terzolo M, Tappero G, Borretta G, et al. High prevalence of colonic polyps in patients with acromegaly. Influence of sex and age. Arch Intern Med 1994;154: 1272–6.

261. Jenkins P, Fairclough P, Richards T, et al. Acromegaly, colonic polyps and carcinoma. Clin Endocrinol 1997;47:17–22.

262. Ron E, Gridley G, Hrubec Z, et al. Acromegaly and gastrointestinal cancer. Cancer 1991;68:1673–7.

263. Barzilay J, Heatley G, Cushing G. Benign and malignant tumors in patients with acromegaly. Arch Intern Med 1991;151:1629–32.

264. Ma J, Pollak MN, Giovannucci E, et al. Prospective study of colorectal cancer risk in men and plasma levels of insulin-like growth factor (IGF)-1 and IGF-binding protein-3. J Natl Cancer Inst 1999;91:620–5.

265. Giovannucci E, Pollak MN, Platz EA. A prospective study of plasma insulin-like growth factor-1 and binding protein-3 and risk of colorectal cancer and adenoma in women. Cancer Epidemiol Biomarkers Prev 2000;9:345–9.

266. Sivaraman L, Leatham MP, Yee J, et al. CYP1A1 genetic polymorphisms and in situ colorectal cancer. Cancer Res 1994;54:3692–5.

267. Kadlubar FF. Biochemical individuality and its implications for drug and carcinogen metabolism: recent insights from acetyltransferase and cytochrome P4501A2 phenotyping and genotyping in humans. Drug Metab Rev 1994;26:37–46.

268. Lang NP, Butler MA, Massengill J, et al. Rapid metabolic phenotypes for acetyltransferase and cytochrome P450A2 and putative exposure to food-borne heterocyclic amines increase the risk for colorectal cancer or polyps. Cancer Epidemiol Biomarkers Prev 1994;3:675–82.

269. Wohlleb JC, Hunter CF, Blass B, et al. Aromatic amine acetyltrasferase as a marker for colorectal cancer: environmental and demographic associations. Int J Cancer 1990;46:22–30.

270. Chen J, Stampfer MJ, Hough HL, et al. A prospective study of N-acetyltransferse genotype, red meat intake, and risk of colorectal cancer. Cancer Res 1998;58:3307–11.

271. Kampman E, Slattery ML, Bigler J, et al. Meat consumption, genetic susceptibility, and colon cancer risk: a United States multicenter case-control study. Cancer Epidemiol Biomarkers Prev 1999;8:15 24.

272. Strange R, Matharoo B, Faulder G, et al. The human glutathione S-transferases: a case-control study of the incidence of the GST1 0 phenotype in patients with adenocarcinoma. Carcinogenesis 1991;12:25–8.

273. Zhong S, Wyllie AH, Barnes D, et al. Relationship between the GSTM1 genetic polymorphism and susceptibility to bladder, breast and colon cancer. Carcinogenesis 1993;14:1821–4.

274. Gertig DM, Stampfer M, Haiman C, et al. Glutathione S-transferase GSTM1 and GSTT1 polymorphisms and colorectal cancer risk: a prospective study. Cancer Epidemiol Biomarkers Prev 1998;7:1001–5.

275. Blount BC, Ames BN. DNA damage in folate deficiency. Baillieres Clin Haematol 1995;8:461–78.

276. Slattery ML, Potter JD, Samowitz W, et al. Methyl-enetetrahydrofolate reductase, diet, and risk of colon cancer. Cancer Epidemiol Biomarkers Prev 1999;8:513–8.

277. Steinmetz KA, Potter JD. Vegetables, fruit, and cancer. II. Mechanisms. Cancer Causes Control 1991;2:427–42.

278. Mehta RG, Liu J, Constantinou A, et al. Cancer chemopreventive activity of brassinin, a phytoalexin from cabbage. Carcinogenesis 1995;16:399–404.

279. Hecht SS. Chemoprevention by isothiocyanates. J Cell Biochem Suppl 1995;22:195–209.

280. Hayes JD, Pulford DJ. The glutathione S-transferase supergene family: regulation of GST and the contribution of the isoenzymes to cancer chemoprotection and drug resistance. Crit Rev Biochem Mol Biol 1995;30:445–60.

281. Zhang Y, Kolm RH, Mannervik B, Talalay P. Reversible conjugation of isothiocyanates with glutathione catalyzed by human glutathione transferases. Biochem Biophys Res Commun 1995;206:748–55.

282. Lin HJ, Probst-Hensch NM, Louie AD, et al. Glutathione transferase null genotype, broccoli, and lower prevalence of colorectal adenomas. Cancer Epidemiol Biomarkers Prev 1998;7:647–52.

283. Lapre JA, Van der Meer R. Diet induced increase in colonic bile acids stimulates lytic activity in fecal water and proliferation of colonic cells. Carcinogenesis 1992;13:41–4.

284. Rafter JJ, Child P, Anderson AM, et al. Cellular toxicity of fecal water depends on diet. Am J Clin Nutr 1987;45:559–63.

285. Stadler J, Yeung KS, Furrer R, et al. Proliferative activity of rectal mucosa and soluble fecal bile acids in patients with normal colons and in patients with colonic polyps or cancer. Cancer Lett 1988;38:315–20.

286. Bayerdorffer E, Mannes GA, Richter WO, et al. Increased serum deoxycholic acid levels in men with colorectal adenomas. Gastroenterology 1993;104:141–51.

287. Cummings JH. The effect of dietary fiber on fecal weight and composition. In: Spiller GA, ed. CRC Handbook of dietary fibre in human nutrition. Boca Raton: CRC Press, 1993. p. 211–80.

288. Alberts DS, Martínez ME, Roe DJ, et al. Lack of effect of a high-fiber cereal supplement on the recurrence of colorectal adenomas. N Engl J Med 2000;342:1156–62.

289. Skraastad O, Reichelt KL. An endogenous colon mitosis inhibitor and dietary calcium inhibit the increased colonic cell proliferation induced by cholic acid. Scand J Gastroenterol 1988;23:801–7.

290. Alberts DS, Ritenbaugh C, Story JA, et al. Randomized, double-blinded, placebo-controlled study of effect of wheat bran fiber and calcium on fecal bile acids in patients with resected adenomatous colon polyps. J Natl Cancer Inst 1996;88:81–92.

291. Alberts DS, Einspahr J, Rees-McGee S, et al. Effects of dietary wheat bran fiber on rectal epithelial cell proliferation in patients with resection for colorectal cancers. J Natl Cancer Inst 1990;82:1280–5.

292. Baron JA, Beach M, Mandel JS, et al. Calcium supplements for the prevention of colorectal adenomas. N Engl J Med 1999;340:101–7.

293. Faivre J, Bonithon-Kopp C, Faculty DE MedicinneCINE. A randomized trial of calcium and fiber supplementation in the prevention of recurrence of colorectal adenomas. Proceedings of American Gastroenterological Association Annual Meeting; 1999. Orlando, FL. p. 1985.

294. Federowski T, Salen G, Tint GS, Mosbach E. Transformation of chenodeoxycholic acid and ursodeoxycholic acid by human intestinal bacteria. Gastroenterology 1979;77:1068–73.

295. Earnest DL, Holubec H, Wali RK, et al. Chemoprevention of azoxymethane-induced colonic carcinogenesis by supplemental dietary ursodeoxycholic acid. Cancer Res 1994;54:5071–4.

296. Pennisi E. Building a better aspirin. Science 1998;280:1191–1192.

297. Earnest DL, Hixon LJ, Alberts DS. Piroxicam and other cyclooxygenase inhibitors: potential for cancer chemoprevention. J Cell Biochem Suppl 1992;161:156–66.

298. Pasricha PJ, Bedi A, O'Connor K, et al. The effects of sulindac on colorectal proliferation and apoptosis in familial adenomatous polyposis. Gastroenterology 1995;109:994–8.

299. Batta AK, Salen G, Pamuken R, et al. Sulindac and its sulfone derivative inhibit colon cancer via modification of intestinal bile acids. Proceedings from The American Gastroenterological Association. Gastroenterology 1996;110:A490.

300. Alberts DS, Hixson L, Ahnen D, et al. Do NSAIDs exert their colon cancer chemoprevention activities through the inhibition of mucosal prostaglandin synthetase? J Cell Biochem Suppl 1995;22:18–23.

301. Hixson LJ, Alberts DS, Krutzsch M, et al. Antiproliferative effect of nonsteroidal antiinflammatory drugs against human colon cancer cells. Cancer Epidemiol Biomarkers Prev 1994;3:433–8.

302. Piazza GA, Kulchak Rahm AL, Krutzsch M, et al. Antineoplastic drugs sulindac sulfide and sulfone inhibit cell growth by inducing apoptosis. Cancer Res 1995;55:3110–6.

303. Gann PH, Manson JE, Glynn RJ, et al. Low-dose aspirin and incidence of colorectal tumors in a randomized trial. J Natl Cancer Inst 1993;85:1220–4.

304. Reddy BS, Rao CV, Seibert K. Evaluation of cyclooxygenase inhibitor for potential chemopreventive properties in colon carcinogenesis. Cancer Res 1996;56:4566–9.

305. Kawamori T, Rao CV, Seibert K, Reddy BS. Chemopreventive activity of celecoxib, a specific cyclooxygenase-2 inhibitor, against colon carcinogenesis. Cancer Res 1998;58:409–12.

306. The Alpha-Tocopherol Beta-Carotene Cancer Prevention Study Group. The effect of vitamin E and beta carotene on the incidence of lung cancer and other cancers in male smokers. N Engl J Med 1994;330:1029–35.

307. Clark LC, Combs GF Jr, Turnbull BW, et al. Effects of selenium supplementation for cancer prevention in patients with carcinoma of the skin. A randomized controlled trial. Nutritional Prevention of Cancer Study Group. JAMA 1996;276:1957–63.

308. MacLennan R, Macrae F, Bain C, et al. Randomized trial of intake of fat, fiber, and beta carotene to prevent colorectal adenomas. J Natl Cancer Inst 1995;87:1760–6.

309. Greenberg ER, Baron JA, Tosteson TD, et al. A clinical trial of antioxidant vitamins to prevent colorectal adenoma. N Engl J Med 1994;331:141–7.

310. Paganelli GM, Biasco G, Brandi G, et al. Effect of vitamin A, C, and E supplementation on rectal cell proliferation in patients with colorectal adenomas. J Natl Cancer Inst 1992;84:47–51.

3

Genetics of Colorectal Carcinoma

TIMOTHY D. JENKINS, MD
ANIL K. RUSTGI, MD

The molecular and genetic basis of colorectal cancer involves the mutation, aberrant expression, or deletion of numerous genes that have only recently been identified. Today, many of the genes responsible for the pathogenesis of colorectal cancer have also been characterized with regard to mechanism of action. Biochemical pathways central to a cell's maintenance of normal growth, proliferation, repair, and death are critically disrupted as a result of alterations in these genes. A clinically evident adenoma or carcinoma is the end manifestation of complex genetic dysregulation at the cellular level.

Molecular genetic discoveries have had a discernible impact in the clinic, where genetic testing for many of the inherited forms of colorectal cancer is available. To date, the most important application of genetic testing has been for risk assessment in family members of a patient affected with an inherited form of colorectal cancer. The stage is now set for advances in the diagnosis and treatment of sporadic colorectal cancer based on an understanding of molecular pathogenetic mechanisms. Translation of basic biomedical research discoveries into treatment is only in its infancy; therapeutic approaches utilizing many different strategies are currently in development. This chapter will review some of the salient features of inherited and sporadic colorectal cancer, namely the oncogenes, tumor suppressor genes, and other genes involved in their pathogenesis. The chapter will conclude with aspects of clinical genetic testing and future directions.

CLASSIFICATION AND CLINICAL FEATURES OF COLORECTAL CANCER

The inherited colorectal cancers had been classified according to their genetic and morphologic clinical features well prior to the discovery and characterization of the genes responsible. Colorectal cancer is associated with several inherited syndromes, including the autosomal dominant adenomatous polyposis syndromes (ADAPS), the autosomal dominant hamartomatous polyposis syndromes (ADHPS), and the hereditary nonpolyposis colorectal cancer syndromes (HNPCC). In addition to these inherited syndromes, there is sporadic colorectal cancer, which accounts for most of the approximately 140,000 new cases per year in the United States.[1] A classification of polyposis and nonpolyposis colorectal cancer is shown in Table 3–1.

The best characterized ADAPS is familial adenomatous polyposis (FAP). Familial adenomatous polyposis is distinguished by the presence of >100 premalignant adenomatous polyps in the colon and by a variety of extracolonic manifestations. Familial adenomatous polyposis and its variants account for less than 1 percent of all colorectal cancers.[2,3] The adenomatous polyps develop between the ages of 5 and 40, typically in early adolescence; colorectal cancer becomes evident in the third to fourth decade of life. Common lesions outside the colon include epidermoid cysts, osteomas, pigmented retinal lesions, desmoid tumors, and gastroduodenal adenomas and carcinomas.[3]

Table 3–1. CLASSIFICATION OF POLYPOSIS AND NONPOLYPOSIS ASSOCIATED COLORECTAL CANCER

Autosomal Dominant Adenomatous Polyposis Syndromes
1. Familial adenomatous polyposis (FAP)
2. Attenuated adenomatous polyposis coli (AAPC)
3. Turcot's syndrome

Autosomal Dominant Hamartomatous Polyposis Syndromes
1. Peutz-Jeghers syndrome
2. Juvenile polyposis
3. Cowden syndrome
4. Neurofibromatosis Type II
5. Ruvalcaba-Myhre-Smith syndrome
6. Devon family syndrome

Hereditary Nonpolyposis Colorectal Cancer (HNPCC) Syndromes
1. HNPCC Type I
2. HNPCC Type II
3. Muir-Torre syndrome

Sporadic Colorectal Cancer

Two other types of adenomatous polyposis have also been described. The first is attenuated adenomatous polyposis coli (AAPC), in which fewer than 100 polyps are found but other characteristics of FAP are present. The second is Turcot's syndrome, which includes malignant tumors of the central nervous system in addition to characteristic multiple colonic adenomas, typically 20 to 100. Although there is evidence that Turcot's syndrome is transmitted in autosomal recessive fashion, the syndrome has been linked to either adenomatous polyposis coli (APC) or DNA mismatch repair gene mutations.[4] Recent reports provide evidence for autosomal dominant transmission, consistent with the other ADAPS.[5]

There are several other ADHPS, two of which predispose to an increased risk of colorectal cancer: Peutz-Jeghers' syndrome and juvenile polyposis. Peutz-Jeghers' syndrome is characterized by mucocutaneous melanin depositions in addition to intestinal hamartomatous polyps. In addition, there is an association with sex-cord tumors. Neoplasms throughout the gastrointestinal tract have the potential to become malignant, presumably arising from an adenomatous element within a hamartoma.

Juvenile polyposis patients may present with rectal bleeding at an early age. These patients are often found to have a few to multiple hamartomatous polyps throughout the colon. Because of the risk for colorectal cancer, such patients should undergo colonoscopic screening or even prophy-

lactic colectomy.[6] Juvenile polyposis patients may also have polyps in the stomach and small intestine. Another ADHPS, Cowden syndrome, is probably not associated with a significant risk for colorectal cancer when compared with the other two syndromes.[6]

HNPCC includes Type I and Type II HNPCC and the Muir-Torre syndrome. Patients with Type I HNPCC are affected only by colorectal adenocarcinomas while Type II patients have extracolonic (particularly endometrial) tumors in addition to colorectal cancer. These syndromes are notable for the absence of large numbers of precursor lesions despite a high risk for cancer. The proximal colon is especially prone to the development of cancer since a distinguishing feature of the syndrome is the presence of up to 100 adenomatous polyps in this location. Multiple primary or metachronous tumors are also common in HNPCC.

The HNPCC syndromes are transmitted in autosomal dominant fashion and account for approximately 5 to 10 percent of all colorectal cancers.[7] One set of criteria for the diagnosis of HNPCC requires that at least three relatives have histologically verified colorectal cancer, that one of those relatives is a first-degree relative of the other two, that at least two successive generations are affected, and that one of the relatives is under the age of 50 when the colorectal cancer is diagnosed. These criteria, the so-called Amsterdam criteria,[8] have been reexamined recently[9] and are summarized along with the Bethesda criteria[10] in Table 3–2. Japanese criteria for HNPCC have also been described.[11] Muir-Torre syndrome is a variant of HNPCC that is characterized by multiple tumors of the skin such as sebaceous adenomas or keratoacanthomas and urinary tract tumors in addition to the colorectal tumors.

Sporadic colorectal cancer describes cancer that occurs in the absence of a family history or in the presence of family history not fulfilling criteria for one of the inherited syndromes. Despite the name, sporadic cases of colorectal cancer undoubtedly entail a significant genetic contribution. Because the risk of colorectal cancer is elevated in family members of a patient affected with colorectal cancer, screening is intensified in these unaffected adults.

MOLECULAR GENETICS OF COLORECTAL CANCER

The development of a colorectal cancer is thought to occur in stages. Normal mucosa yields an adenoma that progresses to become cancer. There is strong experimental evidence that abnormal colonocytes with certain genetic alterations are able to proliferate excessively and acquire additional mutations. Eventually, as this process continues, the cells assume malignant characteristics of invasiveness and metastatic potential.[12]

Early genetic changes, before a mass lesion is grossly visible, can still result in microscopically altered colonic epithelium. This abnormal epithelium, which has the potential to become an adenoma or later a carcinoma, has been described as an aberrant crypt focus (ACF). ACFs can be recognized under magnifying endoscopy and have been shown to regress after treatment with sulindac, similar to the effect of sulindac on adenomas.[13] ACFs have also been found in the early stages of chemically[14] and genetically induced[15] animal models of colorectal cancer.

Adenomas and carcinomas are characterized genetically by alterations that promote growth, invasion, and metastasis of tumor cells. The altered genes include oncogenes (e.g., K-*ras*), tumor suppressor genes (e.g., *APC, p53*), and DNA mismatch repair genes (e.g., *hMSH2, hMLH1*). In addition, there are other genes whose role in tumor formation has not been as clearly delineated (e.g., *COX-2*) but whose expression in altered fashion may contribute to the progression of the tumor sequence. One widely accepted model, first proposed by Vogelstein and colleagues, is that a combination of mutations in these genes is responsible for both the orderly adenoma to carcinoma to metastasis sequence as well as the cellular characteristics of tumors.[16] This model, known as the adenoma to carcinoma sequence, may explain the observation that many years are typically required for an adenoma to progress to cancer. The genetic alterations found in FAP, HNPCC, and sporadic colorectal cancer are summarized in Table 3–3.

K-*ras* and Other Proto-Oncogenes

Mutations that activate the K-*ras* proto-oncogene are common in colon carcinomas, generally present in about 50 percent of such polyps and tumors.[17] K-*ras* is localized near the cell membrane and is responsible for transducing signals from the cell surface

Table 3–2. SUMMARY OF DIAGNOSTIC CRITERIA FOR THE HEREDITARY NONPOLYPOSIS COLORECTAL CANCER SYNDROME

Amsterdam
1. At least three relatives should have histologically verified colorectal cancer
2. One affected relative should be a first-degree relative of the other two
3. At least two successive generations should be affected
4. Colon cancer should be diagnosed under 50 years of age in one relative
5. Familial adenomatous polyposis should be excluded

Amsterdam II
1. At least three relatives with histologically verified HNPCC-associated cancer (colorectal, endometrial, small bowel, ureter, renal pelvis)
2. One affected relative should be a first-degree relative of the other two
3. At least two successive generations should be affected
4. Colon cancer should be diagnosed under 50 years of age in one relative
5. Familial adenomatous polyposis should be excluded

Bethesda
1. Individuals with cancer fulfilling the Amsterdam criteria
2. Individuals with two HNPCC-related cancers
3. Individuals with colorectal cancer and a first-degree relative with colorectal cancer and/or HNPCC-related extracolonic cancer and/or a colonic adenoma (cancer before age 45, adenoma before age 40)
4. Individuals with colorectal or endometrial cancer diagnosed before age 45
5. Individuals with right-sided colon cancer with undifferentiated/solid/cribriform histopathology diagnosed before age 45
6. Individuals with signet-ring cell type colon cancer diagnosed before age 45
7. Individuals with adenomas diagnosed before age 40

ICG
1. Familial clustering of colorectal and/or endometrial cancer
2. Associated cancers of the stomach, ovary, ureter, renal pelvis, brain, small bowel, hepatobiliary tract, skin
3. Development of cancer at an early age
4. Development of multiple cancers
5. Features of colorectal cancer including predilection for the proximal colon, improved survival, multiple colorectal cancers, specific histologic characteristics including mucinous, poorly differentiated, lymphocytic infiltrated tumors
6. Features of colorectal adenomas including number from one to a few, villous growth pattern, high degree of dysplasia, rapid progression from adenoma to carcinoma
7. DNA microsatellite instability
8. Loss of MLH1 or MSH2 protein expression
9. Germline mutation in *hMSH2, hMLH1, hMSH6, hPMS1, hPMS2*

Data from Vasen HF et al.[8]
Vasen HF et al.[9]
Rodriguez-Bigas MA et al.[10]

Table 3–3. COMPARISON OF THE MOLECULAR GENETIC ALTERATIONS TYPICAL OF FAP, HNPCC, AND SPORADIC COLORECTAL CANCER

Familial Adenomatous Polyposis (FAP)
  APC
Hereditary Nonpolyposis Colorectal Cancer (HNPCC)
  hMSH2
  hMLH1
  hMSH6
  hPMS1
  hPMS2
Sporadic Colorectal Cancer
  APC
  ras
  p53
  SMADs
  myc
  src
  SMADs
  COX-2

toward the nucleus. These signals ultimately affect gene transcription, which has the capacity to alter cellular growth and proliferation. A schema of the *ras* signaling pathway is shown in Figure 3–1.

Activating mutations within *ras* tend to occur at a limited number of sites within the coding sequence (codons 12, 13, and 61), simplifying the mutational analysis of clinical specimens.[17] *Ras* mutations have been found to occur in normal epithelium adjacent to a tumor, suggesting that it is an early event in tumorigenesis.[18] Different *ras* mutations have also been found in a single tumor,[18] suggesting that conditions in a tumor that lead to *ras* mutation are not infrequent. Molecular assays have been devised to rapidly analyze *ras* mutations in clinical samples and are now suitable for use in a routine diagnostic laboratory.[19] *Ras* is thus used as a biomarker for tumor development and progression.[20]

The functional consequences of activating *ras* mutations have been demonstrated in many studies. Colon cancer cell lines with activated *ras* display a characteristic tumor phenotype, but when the *ras* gene is disrupted or knocked-out, the cells lose that phenotype.[21] The cells are less able to form tumors in mice, become morphologically altered, and show reduced expression of another oncogene, c-*myc*. Other evidence for the importance of the *ras* pathway in colorectal cancer genetics comes from the development of agents that inhibit the growth of tumors via this pathway. The farnesyl transferase inhibitors (FTIs) inhibit an enzyme critical for activation of functional *ras*. FTIs have been shown in colorectal cancer cell culture and animal models to have potent antiproliferative activity.[22] In chemically induced animal models of colorectal carcinoma, *ras* mutation is also common and appears to play an important role.[23,24]

The signal transduction pathways activated by *ras* are complex, and interactions with tumor suppressor genes have been described. Mutant *ras* has been shown to downregulate the tumor suppressor homeobox gene *CDX-2*.[25] *CDX-2* disruption in mice is lethal in the embryonic state, but mice with a single normal *CDX-2* allele develop intestinal adenomatous polyps, particularly in the proximal colon.[26] The *p16* tumor suppressor gene is inactivated in neoplasms by a number of different mechanisms such as deletion, mutation, or gene silencing by promoter methylation.[27] Activity of *p16* was found to be silenced in a large percentage of colorectal tumor specimens.[28] Activating K-*ras* mutations were highly associated with *p16* promoter methylation in one study, providing a possible link between common *ras* mutations and effects on cellular proliferation.[28]

Two other proto-oncogenes have been associated with colorectal cancer, *src* and *myc*. Activation of *src* and *myc* has been demonstrated in colorectal cancer but the contribution of these genes to overall tumor progression is less clear. *Myc* has been identified as

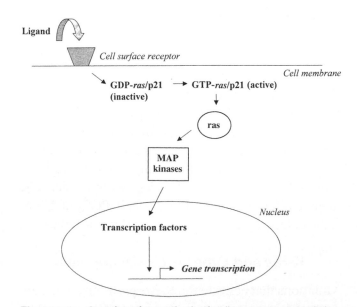

Figure 3–1. Overview of *ras* activation leading to gene transcription.

a target of the *APC* pathway, which will be discussed in the following section.[29] In addition, a truncating mutation in *src* was described that was present in 12 percent of colorectal cancer cases tested. This mutation was capable of promoting the metastatic potential of colorectal cancer cells.[30]

Tumor Suppressor Genes

The FAP tumor suppressor gene locus was identified after studies suggested that genes in the chromosomal region of 5q21 were responsible for polyp and tumor formation. Adenomatous polyposis coli was one of the genes identified that encodes an unusually large protein (310 kilodaltons) that interacts with many other intracellular proteins.[31] The vast majority of APC mutations associated with colon cancer introduce a stop codon, which results in a truncated APC protein. Additionally, some genotypic-phenotypic correlations have emerged, namely that certain mutations within the APC coding sequence are associated with AAPC and extracolonic manifestations such as congenital hypertrophy of the retinal pigment epithelium (CHRPE) and desmoid tumors.

Following the identification of APC as a candidate tumor suppressor gene, animal genetic models of APC mutation successfully recapitulated certain aspects of the human disease. Since a knockout of both alleles of APC is lethal in the embryonic stage, Shibata and colleagues devised a strategy to functionally inactivate both APC alleles in the adult murine colonic epithelium. When mutant APC was activated, the mice developed colonic adenomas extremely rapidly, within about 4 weeks.[32] Many other mutant APC mouse models have confirmed its importance in the neoplastic process.

Recently, some of the mechanisms by which APC exerts its biologic effects have been described. APC has been shown to modulate the effects of an important signal transduction pathway, wnt. A summary of the wnt pathway and the role of APC is shown in Figure 3–2. Mutations of APC that are associated with the polyposis phenotype have been shown to result in the accumulation of β-catenin. β-catenin is usually degraded in the cell, but mutants of APC (or β-catenin) allow its accumulation and subsequent nuclear translocation.[33] The normal function of

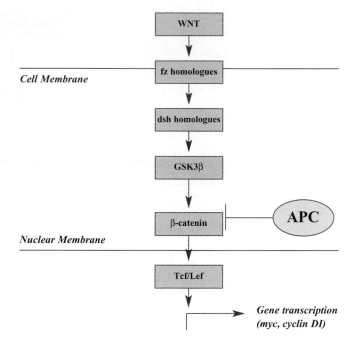

Figure 3–2. APC inhibits the wnt signaling pathway to alter gene transcription, influencing growth and proliferation.

β-catenin is to bind the transcription factors TCF and LEF. The β-catenin/TCF/LEF complex subsequently activates gene transcription. With accumulated β-catenin in the APC deficient cell, transcriptional targets are excessively activated.

Until recently, the transcriptional targets of the β-catenin complex remained undefined. He and colleagues recently showed that expression of the *myc* oncogene is repressed in the presence of normal APC and activated by β-catenin, providing one mechanism for mutant APC to contribute to the earliest stages of transformation.[29] Mutant APC and β-catenin have also been recently shown to activate transcription from the cyclin D1 promoter, leading to excessive amounts of this oncoprotein.[34]

The *p53* tumor suppressor gene is commonly mutated in a number of different cancer types, including colorectal cancer. Among its many diverse functions, wild-type *p53* regulates proliferation by serving as a cell cycle checkpoint, participating in DNA repair, promoting apoptosis in damaged cells, and acting as a transcription factor. Some of the cellular functions of *p53* are illustrated in Figure 3–3.[35]

Primary cultures of colonic epithelial cells have been established from *p53* deficient mice and, on introduction of activated *ras*, these cells acquire a highly malignant potential. Such a model system

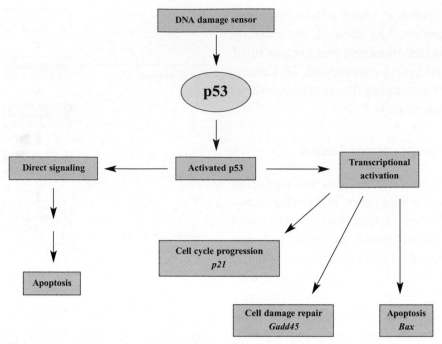

Figure 3–3.   p53 is central to many critical cell regulatory processes.

lends support to the theory of a multistep genetic process in colorectal carcinogenesis.[36] The discovery of mutant *p53* in colon cancers may also have implications for current modes of therapy. One study found that colorectal cancer cells that harbor a mutant *p53* are significantly more resistant to agents such as radiation and 5-fluorouracil, commonly used in the treatment of colorectal cancer.[37]

There is recent evidence that the TGFβ Type II Receptor (TGFβIIR) may act as a tumor suppressor gene in colorectal cancer. TGFβ encompasses a family of growth factors that regulate cellular growth, differentiation, and development in many tissue types.[38] TGFβIIR alleles are susceptible to the acquisition of DNA mismatch repair errors (discussed below), and cells with mutant TGFβIIR are resistant to the growth inhibitory effects of TGFβ.[39,40]

The receptors for the TGFβ family of ligands transduce a signal to the nucleus through a set of proteins known as the SMADs. In the presence of a ligand bound to a receptor, a receptor-associated SMAD (2 or 3) associates with a SMAD4, translocates to the nucleus, and alters gene transcription. Targeted gene deletion of SMAD3 in mice led to the appearance of colorectal adenocarcinomas in one study and also was shown to critically disrupt the TGFβ signaling pathway.[41,42] In some human sporadic colorectal cancers,

SMAD4 is mutated.[43] Activated *ras* has been linked to the TGFβIIR pathway. *Ras* can repress TGFβIIR signaling, disrupting a growth control mechanism in the absence of TGFβIIR or SMAD mutation.[44] A summary of the TGFβIIR-SMAD signaling pathway is shown in Figure 3–4.

The deleted in colon cancer (DCC) gene was first described in 1994 as a gene located on chromosome 18q in a region of common loss of heterozygosity in human colorectal tumors.[45] In a study of 36 cases of sporadic colorectal carcinoma, 26 percent of tumor DNA samples showed loss of heterozygosity at the DCC locus, in addition to 20 percent that had loss of heterozygosity at the APC locus.[46] The DCC gene encodes a protein found in axons of the central and peripheral nervous system, as well as in differentiated cells of the intestine. Colon cancer cells that lose expression of DCC are unable to properly differentiate.[45] There are conflicting data with regard to DCC, and its role in colorectal cancer pathogenesis remains unclear. Using monoclonal antibodies to the immunoglobulin-like domain of DCC, Gotley and colleagues studied normal colonic epithelium, adenomas, and carcinomas and found that DCC was not completely lost in the samples studied.[47] They concluded that the loss of DCC expression is not necessary for tumor progression.

Mismatch Repair Genes

Hereditary nonpolyposis colorectal cancer (HNPCC) is a common inherited disease. Shortly after the recognition that colorectal tumors from families with HNPCC harbored numerous alterations in short repeated DNA sequences,[48] termed microsatellite instability, the search for the genes responsible was successful. Human homologues of the bacterial mismatch repair genes *mutS* and *mutL* were found to be mutated in some HNPCC cases. These genes include *hMLH1*[49] and *hMSH2*[50] and three other genes, *hPMS1, hPMS2,*[51] and *hMSH6. hMLH1* and *hMSH2* are most commonly mutated in HNPCC kindreds.

Further studies confirmed the relevance of mutations of these genes in patients with HNPCC.[52] These genes encode enzymes that repair DNA replication errors: they bind specifically to insertion-deletion loop-type mismatched nucleotides characteristic of DNA microsatellite instability.[53] The HNPCC subtype Muir-Torre syndrome was also found to be associated with a germline truncating mutation in *hMSH2*.[54] In support of the data from human tumors, inactivation of several of the mismatch repair genes in mice also leads to a hereditary predisposition to intestinal and other cancers.[55,56]

Genes involved in cell proliferation and death have been shown to be affected by mutations within the mismatch repair apparatus. In one study of 41 tumors with microsatellite instability, frameshift mutations were commonly found within both alleles of *BAX*, a gene central to the apoptosis pathway.[57] The results showed that mutations in the *BAX* gene may be selected for in the absence of wild-type mismatch repair genes. Another target of microsatellite instability is the TGFβIIR, whose significance in colorectal cancer was previously discussed.

While the persistence of DNA errors throughout cell division has been thought to involve impaired binding of the mismatch repair enzymes to mismatched DNA, it has also been recently shown that mismatch repair proteins can interact with one another. One recent study demonstrated that some germline mutations in *hMLH1* lead to an impaired direct binding of *hMLH1* to *hPMS2*.[58] Impairment of this protein-protein interaction was linked to HNPCC. Thus, the mechanism of the action of mutated DNA mismatch repair enzymes may be more complex than previously envisioned.

Although a germline mutation in a mismatch repair gene allele provides a mechanism for HNPCC, many sporadic cases of colorectal cancer also have microsatellite instability and yet possess wild-type mismatch repair genes. One study found that, despite the wild-type status of these genes, protein levels of the mismatch repair enzymes were

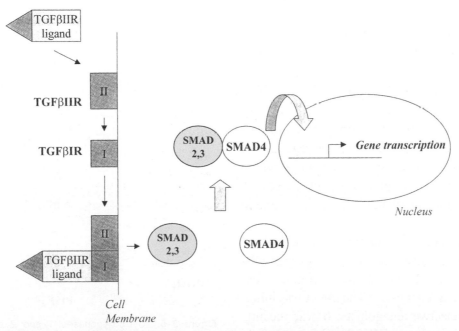

Figure 3–4. The TGFβ signaling pathway acts through SMADs to influence gene transcription.

abnormal. Veigl and colleagues found that the promoters governing repair enzyme expression were methylated. Promoter methylation can reduce expression, and the authors found that treatment with demethylating agents led to normalized expression.[59] The effect of promoter methylation, a type of gene silencing, could be responsible for sporadic cases of colorectal cancer despite wild-type mismatch repair alleles. Somatic mutations of genes commonly altered in sporadic cancer are less commonly mutated in HNPCC, 17 percent for K-ras and 13 percent for p53 in one study.[60] This finding suggests that the pathways responsible for cancer in HNPCC are distinct from those in sporadic colorectal cancer.

Other Genes Imputed in Colorectal Cancer Molecular Pathogenesis

It has been observed for several years that the use of nonsteroidal anti-inflammatory drug (NSAIDs) is associated with a decreased risk of the development of colorectal carcinoma. This subject was recently reviewed by Dubois and colleagues, who found that most studies showed a 40 to 50 percent decreased relative risk in continuous aspirin users.[61] One group of researchers found that, in the elderly, long-term use (greater than 12 months) of non-aspirin NSAIDs decreased the risk of colorectal cancer by almost 50 percent.[62] This study also found that the dose of the drug was not as important as the duration of use.

Because of the epidemiologic and experimental observations regarding NSAIDs and colorectal cancer, it is hypothesized that cyclooxygenase (COX), and particularly the inducible form COX-2, may play a role in the molecular genetic pathogenesis of colorectal carcinoma. The cyclooxygenases regulate the production of arachidonic acid metabolites, which serve as mediators of inflammatory processes. A summary of arachidonate metabolites is illustrated in Figure 3–5.

COX-2 is commonly overexpressed in colorectal cancer. In a tissue culture system, colon cancer cells that overexpress COX-2 were shown to produce factors that promote angiogenesis.[63] The effect was inhibited by COX-2 selective antagonists. It was recently shown that meloxicam, a COX-2 inhibitor, could

inhibit the growth of colon cancer cells that express COX-2 but not the growth of those cells lacking COX-2 expression.[64] A link of COX-2 to DNA mismatch repair has recently been described, as has a link to the TGFβ signaling pathway.[65] Tumors defective in mismatch repair were found to express lower levels of COX-2, a finding that may have implications for the chemoprevention of tumors in HNPCC patients.[66]

The genetic mechanism by which a high-fat diet is associated with an increased risk of colorectal cancer has been investigated recently, leading to a focus on the nuclear receptor peroxisome proliferator-activated receptors (PPARs). The PPARs are activated in response to lipid-derived compounds and fatty acids, and one subtype, PPAR-γ, is expressed at high levels in colon cancer cells and tumors. A ligand for PPAR-γ given to mice predisposed to intestinal neoplasia resulted in significantly increased numbers of tumors in the colon.[67] Similarly, another group showed that activation of PPAR-γ increased the frequency of colon tumors in mice with an APC mutation susceptible to intestinal neoplasia.[68] The animal data are not entirely consistent with human biology, however. In one study, colon

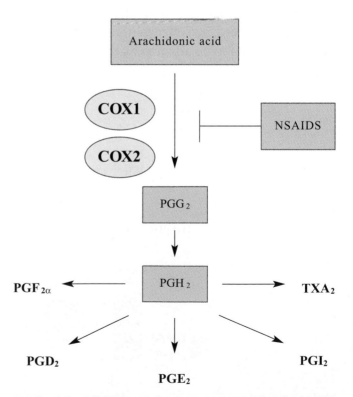

Figure 3–5. Cyclooxygenases 1 and 2 regulate inflammatory mediator production.

cancer cells and transplantable tumors derived from human colorectal cancer showed a decreased growth rate and reversal of characteristics typical of colorectal cancer when treated with a PPAR-γ ligand.[69]

Several other proteins have been shown to play a role in the progression of colorectal cancer. Inducible nitric oxide synthase, which is also overexpressed in colorectal cancers, is significantly upregulated in a chemically induced model of rat colon cancer.[70] Absence of the G protein subunit α_{i2} in mice results in the development of a diffuse colitis followed by adenocarcinoma.[71] Matrix metalloproteinases (MMPs) degrade the extracellular matrix, are important in cell migration, and are thought to play a role in metastasis. In colorectal cancer, the presence of MMP-1 was found to be associated with a poor prognosis, independent of Dukes stage.[72] The PTEN gene encodes a phosphatase that is mutated in Cowden syndrome. Disruption of both PTEN alleles in mice results in early embryonic lethality. Mice homozygous for PTEN show dysplastic changes in the colon characteristic of Cowden syndrome,[73] and colon tumors subsequently developed. The *PPP2R1B* gene, a subunit of a serine/threonine protein phosphatase was shown to be deleted in 15 percent of a sample of primary colon adenocarcinomas. A deletion mutant of *PPP2R1B* was unable to complete the PP2A enzyme and is considered a possible tumor suppressor through its ability to affect cell cycle regulation.[74]

Other as yet unidentified genetic factors probably influence colorectal carcinogenesis as well. The contribution of genetic background to the development of colorectal cancer is shown in mouse studies where different inbred strains are differently susceptible to colorectal cancer.[75] Susceptibility loci have been identified through such studies, including loci that show a strong reciprocal interaction when present concurrently.[75] Studies of genetic background and susceptibility should give additional insight into the mechanisms of sporadic colorectal cancers.

CLINICAL APPLICATION OF MOLECULAR GENETICS

Genetic testing for mutations in genes such as APC and the mismatch repair genes is the most immedi-

ately applicable result of the progress in understanding the molecular genetic events in colorectal cancer. Despite its availability, genetic testing has been mostly limited to the inherited syndromes, which are responsible for a minority of cancer cases. Commercial laboratory facilities capable of rapidly analyzing specimens for common mutations are readily accessible to clinicians. However, personnel trained in the application of genetic testing and counseling of patients regarding the decision to test and consequences of testing are mostly limited to tertiary care referral centers.

One recent study examined factors that predict the utilization of genetic testing by patients at risk for an inherited form of colorectal cancer. It found that increased risk perception, increased perceived ability to cope with unfavorable results, more frequent cancer thoughts, and having already had at least one colonoscopy all predicted an increased utilization of genetic testing.[76] Cultural influences also play a role in utilization of genetic testing and counseling. In Hawaii, persons of Japanese descent at higher risk for colorectal cancer had lower concern for the disease than persons of Hawaiian ancestry at lower risk for the disease.[77]

Many adults are at risk for inherited forms of colorectal cancer despite the absence of a classic family history. It is clear that patients may be at moderate or high risk for colorectal cancer as reflected by a family history of cancer that is not necessarily compatible with known inherited syndromes. Identifying which of these patients are at highest risk prior to the appearance of visible colonic lesions is desirable from the standpoint of designing a screening protocol. One group of investigators has proposed that a molecular genetic phenomenon known as loss of imprinting (LOI) be used to identify a subset of the population at greatest risk for development of cancer.[78] Imprinting, also known as parental imprinting or genomic imprinting, describes the phenomenon that gene expression differs according to the parent from which the gene was inherited. Loss of imprinting occurs when there is loss of this parent-allele specific gene expression and was found in the normal mucosa of patients with microsatellite instability-positive colon tumors (non-HNPCC), suggesting that LOI might serve as a marker predicting cancer development risk.[78] Another area of investigation is the detection of genetic alterations in the stool of patients. Alterations such as mutant *ras*[79] and mutant CD44[80] have been found to predict a higher risk for colorectal cancer.

CONCLUSION

The application of molecular genetics to therapy of colorectal cancer is the next frontier in the management of this disease. Development of animal genetic models of colorectal cancer such as APC mutant mouse models has enabled better understanding of the pathogenetic mechanisms of colorectal cancer. These mouse models also simplify initial testing of chemopreventive agents and other therapies. Gene therapy approaches to the treatment of colorectal cancer, based on information about its molecular pathogenesis, include immunogenic therapy (cytokine or tumor antigen expression to generate tumor immunity) and tumor suppressor gene replacement (with *p53* for example).[81] More precise analytic tools have been developed to dissect the genetic characteristics of a tumor. Using laser microbeam microdissection to isolate and recover cells from archival tumor specimens, a single cell from a colonic adenocarcinoma was recovered and analyzed to detect point mutations in codon 12 of K-*ras* by reverse transcriptase PCR analysis.[82] As advances in molecular genetic understanding and clinical delivery methods converge, early diagnosis, risk stratification, screening, and therapy should progress significantly in the decade to come.

REFERENCES

1. Lieberman D. Endoscopic screening for colorectal cancer. Gastroenterol Clin North Am 1997;26:71–83.
2. Lynch HT, Lynch JF. Genetics of colonic cancer. Digestion 1998;59:481–92.
3. Spigelman AD. Screening modalities in familial adenomatous polyposis and hereditary nonpolyposis colorectal cancer. Gastrointest Endosc Clin N Am 1997; 7:81–6.
4. Suzui M, Yoshimi N, Hara A, et al. Genetic alterations in a patient with Turcot's syndrome. Pathol Int 1998; 48:126–33.
5. Matsui T, Hayashi N, Yao K, et al. A father and son with Turcot's syndrome: evidence for autosomal domi-nant inheritance: report of two cases. Dis Colon Rectum 1998;41:797–801.
6. Giardiello FM, Offerhaus JG. Phenotype and cancer risk of various polyposis syndromes. Eur J Cancer 1995;31A:1085–7.
7. Lynch HT, Smyrk T. An update on Lynch syndrome. Curr Opin Oncol 1998;10:349–56.
8. Vasen HF, Mecklin JP, Khan PM, Lynch HT. The International Collaborative Group on Hereditary Non-Polyposis Colorectal Cancer (ICG-HNPCC). Dis Colon Rectum 1991;34:424–5.
9. Vasen HF, Watson P, Mecklin JP, Lynch HT. New clinical criteria for hereditary nonpolyposis colorectal cancer (HNPCC, Lynch syndrome) proposed by the International Collaborative group on HNPCC. Gastroenterology 1999;116:1453–6.
10. Rodriguez-Bigas MA, Boland CR, Hamilton SR, et al. A National Cancer Institute Workshop on Hereditary Nonpolyposis Colorectal Cancer Syndrome: meeting highlights and Bethesda guidelines. J Natl Cancer Inst 1997;89:1758–62.
11. Fujita S, Moriya Y, Sugihara K, et al. Prognosis of hereditary nonpolyposis colorectal cancer (HNPCC) and the role of Japanese criteria for HNPCC. Jpn J Clin Oncol 1996;26:351–5.
12. Ahnen DJ. The genetic basis of colorectal cancer risk. Adv Intern Med 1996;41:531–52.
13. Takayama T, Katsuki S, Takahashi Y, et al. Aberrant crypt foci of the colon as precursors of adenoma and cancer. N Engl J Med 1998;339:1277–84.
14. Papanikolaou A, Wang QS, Delker DA, Rosenberg DW. Azoxymethane-induced colon tumors and aberrant crypt foci in mice of different genetic susceptibility. Cancer Lett 1998;130:29–34.
15. Steffensen IL, Paulsen JE, Eide TJ, Alexander J. 2-Amino-1-methyl-6-phenylimidazo[4,5-b]pyridine increases the numbers of tumors, cystic crypts and aberrant crypt foci in multiple intestinal neoplasia mice. Carcinogenesis 1997;18:1049–54.
16. Kinzler KW, Vogelstein B. Lessons from hereditary colorectal cancer. Cell 1996;87:159–70.
17. Forrester K, Almoguera C, Han K, et al. Detection of high incidence of K-ras oncogenes during human colon tumorigenesis. Nature 1987;327:298–303.
18. Zhu D, Keohavong P, Finkelstein SD, et al. K-ras gene mutations in normal colorectal tissues from K-ras mutation-positive colorectal cancer patients. Cancer Res 1997;57:2485–92.
19. Ward R, Hawkins N, O'Grady R, et al. Restriction endonuclease-mediated selective polymerase chain reaction: a novel assay for the detection of K-ras mutations in clinical samples. Am J Pathol 1998; 153:373–9.
20. Minamoto T, Esumi H, Ochiai A, et al. Combined analysis of microsatellite instability and K-ras muta-

tion increases detection incidence of normal samples from colorectal cancer patients. Clin Cancer Res 1997;3:1413–7.

21. Shirasawa S, Furuse M, Yokoyama N, Sasazuki T. Altered growth of human colon cancer cell lines disrupted at activated Ki-ras. Science 1993;260:85–8.

22. Lobell RB, Kohl NE. Pre-clinical development of farnesyltransferase inhibitors. Cancer Metastasis Rev 1998;17:203–10.

23. Jackson PE, Cooper DP, O'Connor PJ, Povey AC. The relationship between 1,2-dimethylhydrazine dose and the induction of colon tumours: tumour development in female SWR mice does not require a K-ras mutational event. Carcinogenesis 1999;20:509–13.

24. Erdman SH, Wu HD, Hixson LJ, et al. Assessment of mutations in Ki-ras and p53 in colon cancers from azoxymethane- and dimethylhydrazine-treated rats. Mol Carcinog 1997;19:137–44.

25. Lorentz O, Cadoret A, Duluc I, et al. Downregulation of the colon tumour-suppressor homeobox gene Cdx-2 by oncogenic ras. Oncogene 1999;18:87–92.

26. Chawengsaksophak K, James R, Hammond VE, et al. Homeosis and intestinal tumours in Cdx2 mutant mice. Nature 1997;386:84–7.

27. Liggett WH, Jr., Sidransky D. Role of the p16 tumor suppressor gene in cancer. J Clin Oncol 1998;16:1197–206.

28. Guan RJ, Fu Y, Holt PR, Pardee AB. Association of K-ras mutations with p16 methylation in human colon cancer. Gastroenterology 1999;116:1063–71.

29. He TC, Sparks AB, Rago C, et al. Identification of c-MYC as a target of the APC pathway. Science 1998;281:1509–12.

30. Irby RB, Mao W, Coppola D, et al. Activating SRC mutation in a subset of advanced human colon cancers. Nat Genet 1999;21:187–90.

31. Kinzler KW, Nilbert MC, Su LK, et al. Identification of FAP locus genes from chromosome 5q21. Science 1991;253:661–5.

32. Shibata H, Toyama K, Shioya H, et al. Rapid colorectal adenoma formation initiated by conditional targeting of the Apc gene. Science 1997;278:120–3.

33. Morin PJ, Sparks AB, Korinek V, et al. Activation of beta-catenin-Tcf signaling in colon cancer by mutations in beta-catenin or APC. Science 1997;275:1787–90.

34. Tetsu O, McCormick F. Beta-catenin regulates expression of cyclin D1 in colon carcinoma cells. Nature 1999;398:422–6.

35. Levine AJ. p53, the cellular gatekeeper for growth and division. Cell 1997;88:323–31.

36. Sevignani C, Wlodarski P, Kirillova J, et al. Tumorigenic conversion of p53-deficient colon epithelial cells by an activated Ki-ras gene. J Clin Invest 1998;101:1572–80.

37. Yang B, Eshleman JR, Berger NA, Markowitz SD. Wild-type p53 protein potentiates cytotoxicity of therapeutic agents in human colon cancer cells. Clin Cancer Res 1996;2:1649–57.

38. Massague J. TGF-beta signal transduction. Annu Rev Biochem 1998;67:753–91.

39. Kim YS, Yi Y, Choi SG, Kim SJ. Development of TGF-beta resistance during malignant progression. Arch Pharm Res 1999;22:1–8.

40. Picon A, Gold LI, Wang J, et al. A subset of metastatic human colon cancers expresses elevated levels of transforming growth factor beta1. Cancer Epidemiol Biomarkers Prev 1998;7:497–504.

41. Zhu Y, Richardson JA, Parada LF, Graff JM. SMAD3 mutant mice develop metastatic colorectal cancer. Cell 1998;94:703–14.

42. Datto MB, Frederick JP, Pan L, et al. Targeted disruption of SMAD3 reveals an essential role in transforming growth factor beta-mediated signal transduction. Mol Cell Biol 1999;19:2495–504.

43. Duff EK, Clarke AR. SMAD4 (DPC4)—a potent tumour suppressor? Br J Cancer 1998;78:1615–9.

44. Kretzschmar M, Doody J, Timokhina I, Massague J. A mechanism of repression of TGFbeta/SMAD signaling by oncogenic Ras. Genes Dev 1999;13:804–16.

45. Hedrick L, Cho KR, Fearon ER, et al. The DCC gene product in cellular differentiation and colorectal tumorigenesis. Genes Dev 1994;8:1174–83.

46. Sturlan S, Kapitanovic S, Kovacevic D, et al. Loss of heterozygosity of APC and DCC tumor suppressor genes in human sporadic colon cancer. J Mol Med 1999;77:316–21.

47. Gotley DC, Reeder JA, Fawcett J, et al. The deleted in colon cancer (DCC) gene is consistently expressed in colorectal cancers and metastases. Oncogene 1996;13:787–95.

48. Aaltonen LA, Peltomaki P, Leach FS, et al. Clues to the pathogenesis of familial colorectal cancer. Science 1993;260:812–6.

49. Papadopoulos N, Nicolaides NC, Wei YF, et al. Mutation of a mutL homolog in hereditary colon cancer. Science 1994;263:1625–9.

50. Fishel R, Lescoe MK, Rao MR, et al. The human mutator gene homolog MSH2 and its association with hereditary nonpolyposis colon cancer. Cell 1993;75:1027–38.

51. Nicolaides NC, Papadopoulos N, Liu B, et al. Mutations of two PMS homologues in hereditary nonpolyposis colon cancer. Nature 1994;371:75–80.

52. Leach FS, Nicolaides NC, Papadopoulos N, et al. Mutations of a mutS homolog in hereditary nonpolyposis colorectal cancer. Cell 1993;75:1215–25.

53. Fishel R, Ewel A, Lee S, et al. Binding of mismatched microsatellite DNA sequences by the human MSH2 protein. Science 1994;266:1403–5.

54. Suspiro A, Fidalgo P, Cravo M, et al. The Muir-Torre syndrome: a rare variant of hereditary nonpolyposis colorectal cancer associated with hMSH2 mutation. Am J Gastroenterol 1998;93:1572–4.

55. Edelmann W, Yang K, Kuraguchi M, et al. Tumorigenesis in Mlh1 and Mlh1/Apc1638N mutant mice. Cancer Res 1999;59:1301–7.

56. Edelmann W, Cohen PE, Kneitz B, et al. Mammalian MutS homologue 5 is required for chromosome pairing in meiosis. Nat Genet 1999;21:123–7.

57. Rampino N, Yamamoto H, Ionov Y, et al. Somatic frameshift mutations in the BAX gene in colon cancers of the microsatellite mutator phenotype. Science 1997;275:967–9.

58. Guerrette S, Acharya S, Fishel R. The interaction of the human MutL homologues in hereditary nonpolyposis colon cancer. J Biol Chem 1999;274:6336–41.

59. Veigl ML, Kasturi L, Olechnowicz J, et al. Biallelic inactivation of hMLH1 by epigenetic gene silencing, a novel mechanism causing human MSI cancers. Proc Natl Acad Sci U S A 1998;95:8698–702.

60. Losi L, Ponz de Leon M, Jiricny J, et al. K-ras and p53 mutations in hereditary non-polyposis colorectal cancers. Int J Cancer 1997;74:94–6.

61. DuBois RN, Giardiello FM, Smalley WE. Nonsteroidal anti-inflammatory drugs, eicosanoids, and colorectal cancer prevention. Gastroenterol Clin North Am 1996;25:773–91.

62. Smalley W, Ray WA, Daugherty J, Griffin MR. Use of nonsteroidal anti-inflammatory drugs and incidence of colorectal cancer: a population-based study. Arch Intern Med 1999;159:161–6.

63. Tsujii M, Kawano S, Tsuji S, et al. Cyclooxygenase regulates angiogenesis induced by colon cancer cells. Cell 1998;93:705–16.

64. Goldman AP, Williams CS, Sheng H, et al. Meloxicam inhibits the growth of colorectal cancer cells. Carcinogenesis 1998;19:2195–9.

65. Shao J, Sheng H, Aramandla R, et al. Coordinate regulation of cyclooxygenase-2 and TGF-beta1 in replication error-positive colon cancer and azoxymethane-induced rat colonic tumors. Carcinogenesis 1999;20:185–91.

66. Karnes WE Jr, Shattuck-Brandt R, Burgart LJ, et al. Reduced COX-2 protein in colorectal cancer with defective mismatch repair. Cancer Res 1998;58:5473–7.

67. Saez E, Tontonoz P, Nelson MC, et al. Activators of the nuclear receptor PPARgamma enhance colon polyp formation. Nat Med 1998;4:1058–61.

68. Lefebvre AM, Chen I, Desreumaux P, et al. Activation of the peroxisome proliferator-activated receptor gamma promotes the development of colon tumors in C57BL/6J-APCMin/+ mice. Nat Med 1998;4:1053–7.

69. Sarraf P, Mueller E, Jones D, et al. Differentiation and reversal of malignant changes in colon cancer through PPARgamma. Nat Med 1998;4:1046–52.

70. Rao CV, Kawamori T, Hamid R, Reddy BS. Chemoprevention of colonic aberrant crypt foci by an inducible nitric oxide synthase-selective inhibitor. Carcinogenesis 1999;20:641–4.

71. Rudolph U, Finegold MJ, Rich SS, et al. Ulcerative colitis and adenocarcinoma of the colon in G alpha i2-deficient mice. Nat Genet 1995;10:143–50.

72. Murray GI, Duncan ME, O'Neil P, et al. Matrix metalloproteinase-1 is associated with poor prognosis in colorectal cancer. Nat Med 1996;2:461–2.

73. Di Cristofano A, Pesce B, Cordon-Cardo C, Pandolfi PP. Pten is essential for embryonic development and tumour suppression. Nat Genet 1998;19:348–55.

74. Wang SS, Esplin ED, Li JL, et al. Alterations of the PPP2R1B gene in human lung and colon cancer. Science 1998;282:284–7.

75. van Wezel T, Stassen AP, Moen CJ, et al. Gene interaction and single gene effects in colon tumour susceptibility in mice. Nat Genet 1996;14:468–70.

76. Codori AM, Petersen GM, Miglioretti DL, et al. Attitudes toward colon cancer gene testing: factors predicting test uptake. Cancer Epidemiol Biomarkers Prev 1999;8:345–51.

77. Glanz K, Grove J, Lerman C, et al. Correlates of intentions to obtain genetic counseling and colorectal cancer gene testing among at-risk relatives from three ethnic groups. Cancer Epidemiol Biomarkers Prev 1999;8:329–36.

78. Cui H, Horon IL, Ohlsson R, et al. Loss of imprinting in normal tissue of colorectal cancer patients with microsatellite instability. Nat Med 1998;4:1276–80.

79. Ratto C, Flamini G, Sofo L, et al. Detection of oncogene mutation from neoplastic colonic cells exfoliated in feces. Dis Colon Rectum 1996;39:1238–44.

80. Yamao T, Matsumura Y, Shimada Y, et al. Abnormal expression of CD44 variants in the exfoliated cells in the feces of patients with colorectal cancer. Gastroenterology 1998;114:1196–205.

81. Zwacka RM, Dunlop MG. Gene therapy for colon cancer. Hematol Oncol Clin North Am 1998;12:595–615.

82. Schutze K, Lahr G. Identification of expressed genes by laser-mediated manipulation of single cells. Nat Biotechnol 1998;16:737–42.

4

Colorectal Cancer Prevention and Early Detection

BERNARD LEVIN, MD

We can estimate how many of the 56,300 people who die annually of colorectal cancer whose survival could have been lengthened if their disease had been prevented or detected early: more than 50 percent. Risk of colorectal cancer may be reduced by regular physical activity and appropriate diet, and it can be effectively treated when it is detected early.[1] Only lung cancer, which is expected to take the lives of 156,900 American men and women in 2000, outpaces colorectal cancer in the potential impact prevention strategies could have.[2]

Increased screening and adenoma removal, which prevents progression to invasive cancer, have been credited with the 2.1 percent annual decline in incidence between 1992 and 1996.[2] Early detection translates into a 91.4 percent 5-year relative survival rate for about 37 percent of all cases diagnosed.[1] Another 37 percent are diagnosed when disease is regional, and the survival rate for these cases falls to 66.1 percent. For those remaining cases diagnosed when cancer has metastasized to a distant site, the survival rate is only 8.5 percent.

In the United States, men have higher rates of colorectal cancer incidence and mortality than do women,[3] but mortality rate graph lines tended to intertwine from 1930 to about 1960, when the mortality rate began to decline steadily and in women fell distinctly lower than in men.[1] Cumulative lifetime risk for colorectal cancer is 6 percent.[4] In the United States, a gap exists between overall survival rates by race: the rate for whites (63 percent) sur-

passes that of African Americans (52.5 percent), and researchers blame more than half of the difference on African Americans' more advanced stage of disease at diagnosis.[5]

Globally, incidence of cancer of the colon and rectum is highest in Australia/New Zealand, North America, Western Europe, Northern Europe, and Japan and lowest in Northern, Western, and Middle Africa along with South Central Asia.[3] Worldwide it occurs slightly more frequently in men than in women.

RISK FACTORS

To determine a patient's level of colorectal cancer risk and take an appropriate approach to surveillance, physicians should profile personal and familial health history to identify the patient's level of risk. In asymptomatic persons who have no risk factors other than increased age, routine screening begins at age 50. For those whose risk of having colorectal cancer is higher than average, screening should begin at age 40 or 10 years before the age at which the youngest case in the family was diagnosed, whichever is earlier.[6]

Adversely affecting the risk of colorectal cancer are factors relating to age, family and personal medical history, and diet. Of these, age is the most fundamental in determining risk. Risk increases with age, and almost three-quarters of all cases are diagnosed in those 65 years of age or older. Risk of colon cancer is also higher in those whose family medical history is characterized by familial adenomatous polyposis, including familial polyposis and Gardner's syndrome, or hereditary non-polyposis colorectal cancer (HNPCC), including family cancer syndrome and site-specific inherited colorectal cancer.

Also increasing the risk of colorectal cancer is inflammatory bowel disease (chronic ulcerative colitis or Crohn's disease), intestinal adenomatous polyps (especially if of the villous type or larger than 1 cm), a history of colon cancer, or a history of ovarian or uterine cancer.[7] A history of breast cancer has been found in a retrospective review of 227,165 cases to not be associated with increased risk and was in fact associated with colorectal cancer risk reduction.[8] Obesity has been shown to put men at increased risk.[9,10] Also raising risk is Turcot's syndrome or juvenile polyposis. In addition, dietary animal fats have been linked to an increased risk of colorectal cancer.

Reductions in risk have been associated with fruit and vegetable intake, regular physical activity, estrogen replacement therapy in postmenopausal women,[11,12] and taking acetylsalicylic acid or other nonsteroidal anti-inflammatory drugs including sulindac and proxicam.[13]

SCREENING

General agreement on testing with the fecal occult blood test (FOBT), sigmoidoscopy, a combination of FOBT and sigmoidoscopy, double-contrast barium enema with x-ray studies, or colonoscopy has been reached (Table 4–1) by government, professional, and patient-centered organizations, paving the way for unified educational efforts to improve screening rates.[2,14–16] Also encouraging wider compliance is the U.S. government's Health Care Financing Administration's expansion in January 1998 of Medicare coverage to include routine colorectal cancer screening.[17] The coverage permits annual fecal occult blood testing, with sigmoidoscopy every 4 years for those with average risk. For those at high risk, coverage includes colonoscopy every 2 years. Provider requests for substitution of double-contrast barium enema imaging evaluations for colonoscopy will be honored.

Fecal Occult Blood Test

The FOBT performed annually has demonstrated benefit in reducing mortality from colorectal cancer (for a review, see Towler and colleagues[18]). Testing annually is recommended because randomized trials have shown that testing every 2 years is less effective than testing annually because cost and inconvenience are little affected by frequency and because testing annually may mean detection of disease that, though undetected on previous tests, has not reached a less curable stage.[14] A review of FOBT trials found that reductions in mortality in the annually screened groups ranged from 37 to 14 percent in those studies reporting mortality statistics.[18] One of these trials found that testing annually reduced mortality in the screened group by 33 percent, whereas testing biennially reduced mortality by 5 percent, which was identified as a nonsignificant difference from not screening at all.[19]

The major shortcoming of screening by this method is its high false-positive rate, which means that many disease-free persons will undergo unnecessary colonoscopy with its attendant risks and stresses.[18,20] The likelihood ratio, a test's sensitivity divided by its false-positive rate, is a calculation meant to further refine risk definition and has been identified as substantially better than any other predictors of colorectal cancer risk, including age and family history.[20] It compares the risk of someone who has had the test and had positive results to that of another who has had the test and had negative results. In this ratio, the false-positive rate equals the difference between 100 percent and the specificity rate (or true negative results). For example, sensitivity of FOBT screening divided by its false-positive rate (0.60/1-0.92), using Winawer and colleagues' best estimates for sensitivity and specificity, results in a likelihood of having cancer of 7.5 times that of another whose test result was negative.[14] Calculations of likelihood ratios from studies of FOBT screening indicate a likelihood ratio of 12 for hydrated testing in the Minnesota trial[19] and a likelihood ratio of 50 in the Danish trial,[21] according to Young, Macrae, and St John.[20]

The failure of FOBT screening to produce more consistent and more dramatic mortality reductions needs to prompt development of better tests with

Table 4–1. COLORECTAL CANCER SCREENING RECOMMENDATIONS FOR ASYMPTOMATIC MEN AND WOMEN 50 YEARS OF AGE OR OLDER				
Test	**American Cancer Society**	**Consortium (Winawer 1997)**	**U.S. Preventive Services Task Force (1996)**	**National Comprehensive Cancer Network (2000)**
Fecal occult blood test (FOBT)	Annually plus flexible sigmoidoscopy every 5 years	Annually	Annually	Annually plus flexible sigmoidoscopy every 5 years
			OR	
Sigmoidoscopy	Flexible sigmoidoscopy every 5 years plus FOBT annually	Flexible sigmoidoscopy every 5 years	Flexible or rigid sigmoidoscopy recommended but insufficient evidence to recommend periodicity	Flexible sigmoidoscopy every 5 years plus FOBT annually
			OR	
Combination of FOBT and sigmoidoscopy	FOBT annually plus flexible sigmoidoscopy every 5 years	FOBT annually plus flexible sigmoidoscopy every 5 years	Both "effective" but "insufficient evidence to determine which of these methods is preferable or whether the combination . . . produces greater benefits than either test alone"	FOBT annually plus flexible sigmoidoscopy every 5 years
			OR	
Double-contrast barium enema with x-ray studies	Every 5–10 years	Every 5–10 years	"Insufficient evidence" to recommend for or against routine screening	Every 5 years
			OR	
Colonoscopy	Every 10 years	Every 10 years	"Insufficient evidence" to recommend for or against routine screening	Every 10 years

Data from the American Cancer Society,[2] Winawer et al.,[14] U.S. Preventive Services Task Force,[15] and the National Comprehensive Cancer Network.[16]

lower false-positive rates and improved adenoma and cancer detection capability. But even after such tests come to market, physicians will have to continue helping patients undergoing screening gain perspective on their risks as indicated by the test results and negotiate the emotional and sometimes physical consequences of testing that yields false-positive and false-negative findings.[20]

Flexible Sigmoidoscopy

Recommendations to use sigmoidoscopy to screen for colorectal cancer are based on case-control research and on work showing that colorectal cancer risk is reduced when adenomatous polyps are removed.[22,23] Rigid as well as flexible sigmoidoscopes have been used in research used to support screening with sigmoidoscopy.[14] Flexible sigmoidoscopes, 60 cm in length, have largely replaced screening with the rigid 25-cm scope in most countries because of their increased scope, their greater clarity, and their reputation for better patient tolerance. Of course, the percentage of polyps and cancers detectable by sigmoidoscopy is proportional to the length of the scope. Winawer and colleagues report that when fully inserted, the 60-cm scope can detect 40 to 60 percent of adenomatous polyps and colorectal cancers; the 35-cm scope, 30 to 40 percent; and the 25-cm scope, 20 to 30 percent.[14]

The chief virtues of flexible sigmoidoscopy are its sensitivity and specificity: sensitivity is 96.7 percent for cancer and large polyps and 73.3 percent for small polyps; specificity is 94 percent for cancer and large polyps and 92 percent for small polyps.[14] Also important is its ability to produce direct visualization of the colon and to allow biopsy of suspicious lesions. For these benefits, however, the patient must submit to the associated risk of bowel perforation (2/10,000). The complication rate rises slightly when biopsy or polypectomy is incorporated in the procedure. Patients may also feel inconvenienced or discomforted, but the introduction of flexible sigmoidoscopy was expected to increase compliance with screening practice by reducing discomfort associated with rigid sigmoidoscopy.

Screening intervals must be considered in relation to efficacy and safety and also in relation to such issues as cost, patient acceptability, and availability. For screening sigmoidoscopy, some researchers have found effectiveness to persist as long as 9 to 10 years, though others have reported a shorter protective effect. A panel of experts originally convened by the U.S. government's Agency of Health Care Policy and Research and subsequently sponsored by a consortium of professional, patient, and other nonprofit groups estimated that transformation from polyp to invasive cancer took 10 years.[14] Using a model, the U.S. Preventive Services Task Force (1996) found that the effectiveness of screening sigmoidoscopy was ensured with screening intervals of 10 years, but it based its model on a transformation period of 10 to 14 years.[15]

Despite the advantages offered by sigmoidoscopy, its effectiveness is limited to that part of the colon within reach of its scope. Two other methods facilitate detection in the proximal colon.

Double-Contrast Barium Enema

It was not carefully conducted trials of double-contrast barium enema (DCBE) imaging but general evidence indicating a reduction in colorectal cancer mortality when polyps and cancers were detected early that prompted experts to consider DCBE imaging for colorectal cancer screening. Double-contrast barium enema outperforms the FOBT and extends beyond the reach of sigmoidoscopy, matching the scope of colonoscopy by imaging the entire colon.

Winawer and colleagues[14] reported that DCBE's sensitivity and specificity were better than those of the FOBT and flexible sigmoidoscopy, but recently reported findings comparing barium enema with colonoscopy indicate that barium enema detects about half or fewer of the adenomas detected by colonscopy, the test that has a range it most closely matches. Press deadlines permit only a brief mention (see discussion).

Colonoscopy

Recommendations to use colonoscopy for colorectal screening are based on its supporting role in FOBT trials in which screening produced a reduction in colorectal cancer mortality and on its similarity to sigmoidoscopy, which has proved to be effective. Advantages include its ability to permit visualization of the entire colon and the efficiency afforded by its being both a diagnostic and therapeutic tool. Sensitivity is high in detecting cancers (96.7 percent) and large polyps (85 percent), but lower in detecting small polyps (78.5 percent). Specificity for all measures is 98 percent.[14]

Like the recommendation for performing the test, the recommended interval for the test has been set in part based on experience with sigmoidoscopy. It is also based on the success rate for this procedure and the 10-year estimate for polyp transformation in those with average risk.[14]

RECOMMENDED COLORECTAL CANCER SCREENING GUIDELINES

It is widely agreed that screening for colorectal cancer in asymptomatic adults should begin at age 50.[2,14–16] An age at which to stop screening has not been set, but certainly the onset of other significant disease or diseases is an example of when screening would appropriately end. Also of concern would be the patient's ability or willingness to tolerate the screening procedure and any procedure that logically would be recommended subsequently in follow-up of positive findings.[6] Patient and physician must examine the patient's personal and familial health history to identify the patient's level of risk and therefore the appropriate surveillance strategy (Table 4–2).

Average Risk

Those considered to be at average risk are those who are symptom free and have no personal or family medical history characteristics that would categorize their risk as moderate or high. Anyone with symptoms should undergo a diagnostic work-up. Screening recommendations for those with average risk are

Table 4–2. STRATIFICATION BY RISK OF COLORECTAL CANCER OF ASYMPTOMATIC PERSONS			
Factor	Average (70–80 percentof all cases)	Moderate (15–20 percent of all cases)	High (5–10 percent of all cases)
Age	≥ 50 years	Any	Any
Personal medical history		Adenomatous polyps Colorectal cancer Ovarian or uterine cancer	Inflammatory bowel disease • Chronic ulcerative colitis • Crohn's disease
Family medical history		A first-degree relative < 60 years of age or two or more first-degree relatives of any age with a history of: • adenomatous polyps • colorectal cancer	Family history of: • Familial adenomatous polyposis • Hereditary nonpolyposis colorectal cancer

outlined in Table 4–1. Methods should be selected based on consideration of community screening resources and quality and the patient's medical status. When one test fails to provide sufficient information, another test should serve as a supplement. Although digital rectal examinations are no longer a part of the annual recommendations for screening in asymptomatic adults, they are assumed to be a routine element of sigmoidoscopy, DCBE evaluations, and colonoscopy.

Moderate Risk

Risk for colorectal cancer is higher in those who are symptom free but have a history of adenomatous polyps or of cancer, including ovarian, uterine, or colorectal cancer. Screening in these individuals and those at high risk becomes more aggressive: it may be initiated earlier, be performed more frequently, or become more intensive by the use of more sensitive methods.

Table 4–3 outlines the initial and subsequent tests recommended for preventing or detecting colorectal cancers early in those with factors that put them at moderate or high risk.[24]

High Risk

Higher risk requires higher level testing and associated intervention, making those methods capable of adenoma removal—colonoscopy and flexible sigmoidoscopy—the preferred evaluations for patients with a personal history of inflammatory bowel disease or a family history of familial adenomatous polyposis or HNPCC. Patients with inflammatory

bowel disease can expect colorectal cancer that does develop to be equal to their bowel disease in duration and extent. Screening begins with colonoscopy and biopsy of random sites in the colon. Despite the absence of direct evidence of the effectiveness of this approach, the rationale informing it is that early detection of dysplasia would prompt management likely to lower the risk of invasive carcinoma.

Sigmoidoscopy is an option in screening those with familial adenomatous polyposis, not because the condition is limited but because screening only attempts to obtain an index of the extent of disease, inasmuch as polyps multiply uniformly throughout the colon. The overwhelming number of polyps that develop makes case management by polypectomy an impossibility. Equally stunning is the almost 100 percent likelihood in these cases that colorectal cancer will develop. In these cases, the combination of polyp volume and the ineffectiveness of current therapy to control it almost inevitably requires colectomy. Patient and physician decision making is reduced to determining when to schedule the procedure.

Unlike monitoring in familial adenomatous polyposis, screening in patients who have a family history or have the genetic trait of HNPCC does more than provide a guide to an inevitable outcome. Colonoscopy, the best of the screening evaluations, is necessary because polyps have been found to occur proximally more often than in an even, sporadic pattern throughout the colon. Testing begins earlier and is conducted more frequently because the transformation of HNPCC polyps is faster than that of other polyps. Genetic counseling and testing are necessities. Women with HNPCC have been found

Table 4–3. RECOMMENDED SCREENING AND SURVEILLANCE FOR THOSE AT MODERATE AND HIGH RISK FOR COLORECTAL CANCER

Risk Stratification	Initial Screening	Subsequent Screening or Surveillance Interval
MODERATE RISK		
Personal History		
Adenomatous polyps		
Single, small (< 1 cm) polyps	Colonoscopy at time of polyp diagnosis	Repeat TCE[a] within 3 years of diagnosis. If findings are negative, follow average risk recommendations.
Large (> 1 cm) polyps or multiple polyps of any size	Colonoscopy at time of polyp diagnosis	Repeat TCE within 3 years of initial polyp removal. If findings are negative, repeat TCE every 5 years.
Colorectal cancer Personal history of colorectal cancer and resection of curative intent	TCE within 1 year of resection and perioperative TCE	If normal, TCE in 3 years. If at 3 years normal, TCE every 5 years.
Ovarian or uterine cancer	TCE within 1 year of diagnosis	TCE every 5 years
Family History		
Adenomatous polyps or colorectal cancer First-degree relative < 60 years of age or two first-degree relatives with a history of these	TCE at 40 years of age or 10 years earlier than age at diagnosis of earliest case diagnosed in family	TCE every 5 years
HIGH RISK		
Personal History		
Inflammatory bowel disease	Colonoscopy with biopsy of dysplasia In pancolitis: 8 years after initial diagnosis In colitis on left side: 12–15 years after initial diagnosis	Repeat every 1–2 years
Family History		
Familial adenomatous polyposis	At puberty, endoscopic surveillance, genetic testing counseling, and specialist referral	Consider colectomy if polyposis confirmed or genetic testing positive. Perform endoscopy every 1–2 years.
Hereditary nonpolyposis colon cancer	At 21 years of age, colonoscopy and counseling regarding genetic testing	Colonoscopy every 2 years until age 40 and then annually for patients whose genetic test is positive or for patients who do not undergo genetic testing

Adapted from Byers et al.[24]
[a]TCE, total colon evaluation by colonoscopy or double-contrast barium enema studies.

to be at greater risk of endometrial cancer and should undergo accelerated screening for it.

INITIATIVES AND NEW PROSPECTS FOR BETTER SCREENING AND COMPLIANCE

In 1997, the Centers for Disease Control (CDC) found that as few as 9.2 percent of the residents of one state (95 percent confidence interval = 2.2) had had the FOBT during the preceding year, and the overall average for all states was below 20 percent.[17] The percentage of those surveyed who reported having undergone sigmoidoscopy or proctoscopy within the preceding 5 years was also low: 30.4 percent. These and other earlier studies by the CDC along with other indications of poor screening compliance have prompted it and others to call for increased efforts to encourage colorectal cancer screening.[17,25]

Making testing more comfortable for patients may improve compliance. Under study by radiologists is computed tomographic (CT) colonography, a noninvasive test meant to substitute for colorectal screening's most thorough, most expensive, yet least favorite test: colonoscopy. Sometimes called "virtual colonoscopy," CT colonography, performed on patients who have and have not undergone bowel preparation, is an experimental screening method that relies on sophisticated graphics software to assemble from a 1- to 2-minute CT scan an endoluminal image including surface and volume characteristics.[26,27] Interpretation requires 20 to 40 minutes.[26] A recent workshop report having a larger subject population than that in published reports found that CT colonography sensitivity for polyps ≥ 5 mm was 81.9 to 93.9 percent and concluded that it rivaled conventional colonoscopy.[26] The new method detected all colon carcinomas that had been identified by colonoscopy and pathologic findings.

Making tests more effective is another approach. Fecal occult blood testing has already improved since many of the studies of its screening effectiveness. In the future, stool samples collected for colorectal cancer screening may be searched for gene mutations or loss of DNA heterozygosity rather than occult blood.[6]

Continuing studies of tests will also call for re-evaluation of use. In a recently published comparison of colonoscopy and DCBE for surveillance after polypectomy, Winawer and colleagues[28] found barium enema to be dramatically less effective than previously thought. In comparison with colonoscopic findings, they found that barium enema detected 32 percent of adenomas ≤ 0.5 cm, 53 percent of adenomas 0.6 to 1.0 cm, and 48 percent of those > 1 cm. Their findings prompted them to recognize colonoscopy as a more effective surveillance tool than barium enema after polypectomy. Tests now under way of colonoscopy as a screening measure can also be expected to refine thinking.

Attracting more patients to screening, including those who are less likely to participate, especially minorities and low-income women, is important in reducing mortality, and research indicates that doctor recommendations could spark interest and action in these groups.[17,29] Also important is choosing an appropriate surveillance strategy that matches the patient's risk.[30] Large public campaigns, such as the one organized by the American Digestive Health Foundation and employing multiple organizations whose constituencies are stakeholders in the effort, could benefit thousands at risk.[25] In office practice, efforts can require no technology beyond a telephone: physician input, patient education, and patient reminders by telephone.[31]

REFERENCES

1. American Cancer Society. Special section: Colon & rectum cancer. In: Cancer facts & figures—1999. Atlanta: American Cancer Society, 1999. p. 18–23.
2. American Cancer Society. Cancer facts & figures—2000. Atlanta: American Cancer Society, 2000. p. 4, 10.
3. Parkin DM, Pisani P, Ferlay J. Global cancer statistics. CA Cancer J Clin 1999;49:33–64.
4. Markowitz AJ, Winawer SJ. Screening and surveillance for colorectal cancer. Semin Oncol 1999;26:485–98.
5. Mayberry RM, Coates RJ, Hill HA, et al. Determinants of black/white differences in colon cancer survival. J Natl Cancer Inst 1995;87:1686–93.
6. Bevers T, Levin B. Colorectal cancer: population screening and surveillance. In: McDonald JWD, Burroughs AK, Feagan BG, eds. Evidence based gastroenterology and hepatology. London: BMJ Books, 1999. p. 230–40.
7. Weinberg DS, Newschaffer CJ, Topham A. Risk for colorectal cancer after gynecologic cases. Ann Intern Med 1999;131:189–93.
8. Newschaffer CJ, Topham A, Herzberg T, et al. Colorectal cancer risk is lower in women with previous breast cancer [abstract]. Gastroenterology 2000;118 (Suppl 2):3852.
9. Harvard Center for Cancer Prevention. Harvard report on cancer prevention: causes of human cancer. Cancer Causes Control 1996;7 (Suppl 1):7–15.
10. World Cancer Research Fund. Food, nutrition and the prevention of cancer: a global perspective. Washington, DC: American Institute for Cancer Research, 1997. p. 216–51.
11. Grodstein F, Newcomb PA, Stampfer MJ. Postmenopausal hormone therapy and the risk of colorectal cancer: a review and meta-analysis. Am J Med 1999;106:574–82.
12. Calle EE, Miracle–McMahill HL, Thun MJ, Heath CW. Estrogen replacement therapy and risk of fatal colorectal cancer in a prospective cohort of postmenopausal women. J Natl Cancer Inst 1995;87: 517–23.
13. Thun MJ. NSAID use and decreased risk of gastrointestinal cancers. In: DuBois RN, Giardello, eds. Gastroenterology Clinics of North America: NSAID's, eiconaoids, and the gastroenteric tract. Philadelphia: W B Saunders, 1996. p. 333–48.
14. Winawer SJ, Fletcher RH, Miller L, et al. Colorectal cancer screening: clinical guidelines and rationale. Gastroenterology 1997:12:594–642.
15. U.S. Preventive Task Force. Guide to clinical preventive services. 2nd ed. Baltimore: Williams and Wilkins, 1996.
16. National Comprehensive Cancer Network. NCCN practice guidelines for colorectal screening. Version 1.2000. Rockledge, PA: NCNN, 2000.

17. Screening for colorectal cancer—United States, 1997. MMWR Morb Mortal Wkly Rep 1999;48(February 19):116–21.

18. Towler BP, Irwig L, Glasziou P, et al. Screening for colorectal cancer using the faecal occult blood test, Hemoccult (Cochrane Review). In: The Cochrane Library, Issue 1. Oxford: Update Software, 2000.

19. Mandel JS, Bond JH, Church TR, et al. Reducing mortality from colorectal cancer by screening for fecal occult blood. Minnesota Colon Cancer Control Study. N Engl J Med 1993;328:1365–71.

20. Young GP, Macrae FA, St John DJB. Clinical methods for early detection: basis, use, and evaluation. In: Young GP, Rozen P, Levin B, eds. Prevention and early detection of colorectal cancer. Philadelphia: W B Saunders, 1996. p. 241–70.

21. Kronberg O, Fenger C, Søndergaard O, et al. Initial mass screening for colorectal cancer with fecal occult blood test: a prospective randomised study at Funen in Denmark. Scand J Gastroenterol 1987; 22:677–86.

22. Selby JV, Friedman GD, Quesenberry CP Jr, et al. A case-control study of screening sigmoidoscopy and mortality from colorectal cancer. N Engl J Med 1992;326:653–7.

23. Newcomb PA, Norfleet RG, Storer BE. Screening sigmoidoscopy and colorectal cancer mortality. J Natl Cancer Inst 1992;84:1572–5.

24. Byers T, Levin B, Rothenberger D, ct al. American Cancer Society guidelines for screening and surveillance for early detection of colorectal polyps and cancer: update 1997. CA Cancer J Clin 1997; 47:154–60.

25. Levin B, Bond JH. Colorectal cancer screening: recommendations of the U.S. Preventive Services Task Force. Gastroenterology 1996;111:1381–4.

26. Yee J, Hung RK, Steinauer-Gebauer AM. Prospective comparison of CT colonography and conventional colonoscopy for colorectal polyp detection. Paper presented at the Abdominal Radiology Postgraduate Course 2000 of the Radiological Society of North America, March 13-17, 2000, Kauai, Hawaii.

27. Colon cancer screening: early detection is key. Mayo Clinic Health Oasis. Rochester, MN: Mayo Foundation for Medical Education and Research. Available from: URL: http://www.mayohealth.org/ mayo 9807/htm/colon.htm.

28. Winawer SJ, Stewart ET, Zauber AG, et al. A comparison of colonoscopy and double-contrast barium enema for surveillance after polypectomy. N Engl J Med 2000;342:1766–72.

29. Paskett ED, D'agostino R, Tatum C, et al. Colorectal cancer screening practices among low-income women. Paper presented at the American Cancer Society's 42nd Science Writers Seminar, 26–29 March 2000, Tampa, Florida.

30. Lieberman DA, Garmo PL, Fleischer DE, et al. Colonic neoplasia in patients with nonspecific GI symptoms. Gastrointest Endosc 2000;51:647–51.

31. Anderson J. Clinical practice guidelines: review of the recommendations for colorectal screening. Geriatrics 2000;55:67–73.

5

Pathology and Staging

CAROLYN C. COMPTON, MD, PhD

Pathologic evaluation is a critical component of the management of patients with colorectal cancer, from initial diagnosis through definitive treatment. Pathologic stage of the tumor following resection is the single most powerful prognostic indicator in colorectal cancer, and it typically determines the appropriateness of adjuvant treatment as well. Numerous additional pathologic factors are known to have prognostic significance that is independent of stage and may help to further substratify tumors. In this chapter, the pathologic features of colorectal cancers that predict outcome after surgical resection and have direct bearing on patient care are reviewed.

It should be noted that the pathologic evaluation of a colorectal cancer specimen may be more accurate and complete if the pathologist has knowledge of pertinent clinical and operative data. The principal responsibility for providing essential clinical information lies with the referring clinician(s). In addition, in some cases, orientation of the specimen or indication of anatomic areas of special concern may also be required of the referring clinician (surgeon). Requisition forms for pathology are designed to accommodate clinical information and may serve as the basic means of communication with the pathologist.

DIAGNOSTIC BIOPSY IN COLORECTAL CANCER

Masses or ulcers discovered by rectal examination, imaging, or endoscopic studies that are suspicious for colorectal carcinoma typically require biopsy confirmation as carcinomas before initiating treatment. A number of benign and malignant lesions may mimic colorectal carcinoma and require exclu-

sion on biopsy. Other malignancies that may resemble colon cancer include colorectal lymphomas, carcinoid tumors, gastrointestinal stromal tumors (mural sarcomas), metastatic tumors that exhibit tropism for the gastrointestinal tract (eg, malignant melanoma), and malignancies of adjacent organs that directly invade the colorectum (eg, cancers of the ovary, endometrium, bladder, or prostate). Benign lesions that may mimic colorectal cancer include adenomas, hamartomas, solitary rectal ulcers, stercoral ulcers, endometriomas, and Crohn's disease or diverticular disease with mural stricturing. Multiple biopsies taken from the edges and base of an ulcerating lesion or from the surface of a polypoid mass typically reveal the correct diagnosis. When an obstructing mass is present, however, it may be difficult to pass an endoscope to obtain diagnostic tissue and, in this situation, brush cytology may be useful to confirm the diagnosis. Even when direct access to the tumor is possible, biopsies may fail to reveal a definitive diagnosis if the lesion is extensively ulcerated or otherwise necrotic. In these cases, elevated serum carcinoembryonic antigen (CEA) levels and/or the presence of associated adenomatous epithelium from the edge of the mass increase the certainty that the tumor is a carcinoma.

The type and amount of information that can be derived from a diagnostic biopsy are limited. The presence of carcinoma can be unequivocally established with a successful biopsy, but the histologic type of tumor, the tumor grade, and the presence of invasion may be difficult or even impossible to determine. If the presence of tissue invasion can be identified with certainty, it is never possible to determine the depth of invasion from biopsy material.

PATHOLOGIC EVALUATION OF A MALIGNANT POLYPS

Diagnosis and treatment of colon cancers by endoscopic polypectomy has become commonplace. Most often, the cancer is unsuspected at endoscopy and revealed only on microscopic examination of the polypectomy specimen. Malignant polyps are defined as adenomas containing carcinoma that invades through the muscularis mucosae into the submucosa regardless of the overall proportion of the adenoma that is replaced by cancer (Figure 5–1). They encompass both polypoid carcinomas, in which the entire polyp head is replaced by carcinoma, and adenomas with focal malignancy. By definition, malignant polyps exclude adenomas containing intraepithelial carcinoma or intramucosal carcinoma because these polyps possess no biological potential for metastasis (see *Definition of pTis* below). Polyps containing invasive malignancy represent approximately 5 percent of all adenomas,[1,2] and the chance that any given adenoma will contain an invasive malignancy increases with polyp size. The incidence of invasive carcinoma in adenomas of any histologic type that are greater than 2 cm in size ranges from 35 to 53 percent[3] with villous adenomas having a higher incidence than tubular adenomas of equal size. Therefore, any polyp greater than 2 cm in diameter should be approached with the suspicion that it might harbor an invasive cancer. If technically possible, it is recommended that these polyps be removed in toto in one piece with as great a margin as possible at the base or stalk.

Malignant polyps constitute a form of early colorectal carcinoma that may be cured by endoscopic polypectomy alone.[4-6] Following polypectomy alone, however, the incidence of an unfavorable outcome (i.e., lymph node metastasis or local recurrence from residual malignancy) for malignant polyps varies from about 10 to 20 percent.[7,8] The histopathologic evaluation of malignant polyps removed endoscopically is critical to define polyps with an increased risk of residual or recurrent disease and directly affects the clinical management of the patient.[4] The following histopathologic parameters have been shown to significantly increase the risk of adverse outcome:[9-18]

- High tumor grade (poorly differentiated adenocarcinoma, signet-ring cell carcinoma, small-cell

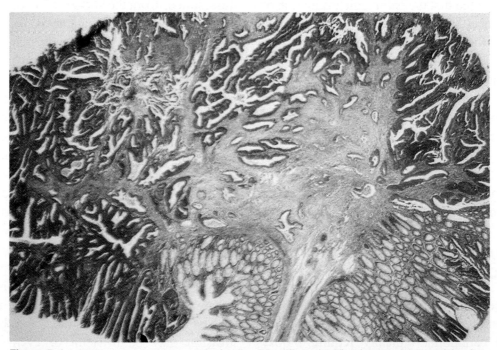

Figure 5–1. Malignant polyp. Low-grade (moderately differentiated) adenocarcinoma arising in a tubulovillous adenoma is seen infiltrating the submucosa of the polyp head where it is associated with a sclerotic stromal response. In the absence of lymphatic invasion, this low-grade cancer, located well above the resection margin of the polyp stalk, would be cured by polypectomy alone and require no further therapy.

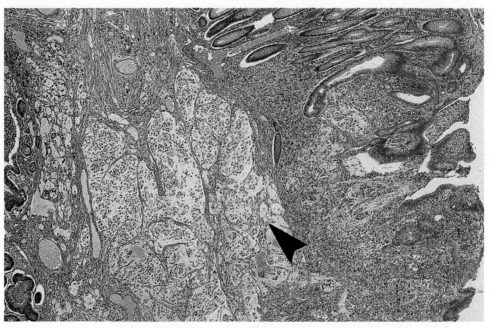

Figure 5–2. Signet-ring cell carcinoma (*arrow*) arising within a tubulovillous adenoma. By convention, this histologic type of carcinoma is classified as high grade (poorly differentiated) and would constitute an adverse prognostic factor for a malignant polyp treated by polypectomy alone.

carcinoma, or undifferentiated carcinoma) (Figures 5–2, 5–3)

- Tumor at or less than 1 mm from the resection margin (Figure 5–4)
- Small (thin-walled) vessel (lymphatic or venular) involvement by tumor (Figure 5–5).

In the presence of one or more of these features, the risk of an adverse outcome following polypectomy alone is estimated to be about 10 to 25 percent.[10,19–22] Therefore, if one or more of these high-risk features are found on pathologic examination of a resected polyp, further therapy may be indi-

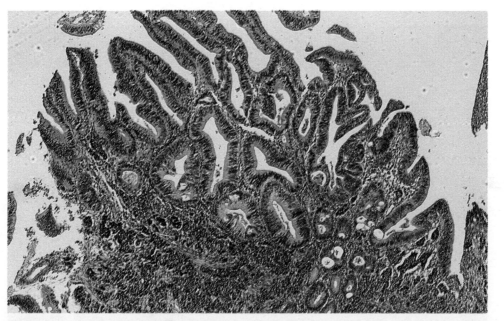

Figure 5–3. Small-cell carcinoma arising within a tubulovillous adenoma. By convention, this histologic type of carcinoma is classified as high grade (undifferentiated) and would constitute an adverse prognostic factor for a malignant polyp treated by polypectomy alone.

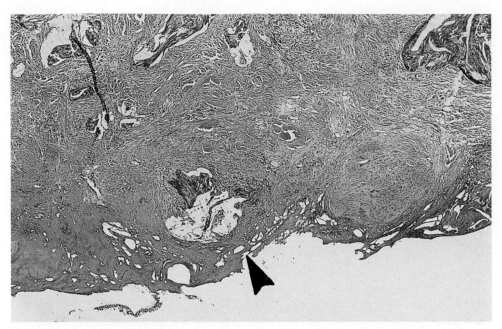

Figure 5–4. Involvement of the cauterized resection of a malignant polyp by invasive carcinoma. Malignant glands are present less than 1 to 2 mm from the resection margin of the polyp base/stalk and are involved by electrocautery artifact (*arrow*). This close approach of tumor to the polyp resection margin is an adverse prognostic factor for a malignant polyp treated by polypectomy alone.

cated. Optimal management is decided on an individual case basis,[23] but segmental resection of the involved colonic segment, local excision (eg, transanal disk excision for a low rectal lesion), or radiation therapy may be considered. In the absence of high-risk features, the chance of adverse outcome is extremely small, and polypectomy alone is considered curative.

In the pathologic assessment of malignant polyps for high-risk features, interobserver variability is greatest in relation to small vessel invasion.[8] This feature may be impossible to diagnose definitively in

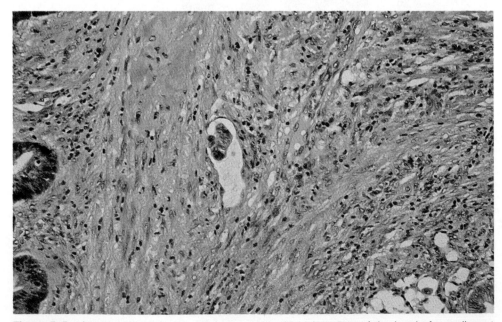

Figure 5–5. Lymphatic invasion by carcinoma within the submucosa of the head of a malignant polyp. A small cluster of carcinoma cells is seen within a thin-walled channel lined by endothelial cells.

some cases and ultimately may be judged as being indeterminate. An absolute diagnosis of vessel invasion is dependent upon finding carcinoma cells within an endothelial-lined space. Contraction artifact in the tissue, tumor-induced stromal sclerosis, or extracellular mucin pools produced by the cancer may all complicate the evaluation of vessel invasion. Examination of additional tissue levels of the specimen, review by a second observer, and/or immunohistochemical staining for endothelial markers (eg, factor VII or CD34) may or may not help to resolve the dilemma. In published cases in which the malignant polyps have lacked definitive evidence of high-risk features but the patients have gone on to die of their disease, lymphatic invasion had been judged (on blinded review) as indeterminate because of a lack of interobserver agreement.[8] Thus, even the suspicion of small vessel invasion may be regarded as ominous.

PATHOLOGIC EVALUATION AND STAGING OF SURGICALLY RESECTED COLORECTAL CANCER

The pathology report of a colorectal cancer resection specimen typically documents the anatomic site of the malignancy, the histologic type, the parameters that determine the local tumor stage, and the histopathologic confirmation of distant metastasis, if applicable. Other features that are reported include those that have additional prognostic or predictive value as well as those that may be important for clinicopathologic correlation or quality control (eg, actual tumor size versus size measurement by imaging techniques). The essential pathologic features of a colorectal cancer and the clinical significance of these findings are reviewed individually below.

Anatomic Site of the Tumor

Documentation of the exact anatomic location of a colorectal carcinoma is a fundamental part of the pathologic assessment. This is performed as part of the gross or macroscopic examination of the specimen. Orientation of the specimen may be difficult in some cases because of distortion of the anatomy by tumor and/or lack of anatomic landmarks that make it possible to differentiate the proximal from the distal

end of the resected segment. In these cases, orientation of the specimen by the surgeon may be required.

Typically, the anatomic site of the tumor is documented by measurement from known landmarks according to general guidelines defining colonic topography. Clinical data may also be helpful in establishing the tumor site in many cases. In general, four major anatomic divisions of the colon are recognized: the right (ascending) colon, the middle (transverse) colon, the left (descending) colon, and the sigmoid colon. The right colon is subdivided into the cecum (peritoneally located and measuring about 6×9 cm) and the ascending colon (retroperitoneally located and measuring 15 to 20 cm long). The descending colon, also located retroperitoneally, is 10 to 15 cm in length. The descending colon becomes the sigmoid colon at the origin of the mesosigmoid, and the sigmoid colon becomes the rectum at the termination of the mesosigmoid. The upper third of the rectosigmoid segment is covered by peritoneum on the front and both sides. The middle third is covered by peritoneum only on the anterior surface. The lower third (also known as the rectum or rectal ampulla) has no peritoneal covering.[24] The rectum is defined clinically as the distal large intestine commencing opposite the sacral promontory and ending at the upper border of the anal canal. When measuring below with a rigid sigmoidoscope, it extends 16 cm from the anal verge. A tumor is classified as rectal if its inferior margin lies less than 16 cm from the anal verge or if any part of the tumor is located at least partly within the supply of the superior rectal artery.[25]

Additional guidelines for assigning a tumor site have been established by the American Joint Committee on Cancer (AJCC).[24] Tumors located at the border between two subsites of the colon (eg, cecum and ascending colon) are registered as tumors of the subsite that is more involved. If two subsites are involved to the same extent, the tumor is classified as an overlapping lesion. Tumors may also be classified as overlapping when anatomic distinction between two subsites is precluded because of tumor distortion of the anatomy. For example, a tumor may be classified as rectosigmoid when differentiation between rectum and sigmoid according to the above guidelines is not possible.[26]

Tumor Size

The tumor dimensions recorded by the pathologist on gross examination of the specimen are considered the definitive determination of tumor size. Although it is recorded as an element of tumor documentation and may be important for quality control purposes (eg, size determinations made via imaging modalities), tumor size is not related to outcome. Eight separate studies have shown that tumor size is of no prognostic significance in colorectal cancer.[27–34]

Tumor Configuration

Tumor configuration is usually recorded as exophytic (fungating), endophytic (ulcerative), diffusely infiltrative (linitis plastica), or annular (Figures 5–6 to 5–9). Exophytic growth may be further defined as pedunculated or sessile. Overlap among these types is common. The clinical significance of tumor configuration is moot. Most studies have failed to demonstrate an independent influence of gross tumor configuration on prognosis.[32,35,36] In three studies, however, exophytic growth proved to be an adverse prognostic factor on multivariate analysis.[37–39] The uncommon linitis plastica configuration (see Figure 5–8) appears to be consistently associated with an unfavorable prognosis,[40] but the prognostic import may be related primarily to the histologic type (signet-ring cell carcinoma) and high grade of carcinomas (see *Tumor Grade* below) that typically exhibit this gross morphology.

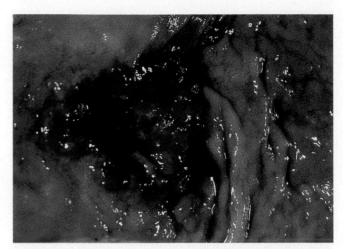

Figure 5–7. Endophytic colonic carcinoma. In this gross photograph, the colon has been opened along the long axis to reveal an ulcerating mass with elevated, irregular borders and a hemorrhagic, cavitated center.

Histologic Type

For consistency and uniformity in reporting, the internationally accepted histologic classification of colorectal carcinomas proposed by the World Health Organization (WHO) (Table 5–1 and Figures 5–12 to 5–17) is recommended by the College of American Pathologists and is usually used in pathology reports.[41,42] It should be noted, however, that medullary carcinoma has been added to the revised WHO classification to be published in 2000. Medullary carcinoma is a distinctive type of non-gland-forming carcinoma that previously would have been classified as an undifferentiated carcinoma. It is composed of uniform polygonal tumor cells that exhibit solid growth in nested, organoid, or trabecu-

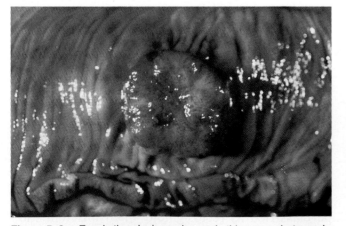

Figure 5–6. Exophytic colonic carcinoma. In this gross photograph, the colon has been opened along the long axis to reveal a fungating mass with a lobulated contour protruding from the mucosal surface.

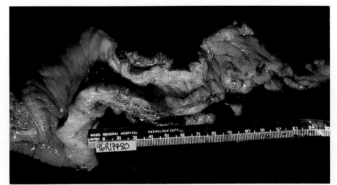

Figure 5–8. Diffusely infiltrative (linitis plastica) colonic carcinoma. The cut edge of the colonic wall shows the diffuse, marked thickening characteristic of linitis plastica, a macroscopic configuration that is usually caused by an underlying signet-ring cell carcinoma.

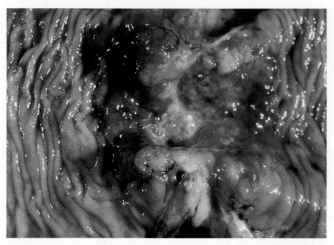

Figure 5–9. Annular colonic carcinoma. The configuration of this carcinoma is characterized primarily by circumferential growth that constricts the colonic lumen.

lar patterns and are characteristically infiltrated by lymphocytes (tumor infiltrating lymphocytes) (Figures 5–10, 5–11). The importance of this unique type is its strong association with microsatellite instability and DNA repair gene dysfunction.

By convention, some histologic types are always assigned a specific histologic grade. For example, signet-ring cell carcinoma, small-cell carcinoma, and undifferentiated carcinoma (histologic type) are all defined as high grade.

Histologic type is always designated in the pathology report, but aside from a few notable exceptions, the histologic type has no prognostic significance.[32,33,35,38,39,43–50] The exceptions include rare types such as signet-ring cell carcinoma and small-cell carcinoma, which are prognostically unfavorable, and medullary carcinoma, which is prognostically favorable.[51] As mentioned above, the latter is a histologic type that was not formerly recognized in the WHO classification (and would have been classified as undifferentiated carcinoma by that system) but is now known to be associated with microsatellite instability and/or the hereditary nonpolyposis colon cancer (HNPCC) syndrome.

To date, no large studies on prognostic factors in colorectal cancer have considered the relationship between the genetic status of the tumor (ie, with or without microsatellite instability), histologic type, and outcome. This shortfall is particularly relevant to mucinous carcinoma, a histologic type representing a high proportion of microsatellite unstable colorectal

cancers but, overall, occurring most frequently without microsatellite instability. Thus, it is not surprising that among all of the histologic types of colonic cancer, the prognostic significance of mucinous carcinoma has been the most controversial. A few studies, largely limited to univariate analyses, have indicated that mucinous adenocarcinoma may be an adverse prognostic factor.[50,52–54] More specifically, mucinous carcinoma has been linked with adverse outcome only if occurring in specific anatomic regions of the bowel (eg, the rectosigmoid)[52,54] or in a specific subset of patients (ie, those less than 45 years of age).[55] In yet other studies, an association with decreased survival has been demonstrated only when mucinous carcinoma and signet-ring cell carcinoma have been grouped together and compared to typical adenocarcinoma.[56–58] However, data of this type may be merely a reflection of the aggressive biologic behavior of signet-ring cell tumors. Only one multivariate analysis has shown mucinous carcinoma to be a stage-independent predictor of adverse outcome,[31] but the study was limited to tumors presenting with large bowel obstruction, which is itself an adverse prognostic factor.

The signet-ring cell type of adenocarcinoma and small-cell (oat-cell) carcinoma are the only histologic types of colonic carcinoma that consistently have been found to have a stage-independent adverse effect on prognosis.[59–61] Small-cell carcinoma is a malignant neuroendocrine carcinoma that is similar histologically and biologically to small-cell (oat-cell) carcinoma of the lung. Less clear is the general prognostic significance of focal neuroendocrine differentiation that may occur as a vari-

Table 5–1. WORLD HEALTH ORGANIZATION CLASSIFICATION OF COLORECTAL CARCINOMA*
Adenocarcinoma in situ/severe dysplasia
Adenocarcinoma (Figure 5–12)
Mucinous (colloid) adenocarcinoma (> 50% mucinous) (Figure 5–13)
Signet-ring cell carcinoma (> 50% signet-ring cells) (Figure 5–14)
Squamous cell (epidermoid) carcinoma
Adenosquamous carcinoma
Small-cell (oat-cell) carcinoma (Figure 5–15)
[Medullary carcinoma] (see Figures 5–10, 5–11)
Undifferentiated carcinoma (Figure 5–16)
Other (eg, papillary carcinoma: Figure 5–17)

*The term "*carcinoma*, NOS" (not otherwise specified) is not part of the WHO classification.

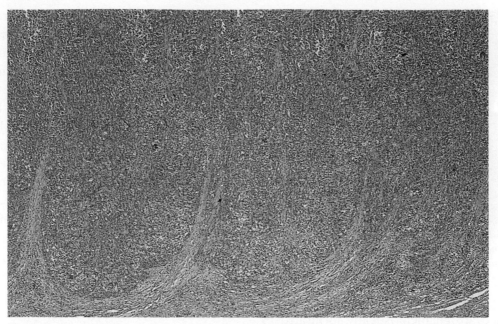

Figure 5–10.   Medullary carcinoma of the colon. This histologic type of colonic carcinoma is characterized at low magnification by solid growth, pushing tumor borders.

able feature in other histologic types of colorectal cancer. Two studies, the most recent of which included a multivariate analysis of 350 cases,[62] have indicated that extensive neuroendocrine differentiation may adversely affect outcome.[62,63]

In summary, based on current evidence, it must be concluded that the only histologic types of colorectal cancer that are prognostically significant are signet-ring cell and small-cell carcinomas (prognostically unfavorable) and medullary carcinoma (prognostically favorable). Mucinous carcinoma, when it is associated with microsatellite instability, is also prognostically favorable, but this association cannot be determined from histopathologic examination alone.

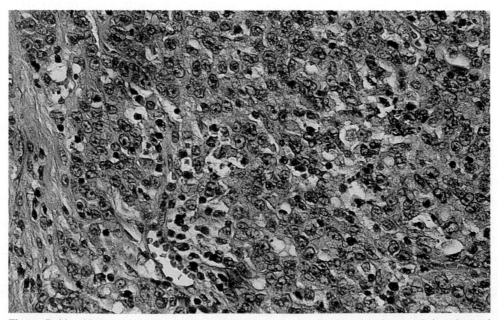

Figure 5–11.   Medullary carcinoma of the colon. At high magnification, the characteristic polygonal cells, nested to an organoid growth pattern, and large numbers of tumor infiltrating lymphocytes of this tumor type are seen.

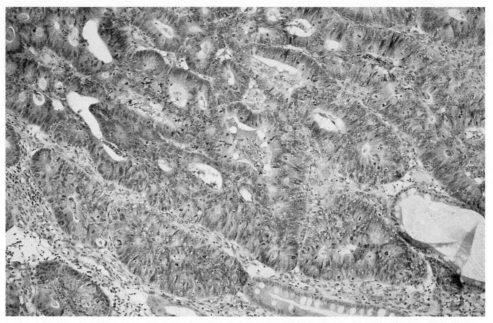

Figure 5–12. Adenocarcinoma of the colon. This histologic type of carcinoma is the most common variety of colon cancer and is characterized by well-formed glands, varying in size and mucin content

Tumor Grade

In general practice, the histologic grading of colorectal cancer, to a large degree, is evaluated subjectively. Although a number of grading systems have been suggested in the literature, a single widely accepted and uniformly employed standard for grading is lacking. Among the suggested grading schemes, the number of grades as well as the criteria for distinguishing among different grades vary markedly. In some systems, grades are defined on the basis of a single microscopic feature, such as the degree of gland formation, and in other systems a large number of features are included in the evalua-

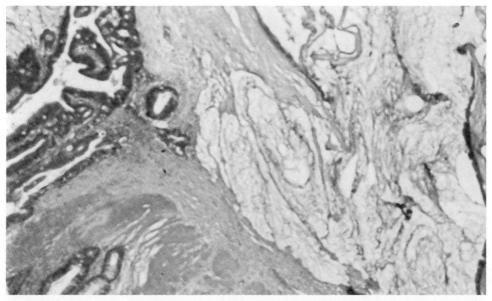

Figure 5–13. Mucinous (colloid) carcinoma of the colon. This histologic type is characterized by the production of large amounts of extracellular mucin. Although any colonic adenocarcinoma may contain foci of mucinous tumor, classification as a mucinous carcinoma requires that more than half of the mass of the neoplasm must be comprised of tumor with mucinous differentiation.

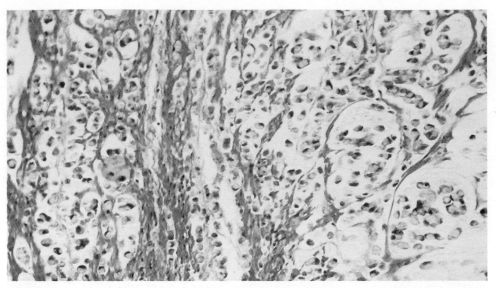

Figure 5–14. Signet-ring cell carcinoma of the colon. This histologic type is characterized by dyshesive cells that contain single, large mucin vacuoles in their cytoplasm. Although any colonic adenocarcinoma may contain foci of signet-ring cell formation, classification as a signet-ring cell carcinoma requires that more than half of the mass of the neoplasm be comprised of signet-ring-type cells.

tion. Irrespective of the complexity of the criteria, however, most systems stratify tumors into three or four grades as follows:

Grade 1—Well differentiated
Grade 2—Moderately differentiated
Grade 3—Poorly differentiated
(Grade 4—Undifferentiated)

Variation in the appearance of individual histologic features may vary widely enough to make implementation of even the simplest grading systems problematic, however, and, ultimately, subjective. Thus, a significant degree of interobserver variability in the grading of colorectal cancer exists.[64] Nevertheless, despite this variability, histologic grade has repeatedly been shown by multivariate

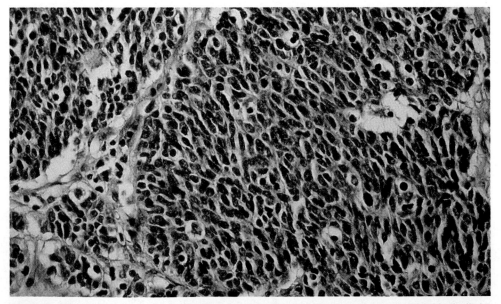

Figure 5–15. Small-cell carcinoma of the colon. This type of tumor is characterized histologically by cells with scanty cytoplasm, a high mitotic rate, and an ovoid to angulated shape. They closely resemble small carcinoma of the lung and, like their pulmonary counterparts, have ultrastructural and immunohistochemical features of neuroendocrine differentiation.

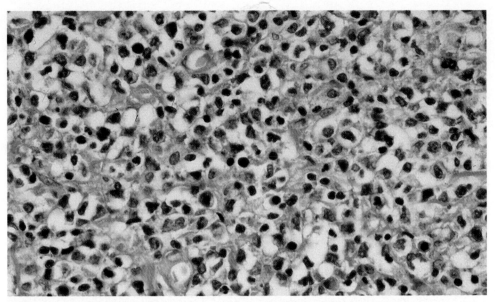

Figure 5–16. Undifferentiated carcinoma of the colon. As its name implies, this histologic type of carcinoma shows little evidence of cellular differentiation. This example shows highly pleomorphic dyshesive cells with no evidence of gland formation or mucin production.

analysis to be a stage-independent prognostic factor.[27,28,30–32,36,37,45,48,65–71] Specifically, it has been demonstrated that high tumor grade is an adverse prognostic factor. It is noteworthy that in the vast majority of studies documenting the prognostic power of tumor grade, the subclassifications have been collapsed to produce a two-tiered stratification for data analysis as follows:

Low Grade: Well differentiated and moderately differentiated (Figure 5–18)
High Grade: Poorly differentiated and undifferentiated (Figure 5–19).

In general practice, a two-tiered grading system based solely on the proportion of gland formation by the tumor (greater or less than 50 percent gland

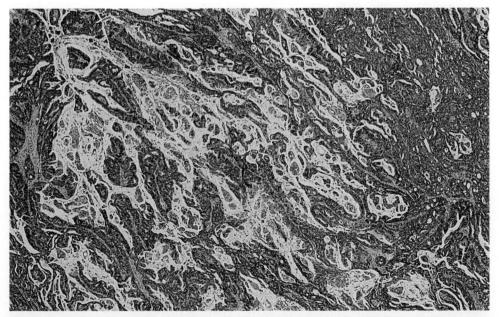

Figure 5–17. Papillary carcinoma of the colon. Carcinomas that form papillations with fibrovascular cores and epithelial tufts (micropapillations) may sometimes occur in the colon and may be classified as papillary carcinomas (histologic type).

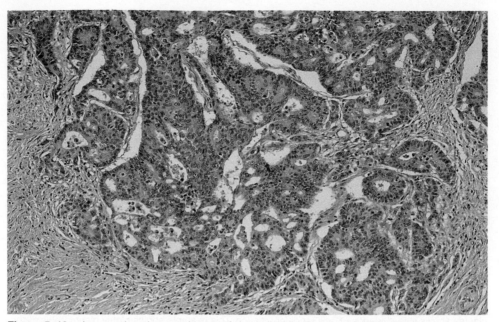

Figure 5–18. Low-grade adenocarcinoma of the colon. Low-grade adenocarcinomas encompass both well-differentiated and moderately differentiated tumors that, respectively, are composed entirely or predominantly of gland-forming cells.

formation) would also be expected to greatly reduce interobserver variability since the widest variations in grading concern the stratification of low-grade tumors into well or moderately differentiated categories.[64] Pathologic identification of poorly differentiated or undifferentiated tumors is more consistent, and interobserver variability in diagnosing high-grade carcinoma is relatively small.[64] Therefore, in light of its proven prognostic value, relative simplicity, and reproducibility, the use of a two-tiered grading system for colorectal carcinoma (ie, low grade and high grade) would be

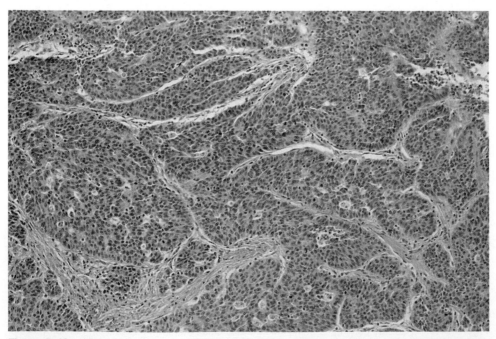

Figure 5–19. High-grade adenocarcinoma of the colon. High-grade carcinomas encompass both poorly differentiated carcinomas and undifferentiated carcinomas that form few or no tumor glands.

advisable. Such a system has been recommended by the colorectal working group of a 1999 Consensus Conference sponsored by the College of American Pathologists.[72]

Pathologic Stage

The best estimation of prognosis in colorectal cancer is related to the anatomic extent of disease determined on pathologic examination of the resection specimen.[40] Although a large number of staging systems have been developed for colorectal cancer over the years, use of the TNM (Tumor, Nodes, Metastasis) Staging System of the AJCC and the International Union Against Cancer (UICC) is recommended by the College of American Pathologists.[24,41] The TNM system is widely used by national, regional, and local tumor registries in the United States, and it is internationally accepted.

In the TNM system, the designation "T" refers to the local extent of the primary tumor at the time of diagnosis, "N" refers to the status of the regional lymph nodes, and "M" refers to distant metastatic disease. The symbol "p" used as a prescript refers to the pathologic determination of the TNM (eg, pT1), as opposed to the clinical determination (designated by the prescript "c"). Pathologic classification is based on gross and microscopic examination of the resection specimen of a previously untreated primary tumor. Assignment of pT requires a resection of the primary tumor or biopsy adequate to evaluate the highest pT category, pN entails removal of nodes adequate to validate lymph node metastasis, and pM implies microscopic examination of distant lesions. Clinical classification (cTMN) is usually determined by imaging techniques carried out before treatment during initial evaluation of the patient or when pathologic classification is not possible.[24] It is the *grouping* of T, N, and M parameters that determines the stage of the tumor and relates to prognosis. Thus, it is inappropriate to use the term "stage" in reference to an individual TNM category (eg, "T stage"). A TNM stage grouping can be constructed using a combination of clinically derived and pathologically derived data (eg, pT1, cN0, cM0). However, when pathologic data become available, they typically replace the corresponding clinically determined parameter. This convention is based on the assumption that pathologically derived data are more accurate.

The definitions of the individual TNM categories and the TNM stage groupings for colorectal carcinoma are shown in Tables 5–2 and 5–3 and Figures 5–20 to 5–23. The corresponding 5-year survival rates for the TNM stages are shown in Table 5–4.[73,74] It is considered the responsibility of the pathologist to assign a pTNM stage grouping when reporting on a colorectal cancer resection specimen. Thus, the pathologically determined T and N categories of the tumor should be explicitly assigned and included in the pathology report. However, the pathologist often lacks knowledge of the status of distant metastatic disease, and assignment of pMX is appropriate in this circumstance. It also may be appropriate to use other staging systems (eg, Dukes' or Modified Astler-Coller classifications) in pathology reporting,

Table 5–2. DEFINITIONS OF TNM CATEGORIES FOR COLORECTAL CARCINOMA

Primary Tumor (T)

TX	Primary tumor cannot be assessed
T0	No evidence of primary tumor
Tis	Carcinoma in situ (intraepithelial or intramucosal carcinoma) (Figure 5–20)
T1	Tumor invades the submucosa (Figure 5–21)
T2	Tumor invades the muscularis propria
T3	Tumor invades through the muscularis propria into the subserosa (Figure 5–22) or into the nonperitonealized pericolic or perirectal tissues
	pT3a – minimal invasion: < 1 mm beyond the border of the muscularis propria
	pT3b – slight invasion: 1 to 5 mm beyond the border of the muscularis propria
	pT3c – moderate invasion: > 5 to 15 mm beyond the border of the muscularis propria
	pT3d – extensive invasion: > 15 mm beyond the border of the muscularis propria (see Figure 5–22)
T4	Tumor directly invades other organs or structures (T4a) or perforates the visceral peritoneum (T4b) (Figure 5–23)

Regional Lymph Nodes (N)

NX	Regional lymph nodes cannot be assessed
N0	No regional lymph node metastasis
N1	Metastasis in 1 to 3 lymph nodes
N2	Metastasis in 4 or more lymph nodes

Distant Metastasis (M)

MX	Presence of distant metastasis cannot be assessed
M0	No distant metastasis
M1	Distant metastasis

Table 5–3. DEFINITION OF TNM STAGE GROUPINGS AND MODIFIED ASTLER-COLLER STAGES

TNM Stage Groupings				Modified Astler-Coller Stages
Stage 0	Tis	N0	M0	Stage A
Stage I	T1	N0	M0	N/A
	T2	N0	M0	Stage B1
Stage II	T3	N0	M0	Stage B2
	T4	N0	M0	Stage B3
Stage III	Any T	N1	M0	Stage C1 (T2); C2 (T3); C3 (T4)
	Any T	N2	M0	Stage C1 (T2); C2 (T3); C3 (T4)
Stage IV	Any T	Any N	M1	Stage D

depending upon institutional tradition, but it is suggested that these are to be used in addition to (not in place of) the TNM stage grouping.

Specific issues related to the assignment of pathologic TNM are discussed in detail below.

Definition of pTis

For colorectal carcinomas, the staging category pTis (carcinoma in situ) includes both malignant cells that are confined within the glandular basement membrane (intraepithelial carcinoma) and those that are invasive into the mucosal lamina propria (intramucosal carcinoma) (Figure 5–20). Carcinoma that extends into but not through the muscularis mucosae also is included in the pTis category. Penetration of the muscularis mucosae and invasion of the submucosa are classified as pT1. High-grade (severe) dysplasia and intraepithelial carcinoma sometimes may be used synonymously, especially in cases of inflammatory bowel disease.[75]

It is noteworthy that for all organ systems other than the large intestine, carcinoma in situ refers exclusively to malignancy that has not yet penetrated

the basement membrane of the epithelium from which it arose, and invasive carcinoma encompasses all tumors that penetrate the underlying stroma. Stromal invasion of any degree is a feature of extreme importance in all non-colorectal sites because of the possible access of tumor cells to stromal lymphatics or blood vessels and the consequent risk of metastasis. In colorectal cancer, however, the designation pTis (ie, carcinoma in situ) is used to refer both to intraepithelial malignancies and to cancers that have invaded the mucosal stroma (intramucosal carcinomas) because the colonic mucosa is biologically unique. In contrast to the mucosa elsewhere in the gastrointestinal tract (or, indeed, in the entire body), tumor invasion of the lamina propria has no associated risk of regional nodal metastasis. Therefore, for the colon and rectum, inclusion of intramucosal carcinoma in the pTis category is justified. Neverthe-

Table 5–4. FIVE-YEAR SURVIVAL RATES FOR THE FIVE TNM STAGES

Stage	Survival Rate
Stage 0, I (Tis, T1; N0; M0)	> 90%
Stage I (T2; N0; M0)	80–85%
Stage II (T3, T4; N0; M0)	70–75%
Stage III (T2; N1-3; M0)	70–75%
Stage III (T3; N1-3; M0)	50–65%
Stage III (T4; N1-3; M0)	25–45%
Stage IV (M1)	< 3%

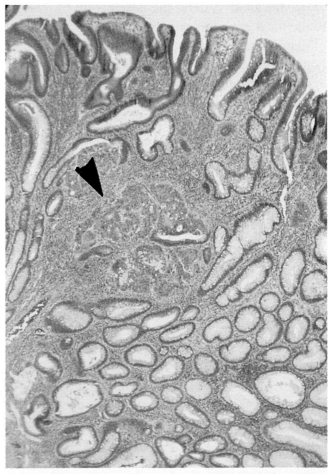

Figure 5–20. Intramucosal carcinoma (pTis). A focus of carcinoma that invades the lamina propria (*arrow*) of the adenoma in which it is arising is classified as carcinoma in situ (pTis) in the TNM staging system.

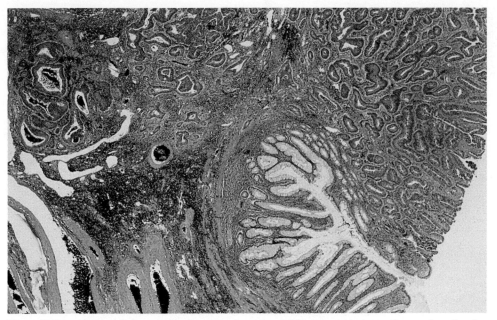

Figure 5–21. Adenocarcinoma invading the submucosa (pT1). Adenocarcinoma is seen invading the submucosa of the head of an adenomatous polyp in which it is arising.

less, the term carcinoma in situ in reference to colorectal cancer can be confusing, depending upon whether it is used to refer to the T category of the TNM staging system or to intraepithelial tumor only, as it does in all other epithelial systems. Therefore, the terms intraepithelial carcinoma and intramucosal carcinoma are preferred descriptive terms for colorectal tumors in the pTis category.[72,76]

Optional Expansion of pT3

The extent of perimuscular invasion has been reported to influence prognosis, whether or not regional lymph node metastasis is present. Thus, optional expansion pT3 has been proposed and is shown in Table 5–2.[26] However, since extramural extension of > 5 mm is the critical subdivision that

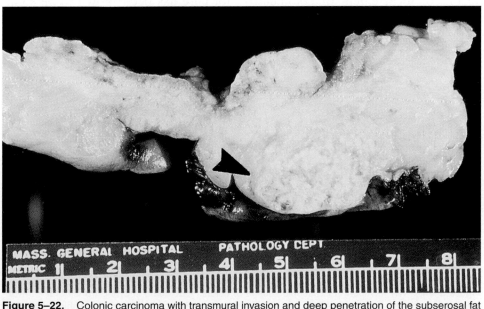

Figure 5–22. Colonic carcinoma with transmural invasion and deep penetration of the subserosal fat (pT3d). This macroscopic view of a transverse section through the tumor at the point of deepest penetration shows extramural extension of more than 15 cm (*arrow*).

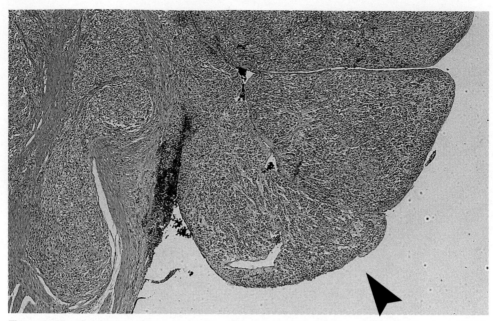

Figure 5–23. Colonic carcinoma with transmural invasion and penetration of the serosal surface (pT4b). A microscopic nodule of tumor is seen penetrating the peritonealized surface of the colon (*arrow*).

has been demonstrated to have an adverse effect on prognosis in most studies, a simpler subdivision of pT3a/b and pT3c/d may be justified.[26] Extramural extension of the tumor within lymphatics or veins does not count as local spread of tumor as defined by pT3 (Figures 5–24, 5–25).[26]

Subclassification of pT4

The highest category of local extent of colorectal tumor, pT4 includes both extension into adjacent organs or structures and penetration of the parietal peritoneum with or without involvement of an adjacent structure (see Figure 5–23). Serosal penetration is a particularly ominous feature. A number of large studies have evaluated serosal penetration as a separate pathologic variable and have demonstrated by multivariate analysis that this feature has independent adverse prognostic significance.[27,32,77,78] The median survival time following surgical resection for cure has been shown to be significantly shorter with pT4 tumors that penetrate the visceral peri-

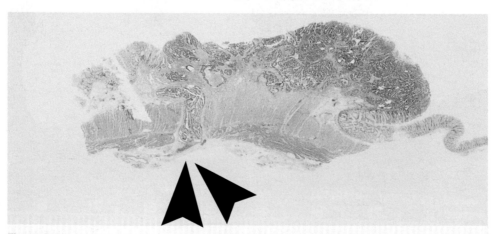

Figure 5–24. Whole mount microscopic section of colonic carcinoma showing transmural intravascular extension. The arrows point to a focus of transmural extension of a carcinoma within a muscular vein. By direct extension, the tumor only shallowly penetrates the inner layer of the muscularis propria and would be classified as pT2 in the TNM classification.

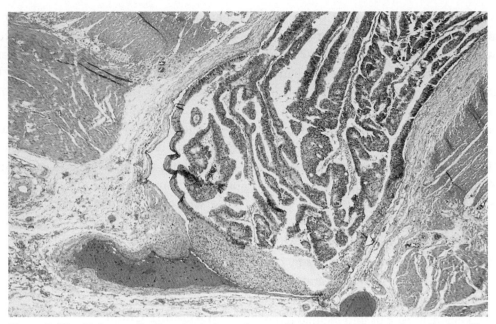

Figure 5–25. High magnification of colonic carcinoma with transmural intravascular extension. The tumor is entirely contained within a muscular vein that is recognized by its endothelial cell lining, smooth muscle wall, and erythrocyte content. Tumor extension within a vascular structure is not classified within the T category of the TNM classification but is noted separately as a stage-independent adverse prognostic factor.

toneum compared with pT4 tumors without serosal involvement, with or without distant metastasis (Table 5–5).[26] A free perforation of a colorectal carcinoma into the peritoneal cavity is also classified as T4b.[26] A more recent study on the importance of local peritoneal involvement in curative resections by Shepherd and colleagues[77] has suggested that the prognostic power of this feature may supersede that of either local extent of tumor (T category) or regional lymph node status (N category).

Although it is undisputedly important, serosal penetration is often difficult to assess histopathologically and may be underdiagnosed for several reasons. Documentation of peritoneal involvement by tumor demands meticulous pathologic analysis and may require extensive sampling and/or serial sectioning. Thus, it can be missed on routine histopathologic examination, a fact that has been emphasized in the literature. It has been shown that cytologic examination of serosal scrapings reveals malignant cells in as many as 26 percent of tumor specimens categorized as pT3 by histologic examination alone.[77,79] In addition, the histopathologic findings associated with peritoneal penetration are heterogeneous, and standard guidelines for their diagnostic interpretation

are lacking. Therefore, interobserver variability in the diagnosis of peritoneal penetration may be substantial, and since most pathologists tend to err on the side of conservative interpretation, underdiagnosis is common.

In the study by Shepherd and colleagues,[77] the spectrum of microscopic features that may be seen with local peritoneal involvement by tumor was recognized and specifically addressed. Three types of local peritoneal involvement were defined and analyzed separately: (1) a mesothelial inflammatory and/or hyperplastic reaction with tumor close to, but not at, the serosal surface; (2) tumor present at the serosal surface with inflammatory reaction, mesothelial hyperplasia, and/or erosion/ulceration; and (3) free tumor cells on the serosal surface (in the

Table 5–5. MEDIAN SURVIVAL TIME FOLLOWING SURGICAL RESECTION FOR CURE		
	5-Year Survival Rate	Median Survival Time (mo)
pT4a,M0	49%	58.2
pT4b,M0	43%	46.2
pT4a,M1	12%	22.7
pT4b,M1	0%	15.5

peritoneum) with underlying ulceration of the visceral peritoneum. All three types of local peritoneal involvement were associated with decreased survival, whereas tumor well clear of the serosal had no independent adverse effect on prognosis.[77] Thus, it has been recommended that, in the definition of T4b, the phrase "involves the visceral peritoneum" be used instead of "penetrates the visceral peritoneum" and that the definition of "involvement" encompass the three types outlined above.[76]

It should be noted that direct invasion of other organs or structures includes invasion of other segments of the colorectum by way of the serosa or mesocolon (eg, invasion of the sigmoid colon by carcinoma of the cecum). In contrast, intramural extension of tumor from one subsite (segment) of the large intestine into an adjacent subsite or into the ileum (eg, for a cecal carcinoma) or anal canal (eg, for a rectal carcinoma) does not affect the pT classification.[26]

Evaluation of Regional Lymph Nodes

All TNM stage-related outcome data are derived from studies in which the pathologic evaluation of the regional lymph nodes has been performed by conventional histologic staining of macroscopically identified lymph nodes. It has been shown that many, if not most, nodal metastases in colorectal cancer are found in small lymph nodes (less than 5 mm in diameter), the criteria for radiologic assessment of lymph node metastasis based on large size notwithstanding.[80] Therefore, aggressive search for all lymph nodes, both small and large, is essential.

There are few universally accepted pathology practice standards for lymph node dissection and examination in colorectal cancer specimens, but typically, all lymph nodes found are submitted for microscopic examination. It has been shown that 12 to 15 negative lymph nodes predict for regional node negativity.[64,72,81] Therefore, 12 regional lymph nodes are regarded as the minimum number to be accepted from a careful lymph node dissection and, if fewer than 12 nodes are found, it has been suggested that additional techniques (ie, visual enhancement techniques such as fat clearing) be considered.[72] However, the actual number of lymph nodes present in any given resection specimen may be limited by anatomic variation, surgical technique, or both. It is recommended that all grossly negative or equivocal lymph nodes be submitted entirely for microscopic examination.[41] For grossly positive lymph nodes, microscopic examination of a representative sample may be adequate for confirmation.

Regional lymph nodes must be examined separately from lymph nodes outside of the anatomic site of the tumor because metastases in any lymph node in the regional nodal group are classified as pN disease whereas all other nodal metastases are classified as pM1. The regional lymph node groups of the anatomic subsites of the colorectum are[24]:

- **Cecum**—anterior cecal, posterior cecal, ileocolic, right colic
- **Ascending Colon**—ileocolic, right colic, middle colic
- **Hepatic Flexure**—middle colic, right colic
- **Transverse Colon**—middle colic
- **Splenic Flexure**—middle colic, left colic, inferior mesenteric
- **Descending Colon**—left colic, inferior mesenteric, sigmoid
- **Sigmoid Colon**—inferior mesenteric, superior rectal sigmoidal, sigmoid mesenteric*
- **Rectosigmoid Colon**—perirectal,* left colic, sigmoid mesenteric, sigmoidal, inferior mesenteric, superior rectal, middle rectal
- **Rectum**—perirectal,* sigmoid mesenteric, inferior mesenteric, lateral sacral, presacral, internal iliac, sacral promontory, superior rectal, middle rectal, inferior rectal

On microscopic examination, tumor in a regional lymph node, whether arriving there via afferent lymphatics or direct invasion through the capsule (Figure 5–26), is regarded as metastatic disease. Microscopic examination of the extramural adipose tissue may reveal discrete nodules of tumor that may represent

---

*Lymph nodes along the sigmoid arteries are considered pericolic nodes and their involvement is classified as pN1 or pN2 according to the number involved. Perirectal lymph nodes include the mesorectal (paraproctal), lateral sacral, presacral, sacral promontory (Gerota), middle rectal (hemorrhoidal), and inferior rectal (hemorrhoidal) nodes. Metastasis in the external iliac or common iliac nodes is classified as pM1.[26]

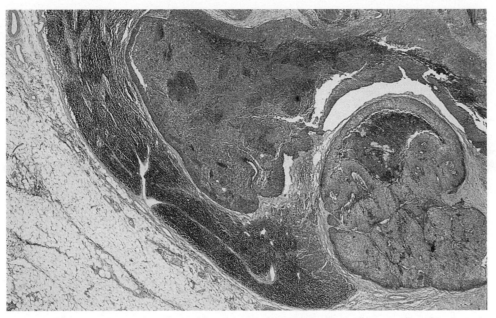

Figure 5–26. Direct extension of tumor into a regional node. Whether malignant cells gain access to regional lymph nodes by direct penetration of the capsule, as shown, or by transmigration within afferent lymphatics, they are classified as regional lymph node metastasis in the TNM classification.

lymph nodes that have been replaced by metastatic tumor but cannot be identified as such with certainty. In order to eliminate arbitrary decisions by different pathologists as to whether or not such nodules are to be interpreted as nodal metastasis, the AJCC/UICC have established the following guidelines. Any extramural tumor nodule within the regional lymph node distribution of the tumor that measures > 3 mm in diameter but lacks histologic evidence of residual lymph node tissue is classified as pN disease. However, tumor nodules measuring ≤ 3 mm in diameter are classified in the pT3 category as discontinuous extramural extension of tumor.[26] Multiple nodules > 3 mm in size should be considered as metastasis in a single lymph node for classification.[24]

The diagnosis of regional lymph node metastasis is limited to the use of conventional pathologic techniques (either gross or histologic). The biologic significance of minute amounts of metastatic tumor, known as micrometastases (tumor measuring ≤ 2.0 mm: Figure 5–27), is controversial. Currently, the data are insufficient to recommend either the routine examination of multiple tissue levels of paraffin blocks or the use of special/ancillary techniques such as immunohistochemistry for epithelial and/or tumor-associated antigens (eg, cytokeratin, carcinoembryonic antigen, etc.) or polymerase chain reaction (PCR) techniques to identify tumor RNA/DNA. All of these methods are costly and some can be difficult to quality control. More importantly, however, the significance of the findings generated from such analyses has yet to be proven.

In one recent study of stage 2 colorectal cancers (N = 26), more than 50 percent of cases showed evidence of micrometastatic disease in "negative" regional lymph nodes analyzed by RT-PCR for CEA.[82] The 5-year survival rate was 50 percent for patients with micrometastatic disease and 91 percent for patients without micrometastasis. However, in a larger study (N = 77) using immunohistochemistry to identify micrometastasis (found in 25% of cases), no difference in the 10-year survival was observed among patients with and without micrometastasis.[83] Clearly, larger statistically robust studies with careful quality control of methodology are required to further define the biologic significance of minute amounts of metastatic tumor in regional nodes and its impact on outcome. Pending definitive studies, it is recommended that any histologically identified focus of tumor that is ≤ 2.0 mm but > 0.2 mm be classified as N1 by the pathologist but be accompanied by a note stating that the biologic significance is unknown.[72,84] Isolated tumor cells, cell clusters that measure ≤ 0.2 mm on H&E stains, or micrometastasis detected only

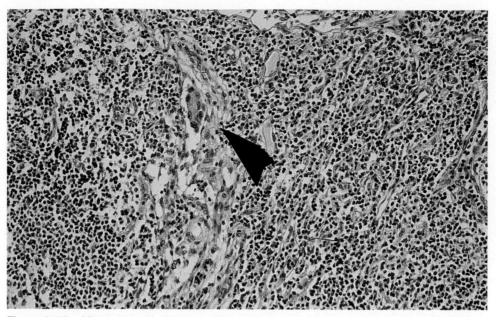

Figure 5–27. Micrometastasis within a regional lymph node. A single minute cluster of malignant cells (*arrow*) is seen in the center of this photomicrograph of a routine histologic section of a regional lymph node. Measuring less than 0.2 mm, this focus would be classified as pN1 but defined as a micrometastasis.

by special studies (immunohistochemical or molecular) should be reported but classified as N0.

Definition of Distant Metastasis

As stated above, metastasis to any nonregional lymph node or metastasis to any distant organ or tissue is categorized as M1 disease. Peritoneal seeding of abdominal organs is also considered M1 disease, as is positive peritoneal fluid cytology. Isolated tumor cells found in the bone marrow are classified as distant micrometastasis, but, like nodal micrometastasis (see above), their significance is as yet unproven.[26]

Multiple tumor foci in the mucosa or submucosa of adjacent bowel (satellite lesions or skip metastasis) are not classified as distant metastasis. Satellite lesions must, however, be distinguished from additional primary tumors in which there is obvious evidence of origin from an overlying adenoma.

Pathologic Staging of Residual Colorectal Carcinoma

By definition, the TNM categories describe the anatomic extent of malignant tumors that have not been previously treated, and the predictive value of the corresponding TNM stage groupings is based solely on data derived from outcome studies of such tumors following complete surgical resection. Tumor that remains in a resection specimen after previous (neoadjuvant) treatment of any type (radiation therapy alone, chemotherapy therapy alone, or any combined modality treatment) is codified by the TNM using a prescript y to indicate the post-treatment status of the tumor.[24] For many therapies, the classification of residual disease has been shown to be a strong predictor of post-treatment outcome. In addition, the ypTNM classification provides a standardized framework for the collection of data needed to accurately evaluate new therapies.

In contrast, a tumor remaining in the patient after primary surgical resection (eg, corresponding to a proximal, distal, or radial resection margin [see below] that is shown to be involved by tumor on pathologic examination) is categorized by a system known as R classification (Table 5–6).[24]

Pathologic Staging of Recurrent Colorectal Carcinoma

In contrast to residual disease, tumor that is locally recurrent after a documented disease-free interval

Table 5–6. R CLASSIFICATION SYSTEM	
RX	Presence of residual tumor cannot be assessed
R0	No residual tumor
R1	Microscopic residual tumor
R2	Macroscopic residual tumor

following surgical resection should be classified according the TNM categories and modified with the prefix r (eg, rpT1). By convention, the recurrent tumor is topographically assigned to the proximal segment of the anastomosis unless the proximal segment is small bowel.[24,26]

Status of Surgical Resection Margins (Proximal, Distal, Radial, and Mesenteric)

The pertinent margins of a colorectal cancer resection specimen include the proximal, distal, and mesenteric margins, and, when appropriate, the radial margin. The radial margin represents the retroperitoneal or perineal adventitial soft tissue margin closest to the deepest penetration of tumor. For all segments of the large intestine that are either incompletely encased (ascending colon, descending colon, upper rectum) or not encased (lower rectum) by peritoneum, the radial mar-

gin is created by blunt dissection of the retroperitoneal or subperitoneal aspect, respectively, at operation.

The radial margin has been demonstrated to be of importance in relation to risk of local recurrence after surgical resection of the rectal carcinomas.[85–88] Multivariate analysis has suggested that tumor involvement of the radial margin (Figure 5–28) is the most critical factor in predicting local recurrence in rectal cancer.[87,88] For this reason, routine assessment of the radial margin is recommended in all applicable colorectal cancers, and measurement of the distance from the tumor to the radial margin, representing the surgical clearance around the tumor, is also suggested.[41,86] It is recommended that the radial resection margin be considered involved if tumor is present ≤ 1 mm from the nonperitonealized surface of the resection specimen. For segments of the colon that are completely encased by a peritonealized (serosal) surface (eg, transverse and sigmoid colon), the mesenteric resection margin may be relevant since tumors may extend to this margin with (pT4) or without (pT3) penetrating the serosal surface. It should be examined when the point of deepest penetration of the tumor is on the mesenteric aspect of the colon. For those tumors limited to an

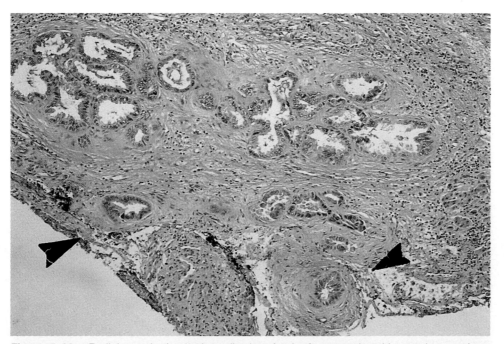

Figure 5–28. Radial margin (nonperitonealized surface) of a rectosigmoid resection specimen involved by tumor. Tumor glands are seen infiltrating the circumferential soft tissue resection margin of the nonperitonealized surface of the resection specimen (*arrows*), a finding that is associated with a significantly increased risk of local recurrence of tumor.

antimesenteric peritonealized aspect of the bowel, the mesenteric margin is not relevant.

Because of its association with local recurrence, involvement of the radial or the mesenteric margin has implications for adjuvant therapy. Whether the primary tumor is classified as pT3 (without serosal penetration) or pT4b (with serosal penetration), resection is considered complete only if all surgical margins are negative, including the radial margin. That is, whether or not the tumor penetrates a serosal surface, resection is considered complete if the resection margins are free of tumor. If a radial or mesenteric margin is involved by tumor, however, adjuvant therapy (eg, local radiation) may be appropriate irrespective of the T category of the tumor.

Venous, Lymphatic, or Perineural Invasion by Tumor

In at least 10 different studies, venous invasion by tumor has been demonstrated by multivariate analysis to have an independent adverse impact on outcome[27,31,32,37–39,55,56,71,89] and by univariate analysis in several additional studies.[43,90–92] Some studies identifying venous invasion as an adverse prognostic factor on univariate analysis have failed, however, to confirm its independent impact on prognosis on multivariate analysis.[39,93] Similarly disparate results have also been reported for lymphatic invasion (Figure 5–29).[34,38,39,45,89,91,93–95] In several studies, vascular invasion as a general feature was found to be prognostically significant by multivariate analysis, but no distinction between lymphatic and venous vessels was made. In other studies, the location of the vascular involvement (eg, invasion of extramural veins: Figure 5–30) has been a strong determinant of prognostic significance.[56,64] Overall, therefore, data from existing studies are difficult to amalgamate. Nevertheless, the importance of venous and lymphatic invasion by tumor is strongly suggested and largely confirmed by the literature.

It is likely that the disparities among existing studies on vessel invasion are directly related to inherent problems related to the pathologic analysis of this feature. Definitive diagnosis of vessel invasion requires the identification of tumor within an endothelial-lined channel. However, assessment of vessel invasion may be difficult and may be complicated by tumor-induced fibrosis and fixation artifact. Interobserver variability may be substantial in the interpretation of small vessel (ie, lymphatic or post-capillary venule) invasion, and large vessel (ie, muscular vein) invasion

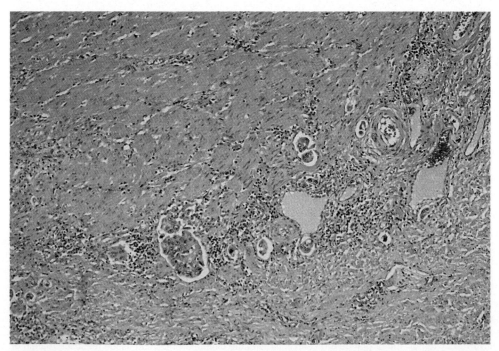

Figure 5–29.   Extramural small vessel (lymphatic) invasion by tumor. Small clusters of tumor cells are seen within thin-walled, endothelial-lined channels in the subserosa.

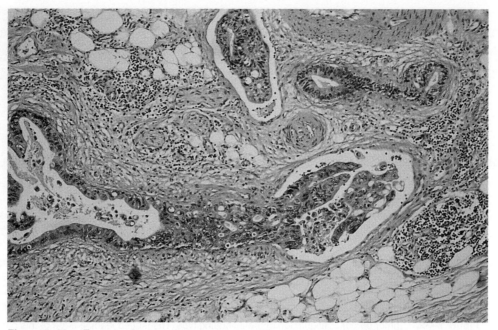

Figure 5–30. Extramural venous invasion by tumor. Tumor is seen within large-bore venous vessels on the extramural soft tissues, a finding associated with increased risk of hepatic metastasis.

with tumor infiltration of the vessel wall and destruction of the vascular architecture may also be difficult to recognize. Special techniques, such as immunohistochemical staining of endothelium or elastic tissue stains of venous walls (Figure 5–31), may increase the ease and accuracy of evaluation. Because these techniques are labor intensive, time consuming, and expensive, however, they are not routinely performed. Additional limitations in the detection of vessel invasion are related to specimen sampling. For example, it has been shown that the reproducibility of detection of extramural venous invasion increases proportion-

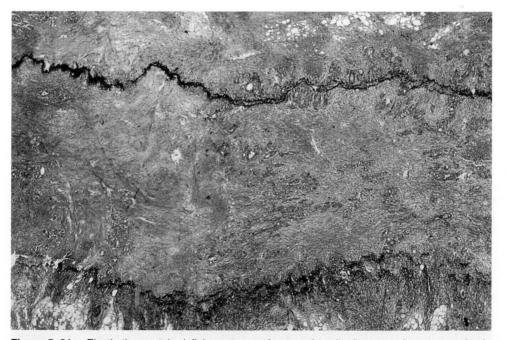

Figure 5–31. Elastic tissue stain defining extramural venous invasion by tumor. An extramural vein that has been infiltrated by tumor is recognized by the black-staining elastin network within its wall. The lumen of the vessel is obliterated by invasive carcinoma.

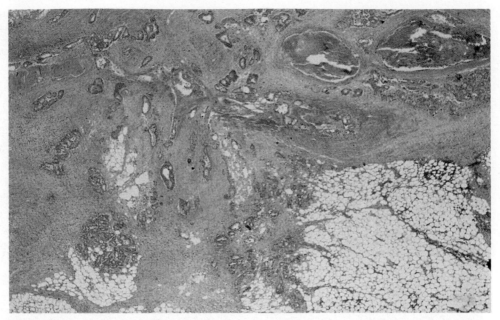

Figure 5–32. Tumor border configuration of the infiltrating type. The jagged leading edge of this carcinoma shows long tongues and irregular buds of tumor that penetrate the extramural soft tissue.

ally from 59 percent with examination of two blocks of tissue at the tumor periphery to 96 percent with examination of five blocks.[64] At present, however, no widely accepted standards or guidelines for the pathologic evaluation of vessel invasion exist, and pathology sampling practices may vary widely on both individual and institutional levels. Complicating this issue is the impact of cost containment on surgical pathology practice, which, in general, has tended to reduce overall sampling of resection specimens. The College of American Pathologists is recommending that at least three blocks (optimally five blocks) of tumor at its point of deepest extent be submitted for microscopic examination.[72]

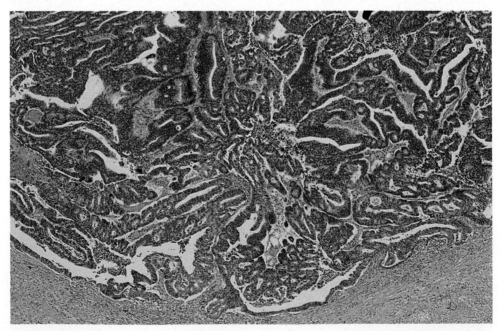

Figure 5–33. Tumor border configuration of the pushing type. The smooth leading edge of this carcinoma bluntly interfaces with the surrounding tissue.

Tumor Border Configuration and Perineural Invasion

For colorectal cancer, the growth pattern of the tumor at the advancing edge (tumor border) has been shown to have prognostic significance that is independent of stage and may predict liver metastasis. Specifically, an irregular, infiltrating pattern of growth (Figure 5–32), as opposed to a pushing border (Figure 5–33), has been demonstrated to be an independent adverse prognostic factor by several univariate[43,56,96,97] and multivariate analyses.[33,46,47,59,77,98,99] Defined as microscopic clusters of undifferentiated cancer cells just ahead of the invasive front of the tumor, irregular growth at the tumor periphery has also been referred to as focal dedifferentiation[95] and tumor budding.[98] It is recommended that pathologic assessment of tumor border configuration be routinely reported in transmurally invasive colorectal tumors.

Jass and colleagues[46] assessed interobserver variability among pathologists evaluating tumor border configuration in general practice (no specific definition provided) and found only a 70 percent (fair) agreement in diagnosis of infiltrating growth pattern. However, concordance was found to improve to 90 percent when diagnostic criteria for defining infiltrating growth were employed (Table 5–7 and Figures 5–34 and 5–35).[46]

Host Lymphoid Response to Tumor

Lymphocytic infiltration of tumor or peritumoral tissue is indicative of a host immunologic response to the invasive malignancy and has been shown by multivariate analysis in several studies to be a favorable prognostic factor.[36,46,56,59] In contrast, other studies have either failed to confirm the prognostic significance of a peritumoral lymphoid reaction[33,100] or demonstrated its significance only by univariate analysis.[43,100–103] The results of these studies are difficult to compare since the histologic criteria for qualitative and quantitative evaluation differ from study to study. Some of the specific features that have been studied include perivascular lymphocytic cuffing in the muscularis propria, perivascular lymphocytic cuffing in the pericolonic fat or subserosa, lymphocytic infiltration at the tumor edge, and a

Table 5–7. INTEROBSERVER VARIABILITY IN EVALUATING TUMOR BORDER CONFIGURATION

Naked Eye Examination of a Microscopic Slide of the Tumor Border
- Inability to define limits of invasive border of tumor and/or
- Inability to resolve host tissue from malignant tissue

Microscopic Examination of the Tumor Border
- Streaming dissection of muscularis propria (dissection of tumor through the full thickness of the muscularis propria without stromal response) (Figure 5–34) and/or
- Dissection of mesenteric adipose tissue by small glands or irregular clusters or cords of cells and/or
- Perineural invasion (Figure 5–35)*

*It should be noted that several studies have shown perineural invasion alone to be an independent indicator of poor prognosis by multivariate analysis.[18,27,31,39,45,90]

transmural Crohn's-like lymphoid reaction (Figure 5–36). In some reports, however, little if any explanation of the criteria used for evaluation of this parameter has been offered. Therefore, although this feature appears promising as a favorable prognostic factor, further studies using comparable criteria are needed for confirmation.

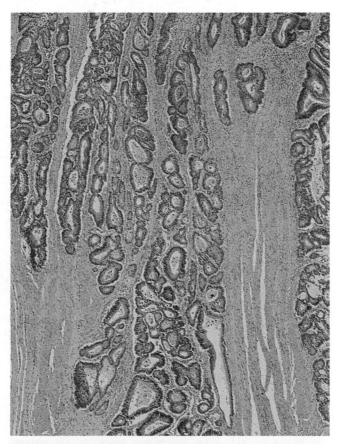

Figure 5–34. Streaming dissection of tumor through the muscularis propria. This microscopic feature is typical of carcinomas with an infiltrating type of tumor border.

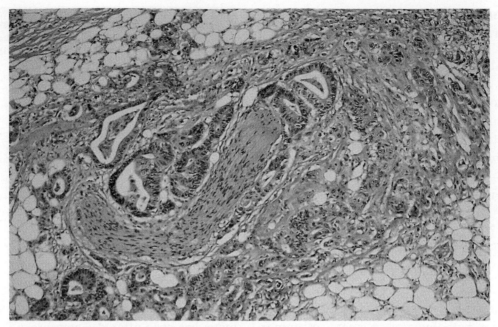

Figure 5–35. Perineural invasion by tumor. Clusters of carcinoma cells are seen within the perineurium of this extramural nerve.

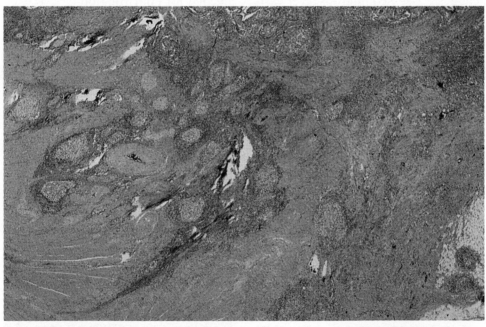

Figure 5–36. Crohn's-like host lymphoid response to tumor. The numerous lymphoid follicles (germinal centers) forming throughout the tissues at the leading edge of the tumor (*seen at top*) constitute a host lymphoid response that resembles that seen in many cases of Crohn's colitis.

REFERENCES

1. Sherlock P, Winawer SJ. Are there markers for the risk of colorectal cancer? N Engl J Med 1984;311:118–9.

2. Itzkowitz SH. Gastrointestinal adenomatous polyps. Semin Gastrointest Dis 1996;7:105–16.

3. Muto T, Bussey HJR, Morson BC. The evolution of cancer of the colon and rectum. Cancer 1975;36:2251–70.

4. Jass JR. Malignant colorectal polyps. Gastroenterology 1995;109:2034–5.

5. Morson BC, Whiteway JE, Jones EA, et al. Histopathology and prognosis of malignant colorectal polyps treated by endoscopic polypectomy. Gut 1984;25:437–44.

6. Wolff WI, Shinya H. Definitive treatment of "malignant" polyps of the colon. Ann Surg 1975;182:516–25.

7. Wilcox GM, Anderson PB, Colacchio TA. Early invasive carcinoma in colonic polyps: a review of the literature with emphasis on the assessment of the risk of metastasis. Cancer 1986;57:160–71.

8. Cooper HS, Deppisch LM, Gourley WK, et al. Endoscopically removed malignant colorectal polyps: clinicopathologic correlations. Gastroenterology 1995;108:1657–65.

9. Cranley JP, Petras RE, Carey WD, et al. When is endoscopic polypectomy adequate therapy for colonic polyps containing invasive carcinoma? Gastroenterology 1986;91:419–27.

10. Cooper HS. Surgical pathology of endoscopically removed malignant polyps of the colon and rectum. Am J Surg Pathol 1983;7:613–23.

11. Cooper HS. The role of the pathologist in the management of patients with endoscopically removed malignant colorectal polyps. Pathol Ann 1988;23:25–43.

12. Cooper HS, Deppisch LM, Kahn EI, et al. Pathology of the malignant colorectal polyp. Hum Pathol 1998; 29:15–26.

13. Cunningham KN, Mills LR, Schuman BM, et al. Long-term prognosis of well-differentiated adenocarcinoma in endoscopically removed colorectal adenomas. Dig Dis Sci 1994;39:2034–7.

14. Haggitt RC, Glotzbach RE, Soffer EE, et al. Prognostic factors in colorectal carcinomas arising in adenomas: implications for lesions removed by endoscopic polypectomy. Gastroenterology 1985;89:328–36.

15. Lipper S, Kahn LB, Ackerman LV. The significance of microscopic invasive cancer in endoscopically removed polyps of the large bowel. A clinicopathologic study of 51 cases. Cancer 1983;52:1691–9.

16. Kyzer S, Begin LR, Gordan PH, et al. The care of patients with colorectal polyps that contain invasive adenocarcinoma. Cancer 1992;70:2044–50.

17. Muller S, Chesner IM, Egan MJ, et al. Significance of venous and lymphatic invasion in malignant polyps of the colon and rectum. Gut 1989;30:1385–91.

18. Volk EE, Goldblum JR, Petras RE, et al. Management and outcome of patients with invasive carcinoma arising in colorectal polyps. Gastroenterology 1995; 109:1801–7.

19. Coverlizza S, Risio M, Ferrari A, et al. Colorectal adenomas containing invasive carcinoma: pathologic assessment of lymph node metastatic potential. Cancer 1989;64:1937–47.

20. Nivatvongs S, Goldberg SM. Management of patients who have polyps containing invasive carcinoma removed via colonoscope. Dis Colon Rectum 1978; 21:8–11.

21. Nivatvongs S, Rojanasakul A, Reiman HM, et al. The risk of lymph node metastasis in colorectal polyps with invasive adenocarcinoma. Dis Colon Rectum 1991;34:323–8.

22. Wilcox GM, Anderson PB, Colacchio TA. Early invasive carcinoma in colonic polyps: a review of the literature with emphasis on the assessment of the risk of metastasis. Cancer 1986;57:160–71.

23. Wilcox GM, Beck JR. Early invasive cancer in adenomatous colonic polyps ("Malignant Polyps"). Evaluation of the therapeutic options by decision analysis. Gastroenterology 1987;92:1159–68.

24. Fleming ID, Cooper JS, Henson DE, et al., editors. AJCC manual for staging of cancer, 5th ed. Philadelphia, PA: Lippincott Raven, 1997.

25. Fielding LP, Arsenault PA, Chapuis PH, et al. Clinicopathological staging for colorectal cancer: an International Documentation System (IDS) and an International Comprehensive Terminology (ICAT). J Gastroenterol Hepatol 1991;6:325–44.

26. Hermanek P, Henson DE, Hutter RVP, et al. TNM supplement. New York: Springer-Verlag, 1993.

27. Chapuis PH, Dent OF, Fisher R, et al. A multivariate analysis of clinical and pathological variables in prognosis after resection of large bowel cancer. Br J Surg 1985;72:698–702.

28. D'Eredita G, Serio G, Neri V, et al. A survival regression analysis of prognostic factors in colorectal cancer. Aust N Z J Surg 1996;66:445–51.

29. Frank R, Saclarides T, Leurgans S, et al. Tumor angiogenesis as a predictor of recurrence and survival in patients with node-negative colon cancer. Ann Surg 1995;222:695–9.

30. Griffin M, Bergstralh E, Coffey R, et al. Predictors of survival after curative resection of carcinoma of the colon and rectum. Cancer 1987;60:2318–24.

31. Mulcahy HE, Skelly MM, Husain A, et al. Long-term outcome following curative surgery for malignant large bowel obstruction. Br J Surg 1996;83:46–50.

32. Newland R, Dent O, Lyttle M, et al. Pathologic determinants of survival associated with colorectal cancer with lymph node metastases. A multivariate analysis of 579 patients. Cancer 1994;73:2076–82.

33. Roncucci L, Fante R, Losi L, et al. Survival for colon and rectal cancer in a population-based cancer registry. Eur J Cancer 1996;32A:295–302.

34. Takebayashi Y, Akiyama S, Yamada K, et al. Angiogenesis as an unfavorable prognostic factor in human colorectal carcinoma. Cancer 1996;78:226–31.

35. Crucitti F, Sofo L, Doglietto G, et al. Prognostic factors in colorectal cancer: current status and new trends. J Surg Oncol 1991;2:76–82.

36. Deans G, Heatley M, Anderson N, et al. Jass' classification revisited. J Am Coll Surg 1994;179:11–7.

37. Freedman L, Macaskill P, Smith A. Multivariate analysis of prognostic factors for operable rectal cancer. Lancet 1984;II:733–6.

38. Michelassi F, Ayala J, Balestracci T, et al. Verification of a new clinicopathologic staging system for colorectal adenocarcinoma. Ann Surg 1991;214:11–8.

39. Michelassi F, Block GE, Vannucci L, et al. A 5- to 21-year follow-up and analysis of 250 patients with rectal adenocarcinoma. Ann Surg 1988;208:379–87.

40. Hermanek P, Sobin LH. Colorectal Carcinoma. In: Hermanek P, Gospodarowicz MK, Henson DE, et al., editors. Prognostic factors in cancer. New York: Springer-Verlag, 1995. p. 64–79.

41. Compton CC. Updated protocol for the examination of specimens removed from patients with carcinomas of the colon and rectum, excluding carcinoid tumors, lymphomas, sarcomas, and tumors of the veriform appendix: a basis for checklists. Arch Pathol Lab Med 2000;124:1016–25.

42. Jass JR, Sobin LH, ed. World Health Organization histological typing of intestinal tumours, 2nd ed. New York: Springer-Verlag, 1989.

43. Carlon C, Fabris G, Arslan-Pagnini C, et al. Prognostic correlations of operable carcinoma of the rectum. Dis Colon Rectum 1985;28:47–50.

44. Green J, Timmcke A, Mitchell W, et al. Mucinous carcinoma—just another colon cancer? Dis Colon Rectum 1993;36:49–54.

45. Hermanek P, Guggenmoos-Holzmann I, Gall FP. Prognostic factors in rectal carcinoma. A contribution to the further development of tumor classification. Dis Colon Rectum 1989;32:593–9.

46. Jass J, Atkin W, Cuzick J, et al. The grading of rectal cancer: historical perspectives and a multivariate analysis of 447 cases. Histopathology 1986;10:437–59.

47. Jass J, Love S, Northover J. A new prognostic classification of rectal cancer. Lancet 1987;I:1303–6.

48. Robey-Cafferty SS, el-Naggar AK, Grignon DJ, et al. Histologic parameters and DNA ploidy as predictors of survival in stage B adenocarcinoma of colon and rectum. Mod Pathol 1990;3:261–6.

49. Spratt J, Spjut H. Prevalence and prognosis of individual clinical and pathologic variables associated with colorectal carcinoma. Cancer 1967;20:1976–85.

50. Umpleby HC, Williamson RC. Carcinoma of the large bowel in the first four decades. Br J Surg 1984;71:272–7.

51. Jesserun J, Romero-Guadarrama M, Manivel JC. Medullary adenocarcinoma of the colon: clinicopathologic study of 11 cases. Hum Pathol 1999;30:843–8.

52. Minsky B, Mies C, Rich T, et al. Colloid carcinoma of the colon and rectum. Cancer 1987;60:3103–12.

53. Secco G, Fardelli R, Campora E, et al. Primary mucinous adenocarcinomas and signet-ring cell carcinomas of colon and rectum. Oncology 1994;51:30–4.

54. Symonds D, Vickery A. Mucinous carcinoma of the colon and rectum. Cancer 1976;37:1891–1900.

55. Heys S, Sherif A, Bagley J, et al. Prognostic factors and survival of patients aged less than 45 years with colorectal cancer. Br J Surg 1994;81:685–8.

56. Harrison J, Dean P, El-Zeky F, et al. From Dukes through Jass: pathological prognostic indicators in rectal cancer. Hum Pathol 1994;25:498–505.

57. Sasaki O, Atkin WS, Jass JR. Mucinous carcinoma of the rectum. Histopathology 1987;11:259–72.

58. Shepherd N, Saraga E, Love S, et al. Prognostic factors in colonic cancer. Histopathology 1989;14:613–20.

59. Halvorsen T, Seim E. Association between invasiveness, inflammatory reaction, desmoplasia and survival in colorectal cancer. J Clin Pathol 1989;42:162–6.

60. Öfner D, Riedmann B, Maier H, et al. Standardized staining and analysis of argyrophilic nucleolar organizer region associated proteins (AgNORs) in radically resected colorectal adenocarcinoma-correlation with tumour stage and long-term survival. J Pathol 1995;75:441–8.

61. Staren ED, Gould VE, Warren WH, et al. Neuroendocrine carcinomas of the colon and rectum: a clinicopathologic correlation. Surgery 1988;104:1080–9.

62. DeBruine A, Wiggers T, Beek C, et al. Endocrine cells in colorectal adenocarcinomas: incidence, hormone profile and prognostic relevance. Int J Cancer 1993;54:765–71.

63. Gaffey M, Mills S, Lack E. Neuroendocrine carcinoma of the colon and rectum. A clinicopathologic, ultrastructural, and immunohistochemical study of 24 cases. Am J Surg Pathol 1990;14:1010–23.

64. Blenkinsopp WK, Stewart-Brown S, Blesovsky L, et al. Histopathology reporting in large bowel cancer. J Clin Pathol 1981;34:509–13.

65. Böttger TC, Potratz D, Stöckle M, et al. Prognostic value of DNA analysis in colorectal carcinoma. Cancer 1993;72:3579–87.

66. Fisher E, Sass R, Palekar A, et al. Dukes' classification revisited. Findings from the National Surgical Adjuvant Breast and Bowel Projects. Cancer 1989;64:2354–60.

67. Jessup JM, Lavin PT, Andrews CW, et al. Sucrase-isomaltase is an independent prognostic marker for colorectal carcinoma. Dis Colon Rectum 1995;38:1257–64.

68. Jessup J, McGinnis L, Steele G, et al. The National Cancer Data Base Report on Colon Cancer. Cancer 1996;78:918–26.

69. Ruschoff J, Bittinger A, Neumann K, et al. Prognostic significance of nucleolar organizing regions (NORs) in carcinomas of the sigmoid colon and rectum. Pathol Res Pract 1990;186:85–91.

70. Scott NA, Wieand HS, Moertel CG, et al. Colorectal cancer. Dukes' stage, tumor site, preoperative plasma CEA level, and patient prognosis related to tumor DNA ploidy pattern. Arch Surg 1987;122:1375–9.

71. Wiggers T, Arends J, Volovics A. Regression analysis of prognostic factors in colorectal cancer after curative resections. Dis Colon Rectum 1988;31:33–41.

72. Compton CC, Fielding LP, Burgart LJ, et al. Prognostic

factors in colorectal cancer: College of American Pathologists consensus statement 2000. Arch Pathol Lab Med 2000;124:979–94.

73. Steele G Jr, Mayer RJ, Podolsky DK, et al. Cancer of the colon, rectum, and anus. In: Osteen RT, editor. Cancer manual. 9th ed. Farmington, MA: American Cancer Society, 1996. p. 399–410.

74. Stower M, Hardcastle J. The results of 1115 patients with colorectal cancer treated over an 8-year period in a single hospital. Eur J Surg Oncol 1985;11:119–23.

75. Sobin LH, Wittekind C, editors. TNM classification of malignant tumours: International Union Against Cancer. 5th ed. New York: John Wiley and Sons, 1997.

76. Compton CC, Fenoglio-Preiser CM, Pettigrew N, et al. American Joint Committee on Cancer Prognostic Factors consensus conference: Colorectal Working Group. Cancer 2000;88:1739–57.

77. Shepherd N, Baxter K, Love S. The prognostic importance of peritoneal involvement in colonic cancer: a prospective evaluation. Gastroenterology 1997; 112:1096–102.

78. Tominaga T, Sakabe T, Koyama Y, et al. Prognostic factors for patients with colon or rectal carcinoma treated with resection only. Five-year follow-up report. Cancer 1996;78:403–8.

79. Zeng Z, Cohen AM, Hajdu S, et al. Serosal cytologic study to determine free mesothelial penetration of intraperitoneal colon cancer. Cancer 1992;70:737–40.

80. Herrera-Ornelas L, Justiniano J, Castillo N, et al. Metastases in small lymph nodes from colon cancer. Arch Surg 1987;122:1253–6.

81. Scott KWM, Grace RH. Detection of lymph node metastases in colorectal carcinoma before and after fat clearance. Br J Surg 1989;76:1165–7.

82. Liefers G-J, Cleton-Jansen A-M, van de Velde CJ, et al. Micrometastases and survival in stage II colorectal cancer. N Engl J Med 1998;339:223–8.

83. Jeffers MD, O'Dowd GM, Mulcahy H, et al. The prognostic significance of immunohistochemically detected lymph node micrometastases in colorectal carcinoma. J Pathol 1994;172:183–7.

84. Hermanek P, Hutter RVP, Sobin LH, et al. Classification of isolated tumor cells and micrometastasis. Cancer 1999;86:2668–73.

85. Adam IJ, Mohamdee MO, Martin IG, et al. Role of the circumferential margin involvement in the local recurrence of rectal cancer. Lancet 1994;344:707–11.

86. Chan K, Boey J, Wong S. A method of reporting radial invasion and surgical clearance of rectal carcinoma. Histopathology 1985;9:1319–27.

87. Quirke P, Scott N. The pathologists role in the assessment of local recurrence in rectal carcinoma. Surg Oncol Clin N Am 1992;3:1–17.

88. Quirke P, Durdy P, Dixon MF, et al. Local recurrence of rectal adenocarcinoma due to inadequate surgical resection. Lancet 1986;II:996–9.

89. Knudsen JB, Nilsson T, Sprechler M, et al. Venous and nerve invasion as prognostic factors in postoperative survival of patients with resectable cancer of the rectum. Dis Colon Rectum 1983;26:613–7.

90. Horn A, Dahl O, Morild I. Venous and neural invasion as predictors of recurrence in rectal adenocarcinoma. Dis Colon Rectum 1991;34:798–804.

91. Lee Y. Local and regional recurrence of carcinoma of the colon and rectum: I. Tumour-host factors and adjuvant therapy. Surg Oncol 1995;4:283–93.

92. Talbot I, Ritchie S, Leighton MH, et al. The clinical significance of invasion of veins by rectal cancer. Br J Surg 1980;67:439–42.

93. Takahashi Y, Tucker S, Kitadai Y, et al. Vessel counts and expression of vascular endothelial growth factor as prognostic factors in node-negative colon cancer. Arch Surg 1997;132:541–6.

94. Minsky B, Mies C, Recht A, et al. Resectable adenocarcinoma of the rectosigmoid and rectum. II. The influence of blood vessel invasion. Cancer 1988;61: 1417–24.

95. Minsky B, Mies C, Rich T, et al. Lymphatic vessel invasion in an independent prognostic factor for survival in colorectal cancer. Int J Radiat Oncol Biol Phys 1989;17:311–8.

96. Ono M, Sakamoto M, Ino Y, et al. Cancer cell morphology at the invasive front and expression of cell adhesion-related carbohydrate in the primary lesion of patients with colorectal carcinoma with liver metastasis. Cancer 1996;78:1179–86.

97. Sinicrope F, Hart J, Brasitus T, et al. Relationship of P-glycoprotein and carcinoembryonic antigen expression in human colon carcinoma to local invasion, DNA ploidy, and disease relapse. Cancer 1994; 74:2908–17.

98. Hase K, Shatney C, Johnson D, et al. Prognostic value of tumor "budding" in patients with colorectal cancer. Dis Colon Rectum 1993;36:627–35.

99. Thynne GS, Weiland LH, Moertel CG, et al. Correlation of histopathologic characteristics of primary tumor and uninvolved regional lymph nodes in Dukes' C colonic carcinoma with prognosis. Mayo Clin Proc 1980;55:243–5.

100. Shirouzu K, Isomoto H, Kakegawa T. Prognostic evaluation of perineural invasion in rectal cancer. Am J Surg 1993;165:233–7.

101. Pihl E, Malahy MA, Khankhanian N, et al. Immunomorphological features of prognostic significance in Dukes' class B colorectal carcinoma. Cancer Res 1977;37:4145–9.

102. Svennevig JL, Lunde OC, Holter J, et al. Lymphoid infiltration and prognosis in colorectal carcinoma. Br J Cancer 1984;49:375–7.

103. Zhou XG, Yu BM, Shen YX. Surgical treatment and late results in 1226 cases of colorectal cancer. Dis Colon Rectum 1983;26:250–6.

6

Endoscopic Management of Colon and Rectal Cancer

WILLIAM R. BRUGGE, MD

Colorectal cancer is an important problem in the United States, with over 130,000 new cases and 55,000 deaths each year. There is strong evidence that screening for colorectal cancer can decrease mortality and incidence of colorectal cancer. Published guidelines recommend that all asymptomatic, average-risk U.S. citizens more than 50 years of age should be encouraged to undergo screening for colorectal cancer. Those at higher risk should be offered more intensive screening and follow-up surveillance. It is estimated that widespread adoption of these recommendations could reduce mortality from colorectal cancer by more than 50 percent. Successful screening and prevention of colon cancer are increasingly being realized through the use of colonoscopy and associated endoscopic procedures.

DIAGNOSTIC TESTS FOR COLON CANCER AND POLYPS

Colonoscopy is the primary diagnostic test for detecting colorectal cancer and its precursors. Current endoscopic techniques provide high-quality digital images of the entire colon using flexible colonoscopes that are capable of diagnosing and removing malignant and premalignant lesions of the colon. The examinations are often performed in the outpatient setting by gastroenterologists or surgeons, and the procedure usually requires 30 to 60 minutes. Patients are prepared with a colonic purge using polyethylene glycol or sodium phosphates.[1] Nursing staff assist by providing anesthesia, patient monitoring, and therapeutic procedures. Intravenous sedation and analgesia are often provided to the patients to improve tolerance.[2]

Colonoscopy is a highly accurate test for detecting and diagnosing colon cancer whether it is performed as a screening or diagnostic test. In a large retrospective series, colonoscopy had an overall sensitivity of 95 percent for detecting colon cancer.[3] The test, however, is dependent on the expertise and training of the endoscopist. When gastroenterologists perform the examination, the sensitivity is 97 percent, compared to 87 percent when practitioners who are not gastroenterologists perform the examination. The most common cause of a missed diagnosis of colon cancer is an incomplete examination of the colon. The miss rates for polyps are higher, particularly for small polyps, and are also dependent on the expertise and training of the endoscopist.[4]

The complications of colonoscopy may be related to the discomfort of the procedure, perforations, or bleeding after polypectomy. The discomfort associated with colonoscopy is variable in intensity and frequency and, in select patients, little or no sedation or analgesia is required.[5] Pelvic adhesions, sigmoid diverticular disease, and a younger age increase the risks of pain associated with colonoscopy. Serious complications consist of bleeding or perforation and occur in less than 0.2 percent of patients.[2] There are, however, no recent large series assessing the risks of colonoscopy using current technology. Bleeding may be noted in up to 2 percent of patients but requires admission or transfusion in less than 0.5 percent of patients.[6] Perforations during diagnostic colonoscopy are most commonly located in the sigmoid colon and usually consist of lacerations that require surgical repair.[7] Small perforations as a result of polyp removal may be managed surgically or medically.

Flexible sigmoidoscopy uses a small diameter fiberoptic or video scope, similar to colonoscopes, but the examination is limited to the left colon and often to the sigmoid colon.[8] Flexible sigmoidoscopy may be performed by a wide range of health care providers using less expensive equipment. Although the preparation for sigmoidoscopy is similar to colonoscopy, the procedure is quite different. Since the examination lasts only a few minutes and there is much less discomfort, intravenous sedation is rarely used. Without the need for intravenous sedation, there is little need for nursing assistance, and the cost is considerably less.[9] Although polyps may be removed during flexible sigmoidoscopy, this should be done only after the entire colon has been examined by colonoscopy.

Barium enemas can also be used as a screening test or, more commonly, as a diagnostic test. In the past, barium enemas were more often employed than colonoscopy in the diagnostic evaluation of colon cancer. Barium enemas are not, however, as sensitive as colonoscopy for the detection of colon cancer. The use of double-contrast barium enemas will improve the diagnostic rate only slightly, from 82 to 85 percent. The cancers found by barium enemas are larger and more advanced than the cancers diagnosed with colonoscopy. When an abnormality is seen on barium enema, colonoscopy is often used to diagnose or remove the lesion.

DIAGNOSTIC FINDINGS ON COLONOSCOPY

There is a wide range of endoscopic findings that diagnose colon cancer with colonoscopy (Figure 6–1). The most common lesion is a large, irregular mucosal mass that may obstruct the lumen of the colon. This endoscopic finding is nearly always diagnostic of colon cancer. In this setting, endoscopic biopsies are superfluous, but often done to provide a conclusive tissue diagnosis. Other endoscopic findings that suggest a malignancy are large irregular polyps, villous lesions, and small flat-mass lesions.

Adenomas are the most common premalignant finding encountered during colonoscopy. Adenomas range in size from 2 mm to several centimeters and, when they appear on a stalk, they are referred to as pedunculated polyps (Figure 6–2). They are readily

removed during colonoscopy using cautery applied through a snare. Polypectomy is performed for two reasons, for diagnostic purposes and for the prevention of malignant transformation of a polyp. The ability of colonoscopy to detect adenomas is dependent on the size of the adenoma and colonoscopic techniques. The overall miss rate for detecting all adenomas is approximately 24 percent.[10] For adenomas larger than 1 cm, the miss rate is less than 6 percent. The missed adenomas tend to be in the right colon where the accumulation of stool may obscure the presence of a polyp.

The origin of colon polyps is not well understood. Endoscopically, a precursor to the adenoma has been identified using magnifying endoscopy. Aberrant crypt foci are commonly seen in patients with adenomas, and the number of foci and dysplastic changes are more common in patients with colon cancer.[11] Although clinical significance of aberrant crypt foci has not been determined, the number of aberrant crypts is reduced by the use of aspirin.[11] The use of spray dyes on the colon mucosa during magnification colonoscopy may assist in the detection of small adenomas or flat cancers.[12] This technique can also assist in making the diagnosis of polyposis syndromes because of the ability to visualize small mucosal polyps.[13]

Small adenomas in the left colon may be an early indicator of colon cancer. Nearly one-third of patients with a left-sided small adenoma have a right-sided adenoma and 6 percent have a colon malignancy.[14] The presence of a large adenoma in the left colon increases the risk of an adenoma on the right colon by 57 percent. The current recommendation is for all patients with the finding of a left-sided adenoma to undergo a colonoscopy. However, patients with a single diminutive adenoma less than 5 mm in the left colon rarely have a significant right-sided lesion.[15] The risk of a right-sided lesion is increased by age, having more than one polyp, and a family history of colon cancer.[16]

Malignant polyps are polyps resected with histologic evidence of malignancy within the polyp (Figure 6–3). Those with a favorable histology, grade I or II carcinoma with negative resection margins, have a good prognosis, and surgical resection is often not required. In contrast, patients with advanced malignant polyps should undergo surgical resection (Figure 6–4). Some of the criteria used to predict residual malignancy include high-grade adenocarcinoma, lymphatic invasion, or stalk invasion.[17] As many as 42 percent of patients with advanced malignant polyps will have evidence of metastases, will have residual malignancy at the resection site, or will develop recurrent malignancy.[18]

Large, flat, villous tumors are a challenge to the endoscopist. Endoscopically, they are seen as a carpet-like lesion often covering a large surface area. They are difficult to remove endoscopically, and superficial biopsies may miss areas of malignancy. The risk of malignancy is between 2 and 50 percent

in these types of polyps and, despite numerous biopsies, documentation of malignancy may not be possible[19]; therefore, surgical or aggressive endoscopic excision is often recommended for apparently benign villous adenomas.

Hyperplastic polyps are small benign polypoid lesions that are commonly encountered in the rectum (Figure 6–5). They rarely grow larger than 5 mm in diameter or cause bleeding. Because there is essentially no potential for malignant degeneration, they are often not removed except for diagnostic purposes. It is difficult to accurately differentiate between adenomas and hyperplastic polyps based on the endoscopic appearance. The confusion between

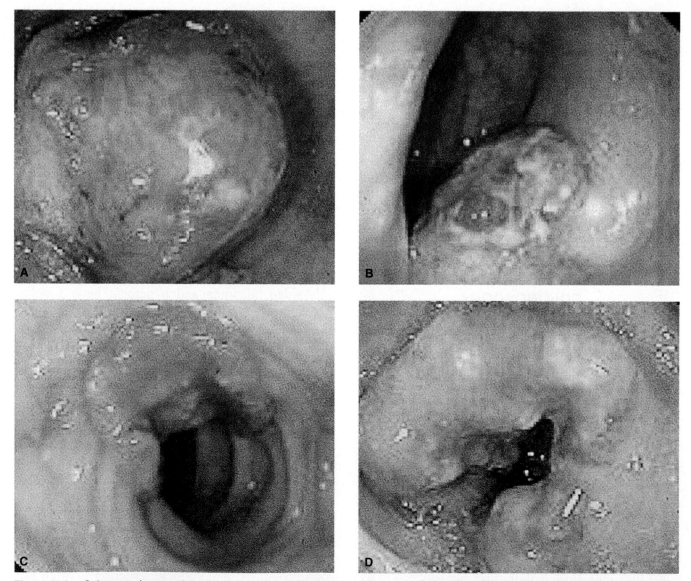

Figure 6–1. Colonoscopic examples of colon cancers. *A,* Early but invasive colon cancer. *B,* Colon cancer invading the wall of the colon. *C,* Flat colon cancer involving half of the circumference of colon lumen. *D,* Circumference colon cancer.

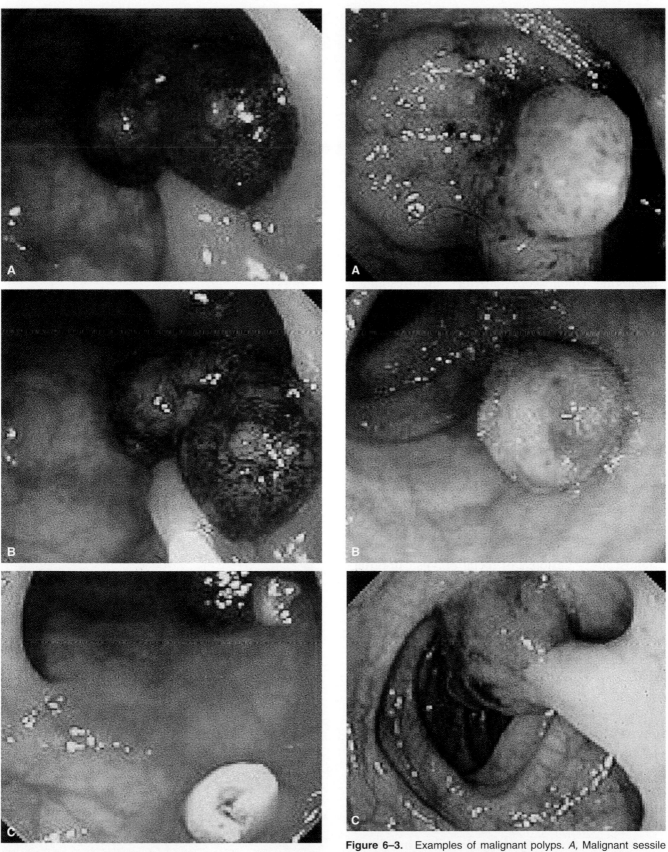

Figure 6–2. Pedunculated adenomatous polyp. *A,* Colonoscopic view of a 1-cm adenoma with a stalk. *B,* Placement of a snare for polyp resection. *C,* Polypectomy site.

Figure 6–3. Examples of malignant polyps. *A,* Malignant sessile polyp that could not be resected endoscopically. *B,* Small adenoma that when resected contained carcinoma in situ in the short stalk. *C,* Malignant pedunculated polyp without invasion of the stalk.

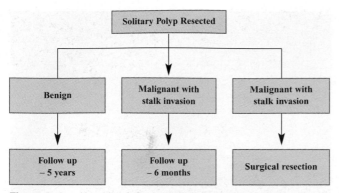

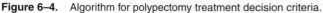

Figure 6–4. Algorithm for polypectomy treatment decision criteria.

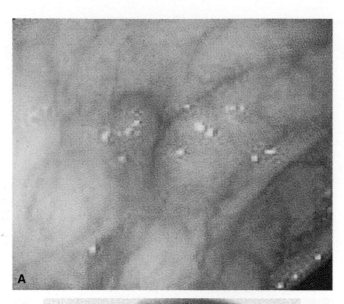

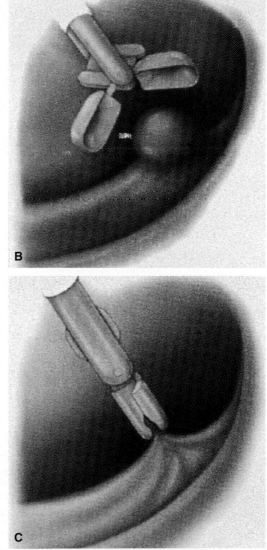

these types of polyps often requires biopsies or polyp removal, a time-consuming and costly requirement. Magnifying colonoscopy provides high-resolution images of polyps and their surface characteristics and may improve the ability to diagnose adenomas.[20] Recently, fluorescence endoscopic imaging has been used in an attempt to differentiate between adenomas and hyperplastic polyps. The rate of decay of laser-induced autofluorescence can distinguish adenomas from nonadenomas.[21] With the use of photosensitizers, 77 percent of hyperplastic polyps can be correctly differentiated from adenomas.[22] More advanced imaging techniques have been reported to diagnose adenomas and detect dysplasia within a polyp.[23] The presence of hyperplastic polyps in the rectum is not highly predictive of proximal adenomas and should not be the sole indication for colonoscopy.[24,25] Biopsy of rectal polyps can differentiate between adenomas and hyperplastic polyps, and the finding of a rectal adenoma is a frequent basis for proceeding with colonoscopy.[26] Although patients with hyperplastic polyps do not require colonoscopy, there are reports that patients with hyperplastic polyps are more likely to develop adenomas in the future.[27]

Flat adenomas are an unusual type of colonic tumor. These tumors are often small, flat, translucent, and not easily seen with traditional colonoscopy.[28] Recently, the use of dye sprays in combination with high-resolution video endoscopy has enabled endoscopists to identify and diagnose these lesions. Although they were originally identified in Japan, they are more frequently being described in Western countries in association with hereditary nonpolyposis colon cancer.[28] The risk of malignancy is propor-

Figure 6–5. Hyperplastic polyp. *A,* Colonoscopic view of a small, smooth, hyperplastic polyp. *B,* Forceps biopsy of a hyperplastic polyp. *C,* Endoscopic removal is often achieved with forceps biopsy.

tional to the size of the polyp. Lesions greater than 1 cm have a 2 percent risk of adenocarcinoma while 12 percent have high-grade dysplasia. These polyps are commonly missed on routine examination.[29] The finding of a central depression is associated with invasive malignancy.[29,30]

Carcinoid tumors occur commonly in the rectum (Figure 6–6). They are usually small and smooth, and often are confused with adenomas. They are readily diagnosed with histology of the resected polyp. If the tumor is superficial and completely resected, the prognosis is very good.[31]

ENDOSCOPIC DETECTION OF COLON CANCER

The endoscopic screening of large populations for colorectal cancers has traditionally been done with flexible sigmoidoscopy. The technique is widely available in the United States and is relatively simple and inexpensive. The examinations, however, are limited to the lower 30 cm of the colon in 33 percent of patients because of pain or difficulty in passage of the sigmoidoscope through the sigmoid colon.[8] The examination may be performed by a physician or a trained nurse practitioner with similar miss rates for adenomas.[32] This type of screening is limited by the concerns over undetected right-sided colon cancer.[16] Although flexible sigmoidoscopy may be used in conjunction with stool occult blood testing, it should not be the sole test used to evaluate patients with occult bleeding.

Colonoscopy is often performed in patients who have been identified as being at high risk for development of colorectal cancer. Several risk factors have been identified, including family history, age, and a history of left-sided polyps. Left-sided polyps are often used as predictors of right-sided polyps. Hyperplastic polyps in the left colon are not highly predictive of adenomas or malignancies in the right colon. The use of a left-sided adenoma as a sign of right-sided cancer has recently been examined by Rex and colleagues.[25] In patients with right-sided cancers, only 34 percent had left-sided lesions.[33] In fact, only 25 percent had any adenomas. Other studies have also documented that a significant percentage of patients with proximal colon cancers have no left-sided sen-

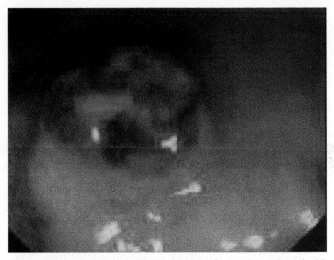

Figure 6–6. Rectal carcinoid. An example of a small rectal carcinoid.

tinel findings.[34] The size, number, and presence of atypia in left-sided polyps is predictive of right-sided adenomas or advanced polyps in some studies and not in others.[35,36] For advanced adenomas in the right colon, only 16 percent of patients were found to have an index lesion within reach of the sigmoidoscope.[37] These observations have led to increasing use of screening colonoscopy after the age of 50 in low-risk populations. With the recent reductions in the cost of colonoscopy, this strategy may become cost effective.[38] The use of colonoscopy will also reduce the need for additional examinations of the colon.

The size, configuration, and presence of atypia in polyps are risk factors for the development of colon cancer and should serve as identifiable risk for determining the frequency of follow-up colonoscopy.[39] The risk of recurrent polyps is increased in those patients with more than three polyps or a tubulovillous histology.[40] Surveillance colonoscopy after polypectomy can be performed at 3 years without risk to the patient.[41] After resection of a benign adenoma in an average-risk patient, follow-up colonoscopy is currently recommended at 5-year intervals.[42] If there are multiple adenomas, follow-up colonoscopy is recommended at 3-year intervals. Malignant polyps will require surveillance at closer intervals.

The effectiveness of widespread use of colonoscopic polypectomy has been examined with the National Polyp Study.[43] The rate of colon cancer over a 6-year period in a group of patients undergoing periodic colonoscopy for the finding of polyps was compared to groups of patients not undergoing colonoscopic polypectomy. The frequency of colon cancer was reduced 88 to 90 percent through the use of colonoscopy and polypectomy. Compared to a general population of low-risk patients not undergoing colonoscopy, the rate of colon cancer was reduced by 76 percent. Similar reductions in the rate of colon cancer have been reported in the United States veteran population undergoing colonoscopies.[44] In the United Kingdom, a threefold increase in the incidence of rectal cancer was observed in patients undergoing incomplete resection of rectal adenomas during rigid sigmoidoscopy compared to the general population.[45] With widespread use of colonoscopy and polypectomy, rectal cancers have been diagnosed at an earlier stage in France, and there has been a dramatic improvement in the survival rate.[46]

The effectiveness of colonoscopic surveillance in high-risk groups has been examined in several different populations. The effectiveness of surveillance colonoscopy in patients with hereditary polyposis was compared to prophylactic colectomy.[47] In patients with hereditary nonpolyposis colorectal cancer (HNPCC), colonoscopy was found to increase life expectancy by 13.5 years using a decision analysis model. When quality of life measures were used, colonoscopy was found to offer the optimal approach to reducing the risk of malignancy in HNPCC. In addition, the use of colonoscopic surveillance was found to be cost effective in patients diagnosed with mutated mismatch repair gene associated with HNPCC.[48] In patients at risk for familial adenomatous polyposis (FAP), decision analysis has demonstrated that sigmoidoscopy is more cost effective than genotyping for establishing a diagnosis if small numbers of high-risk family members are examined.[49] Sigmoidoscopy is also the preferred technique for following patients with FAP in whom a subtotal colectomy has been performed.[50] Similar findings of effectiveness for surveillance have also been demonstrated in high-risk patients with chronic ulcerative colitis.[51] Adenomas detected in patients with ulcerative colitis can be resected endoscopically without fear of underlying malignancy.[52] Malignancies found arising in the setting of colonoscopy tend to be smaller, less invasive, and

associated with better survival than those patients not undergoing surveillance colonoscopy.[53,54]

A family history of adenomas or cancer has recently been examined as a risk factor for colon cancer. The risk of cancer varies with the age of diagnosis in the relative. In a recent study, 12 percent of patients who had relatives with colon cancer had adenomas, 25 percent of which were proximal and not detectable with sigmoidoscopy.[55] Colonoscopic surveillance in patients with a first-degree relative who has an adenoma has been retrospectively examined.[56] The risk of colorectal cancer discovered during colonoscopy was 1.7 times that of patients without a family history of an adenoma. When a first-degree relative of less than 50 years had an adenoma, the relative risk was even greater, 4.3 times. For further discussion of colon and rectal cancer screening, refer to Chapter 4 "Colorectal Prevention and Early Detection."

Iron deficiency anemia and occult bleeding are risk factors for colon cancer and should be evaluated with colonoscopy, particularly in elderly patients. In a recent series, 32 percent of patients were found to have a colonic lesion at the time of colonoscopy.[57] In contrast, the yield of colonoscopy in premenopausal women with iron deficiency anemia and no evidence of chronic blood loss is very low.[58]

The accuracy of colonoscopy for the detection of polyps has been examined using several techniques. Tandem colonoscopy, repeating colonoscopy immediately after an initial examination, will detect a significant number of polyps, although usually small. Follow-up colonoscopy by the same endoscopist or a different one will detect an additional 8 or 11 percent of polyps.[4] Most of the polyps missed during colonoscopy are less than 1 cm in diameter and without evidence of malignancy.

The current recommendations of the American Cancer Society for screening in average-risk individuals is (1) fecal occult blood testing every year combined with flexible sigmoidoscopy every 5 years, (2) double-contrast barium enema every 5 to 10 years, or (3) colonoscopy every 10 years. A digital rectal examination should be performed at the same time as sigmoidoscopy, colonoscopy, or double-contrast barium enema. The recommendations for moderate- and high-risk patients are listed in Table 6–1.

STAGING OF COLON CANCER WITH ENDOSCOPIC TECHNIQUES

Endoscopic ultrasound probes can provide local tumor and nodal staging of rectal cancers[59,60] (Figure 6–7). The technique is particularly effective for the staging of superficial malignancies where the accuracy rate is more than 90 percent.[61–63] Advanced malignancies are staged with much lower accuracy rates. The sensitivity for detecting lymph node metastases is 85 percent, but compromised by a low specificity rate of 72 percent. Furthermore, the accuracy of endoscopic ultrasound staging (EUS) for accurately staging small (<5 mm) malignant nodes is poor.[64] Rectal EUS has also been used to document the tumor response to neoadjuvant chemoradiation.[65] Ultrasound staging can also be performed using laparoscopic ultrasound instruments, which determine the depth of invasion and the presence of lymph nodes in the peritoneal cavity.[66]

In large comparative trials, EUS has produced staging accuracy rates that have surpassed CT scanning and magnetic resonance imaging (MRI) using rectal coils.[67,68,69] Endoscopic ultrasound staging is also less expensive than MRI of rectal cancers.[67] Lymph node staging was comparable with all techniques. EUS has many advantages, including ease of use, small diameter, and low cost. The use of EUS to improve the preoperative staging of rectal cancer will improve the selection of patients for sphincter preserving surgery.[70]

Endoscopic ultrasound can also be used to determine the depth of malignant invasion of a malignant polyp after resection. This may be useful when

Table 6–1. AMERICAN CANCER SOCIETY RECOMMENDATIONS FOR COLON CANCER SCREENING IN MODERATE- AND HIGH-RISK PATIENTS

Risk Category	Recommendation	Age to Begin	Interval
Moderate Risk			
People with single, small (< 1 cm) adenomatous polyps	Colonoscopy diagnosis	At time of initial polyp diagnosis	TCE within 3 years after initial polyp removal; if normal, colonoscopy every 5–10 years
People with large (≥ 1 cm) or multiple adenomatous polyps of any size	Colonoscopy diagnosis	At time of initial polyp diagnosis	TCE within 3 years after initial polyp removal; if normal, TCE every 5 years
Personal history of curative-intent resection of colon cancer	TCE	Within 1 year after resection	If normal, TCE in 3 years; if still normal, TCE every 5 years
Colorectal cancer or adenomatous polyps in first-degree relative younger than age 60 or in two or more first-degree relatives of any age	TCE	Age 40 or 10 years before the youngest case in the family, whichever is earlier	Every 5 years
Colorectal cancer in other relatives (not included above)	Colonoscopy every 5 to 10 years; may consider beginning screening before age 50		
High Risk			
Family history of familial adenomatous polyposis	Early surveillance with endoscopy, counseling to consider genetic testing, and referral to a specialty cancer center	Puberty	If genetic test positive, or polyposis confirmed, consider colectomy; otherwise endoscopy every 1 to 2 years
Family history of hereditary nonpolyposis colon cancer	Colonoscopy and counseling to consider genetic testing	Age 21	If genetic test positive, or if patient has not had genetic testing, colonoscopy every 2 years till age 40, then every year
Inflammatory bowel disease	Colonoscopies with biopsies for dysplasia	8 years after start of pancolitis; 12 to 15 years after the start of left-sided colitis	Every 1 to 2 years

TCE = total colon evaluation.

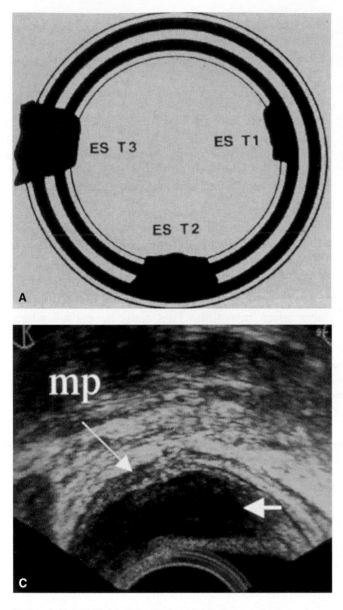

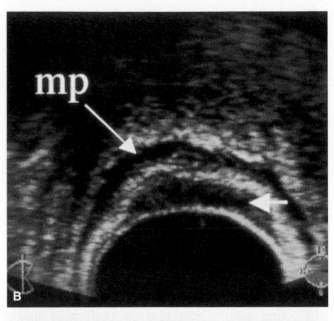

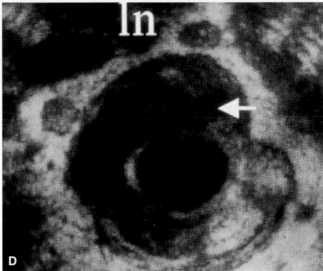

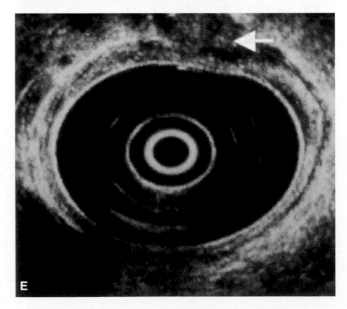

Figure 6–7.   Rectal cancer staging. *A,* Ultrasound staging schema for rectal cancer. *B,* Rectal ultrasound example of T1 cancer (arrow points to mass; mp: muscularis propria). *C,* Rectal ultrasound example of T2 cancer (arrow points to mass; mp: muscularis propria). *D,* Rectal ultrasound example of T3 cancer (arrow points to mass, note adjacent lymph nodes, ln). *E,* Rectal ultrasound example of recurrent cancer (arrow points to mass).

deciding whether surgical resection of the polypectomy site is necessary.[71] Similarly, EUS can document rectal cancer recurrence with sensitivities greater than rectal examinations or sigmoidoscopy.[72,73] Lymph node metastases can also be documented using EUS-guided biopsies.[68] Through the use of endosonography in the colon, malignant recurrences at an anastomosis can be diagnosed using the finding of an irregular hypoechoic mass.[74]

Carcinoid tumors can also be staged with linear array EUS.[75] The staging of carcinoids is particularly important and has a direct bearing on the treatment. Carcinoids localized to the rectal mucosa or submucosa can be treated with local or endoscopic excision.[31] Linear array endosonography and guided lymph node biopsies can accurately detect malignant nodes associated with the primary tumor with an overall staging accuracy of 90 percent.[75] The prognosis for small rectal carcinoids is excellent.[76]

ENDOSCOPIC MANAGEMENT OF COLON CANCER

Endoscopic removal of colon or rectal cancers is performed with either electrocautery or laser treatments (see Figure 6–2). Snare resection is the most commonly used technique for polyp removal and is ideal for pedunculated polyps. The stalk is transected with cautery and the polyp is retrieved. The complication rate of this technique is low, with bleeding being the most common complication.

Large sessile polyps at high risk for malignancy may have to be resected using piecemeal techniques[77] (Figure 6–8). This technique requires several snare excisions through the polyp and has a complication rate of 3 percent. Although 88 percent of patients will have a successful resection, malignant recurrence and the need for surgical resection are not uncommon. Incompletely resected malignant polyps or malignant polyps with malignancy present at the resection site should be surgically removed.[18] Polyps with unfavorable histology (poorly differentiated carcinoma) are associated with a greater chance of recurrence of metastasis.[17] Community pathologists have a significant rate of misdiagnosis on polyp specimens and will miss 31 percent of the findings of dysplasia.[78] Therefore, polyps with sus-

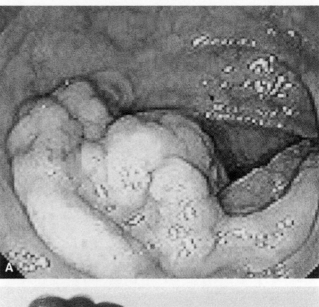

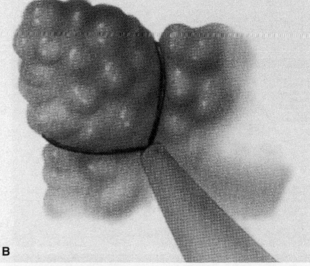

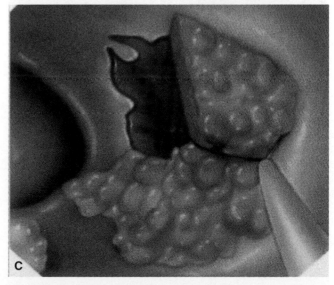

Figure 6–8.   Piecemeal polypectomy of a sessile polyp. *A,* Colonoscopic view of a large sessile villous adenoma. *B,* Snare resection of a portion of the sessile polyp. *C,* Piecemeal removal of a sessile polyp.

picious pathology should be carefully reviewed by experienced pathologists. Polyps requiring surgical removal should be marked with india ink injection during colonoscopy.[79] The tattooing enables the surgeon to readily identify the site of the polyp at the time of resection.

Piecemeal resection can also be used for large benign sessile adenomas. Injection of saline under the sessile polyps enables the endoscopist to minimize the risk of bleeding and perforation through the muscularis propria.[80] A success rate of 81 percent is achieved with localized adenomas and is higher than

the rates seen with laser ablation of sessile adenomas. Recurrence of adenomatous tissue after piecemeal resection of large polyps has been reported in 10 to 20 percent of patients.[81] Recurrence of benign adenomas may be effectively treated with superficial tissue coagulation.[82] The technique appears to be particularly useful in large, flat, benign adenomas.[83] The approach can also be used successfully for rectal carcinoids.[84]

Superficial colonic malignancies can be resected endoscopically. Saline injection under the tumor and demonstration of the lift sign indicates a tumor that is localized to the mucosa or submucosa.[85] This technique should be used only in patients that are not surgical candidates or when the superficial nature of the malignancy has been well established with staging.

Advanced or unresectable rectal cancers can be treated endoscopically for palliation or attempt at local control.[86] Through laser fulguration of malignant tissue, noncircumferential rectal tumors can be eliminated for periods of up to 36 months.[87] The use of chemotherapy and radiation in conjunction with cautery may provide prolonged tumor ablation.[88] Fulguration is particularly effective in patients with small recurrences after surgical resection. Rectal tumors can also be injected with chemotherapeutic agents with good local tumor response.[89] Complication rates of approximately 10 percent are noted after fulguration and include strictures, bleeding, and fistulas.[90] The use of lasers for large benign rectal villous adenomas may be less costly than surgical resection.[91] Endoscopically placed stents may improve the long-term patency of a malignant stricture after laser fulguration[92] (Figure 6–9).

CONCLUSION

Effective screening for colon cancer, using colonoscopy to detect and remove premalignant polyps and early cancers, can reduce the incidence and mortality of colon cancer.

REFERENCES

1. Hsu CW, Imperiale TF. Meta-analysis and cost comparison of polyethylene glycol lavage versus sodium phosphate for colonoscopy preparation. Gastrointest Endosc 1998;48:276–82.

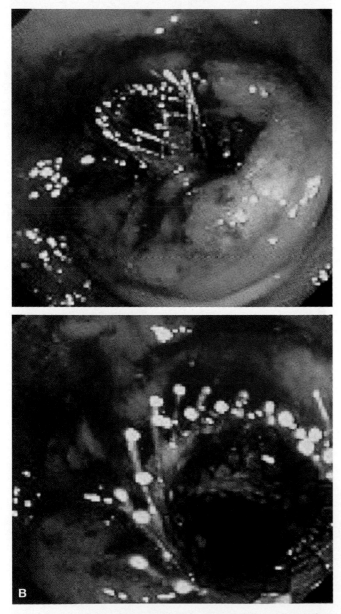

Figure 6–9.   Colon cancer stenting. An expandable metal stent has been placed into the lumen of a circumferential malignancy. Note protruding wire tips of metal wall stent.

2. Eckardt VF, Kanzler G, Schmitt T, et al. Complications and adverse effects of colonoscopy with selective sedation. Gastrointest Endosc 1999;49:560–5.

3. Rex DK, Rahmani EY, Haseman JH, et al. Relative sensitivity of colonoscopy and barium enema for detection of colorectal cancer in clinical practice. Gastroenterology 1997;112:17–23.

4. Bensen S, Mott LA, Dain B, et al. The colonoscopic miss rate and true one-year recurrence of colorectal neoplastic polyps. Polyp Prevention Study Group. Am J Gastroenterol 1999;94:194–9.

5. Rex DK, Imperiale TF, Portish V. Patients willing to try colonoscopy without sedation: associated clinical factors and results of a randomized controlled trial. Gastrointest Endosc 1999;49:554–9.

6. Zubarik R, Fleischer DE, Mastropietro C, et al. Prospective analysis of complications 30 days after outpatient colonoscopy. Gastrointest Endosc 1999; 50:322–8.

7. Orsoni P, Berdah S, Verrier C, et al. Colonic perforation due to colonoscopy: a retrospective study of 48 cases. Endoscopy 1997;29:160–4.

8. Stewart BT, Keck JO, Duncan AV, et al. Difficult or incomplete flexible sigmoidoscopy: implications for a screening programme. Aust N Z J Surg 1999; 69:19–21.

9. Wallace MB, Kemp JA, Meyer F, et al. Screening for colorectal cancer with flexible sigmoidoscopy by nonphysician endoscopists. Am J Med 1999;107: 214–8.

10. Rex DK, Cutler CS, Lemmel GT, et al. Colonoscopic miss rates of adenomas determined by back-to-back colonoscopies. Gastroenterology 1997;112:24–8.

11. Takayama T, Katsuki S, Takahashi Y, et al. Aberrant crypt foci of the colon as precursors of adenoma and cancer. N Engl J Med 1998;339:1277–84.

12. Fleischer DE. Chromoendoscopy and magnification endoscopy in the colon. Gastrointest Endosc 1999;49:S45–9.

13. Wallace MH, Frayling IM, Clark SK, et al. Attenuated adenomatous polyposis coli: the role of ascertainment bias through failure to dye-spray at colonoscopy. Dis Colon Rectum 1999;42:1078–80.

14. Read TE, Read JD, Butterly LF. Importance of adenomas 5 mm or less in diameter that are detected by sigmoidoscopy. N Engl J Med 1997;336:8–12.

15. Wallace MB, Kemp JA, Trnka YM, et al. Is colonoscopy indicated for small adenomas found by screening flexible sigmoidoscopy? Ann Intern Med 1998;129: 273–8.

16. Levin TR, Palitz A, Grossman S, et al. Predicting advanced proximal colonic neoplasia with screening sigmoidoscopy. JAMA 1999;281:1611–7.

17. Volk EE, Goldblum JR, Petras RE, et al. Management and outcome of patients with invasive carcinoma arising in colorectal polyps. Gastroenterology 1995;109:1801–7.

18. Netzer P, Forster C, Biral R, et al. Risk factor assessment of endoscopically removed malignant colorectal polyps. Gut 1998;43:669–74.

19. Detry R, Kartheuser A, Hermans BP, et al. Colorectal villous tumors accuracy of the preoperative biopsies. Acta Gastroenterol Belg 1999;62:9–12.

20. Togashi K, Konishi F, Ishizuka T, et al. Efficacy of magnifying endoscopy in the differential diagnosis of neoplastic and non-neoplastic polyps of the large bowel. Dis Colon Rectum 1999;42:1602–8.

21. Mycek MA, Schomacker KT, Nishioka NS. Colonic polyp differentiation using time-resolved autofluorescence spectroscopy. Gastrointest Endosc 1998;48: 390–4.

22. Eker C, Montan S, Jaramillo E, et al. Clinical spectral characterisation of colonic mucosal lesions using autofluorescence and delta aminolevulinic acid sensitisation. Gut 1999;44:511–8.

23. Wang TD, Crawford JM, Feld MS, et al. In vivo identification of colonic dysplasia using fluorescence endoscopic imaging. Gastrointest Endosc 1999;49: 447–55.

24. Sciallero S, Costantini M, Bertinelli E, et al. Distal hyperplastic polyps do not predict proximal adenomas: results from a multicentric study of colorectal adenomas. Gastrointest Endosc 1997;46:124–30.

25. Rex DK, Chak A, Vasudeva R, et al. Prospective determination of distal colon findings in average-risk patients with proximal colon cancer. Gastrointest Endosc 1999;49:727–30.

26. Provenzale D, Garrett JW, Condon SE, Sandler RS. Risk for colon adenomas in patients with rectosigmoid hyperplastic polyps. Ann Intern Med 1990; 113:760–3.

27. Croizet O, Moreau J, Arany Y, et al. Follow-up of patients with hyperplastic polyps of the large bowel. Gastrointest Endosc 1997;46:119–23.

28. Jaramillo E, Watanabe M, Slezak P, Rubio C. Flat neoplastic lesions of the colon and rectum detected by high-resolution video endoscopy and chromoscopy. Gastrointest Endosc 1995;42:114–22.

29. Tada S, Iida M, Matsumoto T, et al. Small flat cancer of the rectum: clinicopathologic and endoscopic features. Gastrointest Endosc 1995;42:109–13.

30. Saitoh Y, Obara T, Watari J, et al. Invasion depth diagnosis of depressed type early colorectal cancers by combined use of videoendoscopy and chromoendoscopy. Gastrointest Endosc 1998;48:362–70.

31. Matsumoto T, Iida M, Suekane H, et al. Endoscopic ultrasonography in rectal carcinoid tumors: contribution to selection of therapy. Gastrointest Endosc 1991;37:539–42.

32. Schoenfeld P, Lipscomb S, Crook J, et al. Accuracy of polyp detection by gastroenterologists and nurse endoscopists during flexible sigmoidoscopy: a randomized trial. Gastroenterology 1999;117:312–8.

33. Rex DK, Chak A, Vasudeva R, et al. Prospective determination of distal colon findings in average-risk patients with proximal colon cancer. Gastrointest Endosc 1999;49:727–30.

34. Schoen RE, Corle D, Cranston L, et al. Is colonoscopy needed for the nonadvanced adenoma found on sigmoidoscopy? The Polyp Prevention Trial. Gastroenterology 1998;115:533–41.

35. Sciallero S, Bonelli L, Aste H, et al. Do patients with rectosigmoid adenomas 5 mm or less in diameter need total colonoscopy? Gastrointest Endosc 1999;50:314–21.

36. Collett JA, Platell C, Fletcher DR, et al. Distal colonic neoplasms predict proximal neoplasia in average-risk, asymptomatic subjects. J Gastroenterol Hepatol 1999;14:67–71.

37. Netzer P, Buttiker U, Pfister M, et al. Frequency of advanced neoplasia in the proximal colon without an index polyp in the rectosigmoid. Dis Colon Rectum 1999;42:661–7.

38. Khullar SK, DiSario JA. Colon cancer screening. Sigmoidoscopy or colonoscopy. Gastrointest Endosc Clin N Am 1997;7:365–86.

39. Bertario L, Russo A, Sala P, et al. Risk of colorectal cancer following colonoscopic polypectomy. Tumori 1999;85:157–62.

40. van Stolk RU, Beck GJ, Baron JA, et al. Adenoma characteristics at first colonoscopy as predictors of adenoma recurrence and characteristics at follow-up. The Polyp Prevention Study Group. Gastroenterology 1998;115:13–8.

41. Winawer SJ, Zauber AG, O'Brien MJ, et al. Randomized comparison of surveillance intervals after colonoscopic removal of newly diagnosed adenomatous polyps. The National Polyp Study Workgroup. N Engl J Med 1993;328:901–6.

42. American Society for Gastrointestinal Endoscopy. ASGE guidelines for clinical application. The role of colonoscopy in the management of patients with colonic polyps neoplasia. Gastrointest Endosc 1999;50:921–4.

43. Winawer SJ, Zauber AG, Ho MN, et al. Prevention of colorectal cancer by colonoscopic polypectomy. The National Polyp Study Workgroup. N Engl J Med 1993;329:1977–81.

44. Muller AD, Sonnenberg A. Prevention of colorectal cancer by flexible endoscopy and polypectomy. A case-control study of 32,702 veterans. Ann Intern Med 1995;123:904–10.

45. Atkin WS, Morson BC, Cuzick J. Long-term risk of colorectal cancer after excision of rectosigmoid adenomas. N Engl J Med 1992;326:658–62.

46. Finn-Faivre C, Maurel J, Benhamiche AM, et al. Evidence of improving survival of patients with rectal cancer in France: a population based study. Gut 1999;44:377–381.

47. Syngal S, Weeks JC, Schrag D, et al. Benefits of colonoscopic surveillance and prophylactic colectomy in patients with hereditary nonpolyposis colorectal cancer mutations. Ann Intern Med 1998;129:787–96.

48. Vasen HF, van Ballegooijen M, Buskens E, et al. A cost-effectiveness analysis of colorectal screening of hereditary nonpolyposis colorectal carcinoma gene carriers. Cancer 1998;82:1632–7.

49. Cromwell DM, Moore RD, Brensinger JD, et al. Cost analysis of alternative approaches to colorectal screening in familial adenomatous polyposis. Gastroenterology 1998;114:893–901.

50. Matsumoto T, Iida M, Tada S, et al. Early detection of nonpolypoid cancers in the rectal remnant in patients with familial adenomatous polyposis/Gardner's syndrome. Cancer 1994;74:12–5.

51. Karlen P, Kornfeld D, Brostrom O, et al. Is colonoscopic surveillance reducing colorectal cancer mortality in ulcerative colitis? A population based case control study. Gut 1998;42:711–4.

52. Engelsgjerd M, Farraye FA, Odze RD. Polypectomy may be adequate treatment for adenoma-like dysplastic lesions in chronic ulcerative colitis. Gastroenterology 1999;117:1288–94; discussion 1488–91.

53. Garas G, Choi PM, Nugent FW, et al. Colonoscopic surveillance in ulcerative colitis. Colonoscopic surveillance reduces mortality from colorectal cancer in ulcerative colitis. Gut 1999;44:580.

54. Karlen P, Kornfeld D, Brostrom O, et al. Is colonoscopic surveillance reducing colorectal cancer mortality in ulcerative colitis? A population based case control study. Gut 1998;42:711–4.

55. Hunt LM, Rooney PS, Hardcastle JD, Armitage NC. Endoscopic screening of relatives of patients with colorectal cancer. Gut 1998;42:71–5.

56. Ahsan H, Neugut AI, Garbowski GC, et al. Family history of colorectal adenomatous polyps and increased risk for colorectal cancer. Ann Intern Med 1998;128:900–5.

57. Joosten E, Ghesquiere B, Linthoudt H, et al. Upper and lower gastrointestinal evaluation of elderly inpatients who are iron deficient. Am J Med 1999;107:24–9.

58. Kepczyk T, Cremins JE, Long BD, et al. A prospective, multidisciplinary evaluation of premenopausal women with iron-deficiency anemia. Am J Gastroenterol 1999;94:109–15.

59. Tio TL, Coene PP, van Delden OM, Tytgat GN. Colorectal carcinoma: preoperative TNM classification with endosonography. Radiology 1991;179:165–70.

60. Roubein LD, David C, DuBrow R, et al. Endoscopic ultrasonography in staging rectal cancer. Am J Gastroenterol 1990;85:1391–4.

61. Kaneko K, Boku N, Hosokawa K, et al. Diagnostic utility of endoscopic ultrasonography for preoperative rectal cancer staging estimation. Jpn J Clin Oncol 1996;26:30–5.

62. Massari M, De Simone M, Cioffi U, et al. Value and limits of endorectal ultrasonography for preoperative staging of rectal carcinoma. Surg Laparosc Endosc 1998;8:438–44.

63. Boyce GA, Sivak MV Jr, Lavery IC, et al. Endoscopic ultrasound in the pre-operative staging of rectal carcinoma. Gastrointest Endosc 1992;38:468–71.

64. Spinelli P, Schiavo M, Meroni E, et al. Results of EUS in detecting perirectal lymph node metastases of rectal cancer: the pathologist makes the difference. Gastrointest Endosc 1999;49:754–8.

65. Adams DR, Blatchford GJ, Lin KM, et al. Use of pre-operative ultrasound staging for treatment of rectal cancer. Dis Colon Rectum 1999;42:159–66.

66. Goletti O, Celona G, Galatioto C, et al. Is laparoscopic sonography a reliable and sensitive procedure for staging colorectal cancer? A comparative study. Surg Endosc 1998;12:1236–41.

67. Kim NK, Kim MJ, Yun SH, et al. Comparative study of transrectal ultrasonography, pelvic computerized tomography, and magnetic resonance imaging in preoperative staging of rectal cancer. Dis Colon Rectum 1999;42:770–5.

68. Meyenberger C, Huch Boni RA, Bertschinger P, et al. Endoscopic ultrasound and endorectal magnetic resonance imaging: a prospective, comparative study for preoperative staging and follow-up of rectal cancer. Endoscopy 1995;27:469–79.

69. Kulling D, Feldman DR, Kay CL, et al. Local staging of anal and distal colorectal tumors with the magnetic resonance endoscope. Gastrointest Endosc 1998;47:172–8.

70. Hildebrandt U, Feifel G. Importance of endoscopic ultrasonography staging for treatment of rectal cancer. Gastrointest Endosc Clin N Am 1995;5:843–9.

71. Kruskal JB, Sentovich SM, Kane RA. Staging of rectal cancer after polypectomy: usefulness of endorectal US. Radiology 1999;211:31–5.

72. Romano G, Belli G, Rotondano G. Colorectal cancer. Diagnosis of recurrence. Gastrointest Endosc Clin N Am 1995;5:831–41.

73. Ramirez JM, Mortensen NJ, Takeuchi N, Humphreys MM. Endoluminal ultrasonography in the follow-up of patients with rectal cancer. Br J Surg 1994;81:692–4.

74. Giovannini M, Bernardini D, Seitz JF, et al. Value of endoscopic ultrasonography for assessment of patients presenting elevated tumor marker levels after surgery for colorectal cancers. Endoscopy 1998;30:469–76.

75. Yoshikane H, Tsukamoto Y, Niwa Y, et al. Carcinoid tumors of the gastrointestinal tract: evaluation with endoscopic ultrasonography. Gastrointest Endosc 1993;39:375–83.

76. Matsui K, Iwase T, Kitagawa M. Small, polypoid-appearing carcinoid tumors of the rectum: clinicopathologic study of 16 cases and effectiveness of endoscopic treatment. Am J Gastroenterol 1993;88:1949–53.

77. Walsh RM, Ackroyd FW, Shellito PC. Endoscopic resection of large sessile colorectal polyps. Gastrointest Endosc 1992;38:303–9.

78. Rex DK, Alikhan M, Cummings O, Ulbright TM. Accuracy of pathologic interpretation of colorectal polyps by general pathologists in community practice. Gastrointest Endosc 1999;50:468–74.

79. McArthur CS, Roayaie S, Waye JD. Safety of preoperation endoscopic tattoo with india ink for identification of colonic lesions. Surg Endosc 1999;13:397–400.

80. De Palma GD, Caiazzo C, Di Matteo E, et al. Endoscopic treatment of sessile rectal adenomas: comparison of Nd:YAG laser therapy and injection-assisted piecemeal polypectomy. Gastrointest Endosc 1995;41:553–6.

81. Binmoeller KF, Bohnacker S, Seifert H, et al. Endoscopic snare excision of "giant" colorectal polyps. Gastrointest Endosc 1996;43:183–8.

82. Zlatanic J, Waye JD, Kim PS, et al. Large sessile colonic adenomas: use of argon plasma coagulator to supplement piecemeal snare polypectomy. Gastrointest Endosc 1999;49:731–5.

83. Kanamori T, Itoh M, Yokoyama Y, Tsuchida K. Injection-incision–assisted snare resection of large sessile colorectal polyps. Gastrointest Endosc 1996;43:189–95.

84. Higaki S, Nishiaki M, Mitani N, et al. Effectiveness of local endoscopic resection of rectal carcinoid tumors. Endoscopy 1997;29:171–5.

85. Ishiguro A, Uno Y, Ishiguro Y, et al. Correlation of lifting versus non-lifting and microscopic depth of invasion in early colorectal cancer. Gastrointest Endosc 1999;50:329–33.

86. Dohmoto M, Hunerbein M, Schlag PM. Palliative endoscopic therapy of rectal carcinoma. Eur J Cancer 1996;32A:25–9.

87. Escourrou J, Delvaux M, Buscail L, et al. Nd:YAG laser in treatment of rectal cancer. Are there features predicting a curative result? Dig Dis Sci 1994;39:464–72.

88. Graham RA, Hackford AW, Wazer DE, et al. Local excision of rectal carcinoma: a safe alternative for more advanced tumors? Postsurgical surveillance of colon cancer: preliminary cost analysis of physician examination, carcinoembryonic antigen testing, chest x-ray, and colonoscopy. J Surg Oncol 1999;70:235–8.

89. Hagiwara A, Hirata Y, Takahashi T. A pilot study of fiberscopy-guided local injection of anti-cancer drugs bound to carbon particles for control of rectal cancer. Anticancer Drugs 1998;9:363–7.

90. Hyser MJ, Gau FC. Endoscopic Nd:YAG laser therapy for villous adenomas of the colon and rectum. Am Surg 1996;62:577–81.

91. Brunetaud JM, Maunoury V, Cochelard D, et al. Endoscopic laser treatment for rectosigmoid villous adenoma: factors affecting the results. Gastroenterology 1989;97:272–7.

92. Tack J, Gevers AM, Rutgeerts P. Self-expandable metallic stents in the palliation of rectosigmoidal carcinoma: a follow-up study. Gastrointest Endosc 1998;48:267–71.

7

Diagnostic Radiology of Colon and Rectal Cancer

MARK L. MONTGOMERY, MD
PETER R. MUELLER, MD

Evaluating colorectal neoplasms by means of radiographic imaging continues to play a major role in detecting and staging cancer of the lower gastrointestinal tract. A variety of imaging modalities can be used in staging, detection, and follow-up of patients with colorectal carcinoma. The diagnosis of colon cancer has traditionally been made on the basis of barium enema and/or colonoscopy. Computed tomography (CT) scanning is typically used in the evaluation of patients with known colonic neoplasms or in the detection of colorectal tumors in patients with nonspecific abdominal complaints. Virtual colonoscopy is a relatively new method of imaging colonic mucosa that uses virtual-reality software and CT. Magnetic resonance imaging (MRI) is extremely helpful in detection and characterization of suspected hepatic metastases, particularly in the setting of a negative CT scan. MRI is also effective in the staging of tumor for local extension. Transrectal ultrasonography has become popular in staging tumors for local extension because of its ability to demonstrate the various layers of the colon wall. Positron emission tomography (PET) is helpful in following patients with colorectal neoplasms and gauging therapeutic treatment responses.

BARIUM ENEMA

Barium enema continues to be a safe, accurate, and effective means of diagnosing colonic polyps and cancer. Polyps measuring 1 cm in diameter have a 10 percent chance of harboring malignancy.[1,2] The sensitivity of a colonic examination is therefore judged on its ability to detect lesions of this size. The sensitivity of detecting 1-cm polyps has been reported in the 90 to 95 percent range by barium enema.[3,4] Single-contrast and double-contrast barium enema studies have reported equal sensitivity in the detection of 1-cm polyps. Double-contrast studies, however, more frequently detect smaller polyps with greater reliability.[5]

Adequate bowel preparation is required before performing a barium enema. As in CT and virtual colonoscopy, the presence of fecal material is the most common reason for false-positive findings.[6] At our institution, patients arc instructed to eat a nonresidue diet 24 hours before the examination and then drink a solution of magnesium citrate. Magnesium citrate, magnesium hydroxide, and sodium phosphate are hyperosmolar solutions that act as laxatives by drawing fluid into the bowel lumen and promoting peristalsis. Adequate fluid intake during this process is important to prevent dehydration. Bisacodyl tablets are recommended at bedtime to increase bowel peristalsis. The morning of the examination, the patient is instructed not to eat or drink and to administer a suppository.

The selection of single- or double-contrast barium enema depends largely on the patient's ability to cooperate with the examination. Elderly patients who are unable to maneuver themselves on the fluoroscopic table are typically not candidates for double-contrast studies. Double contrast, however, is preferred by most gastrointestinal radiologists because of the more reliable detection of small lesions (< 1 cm).[5] Performing meticulous compression throughout the colon during single-contrast examination has been touted as equally effective in lesion detection.[7] Barium enema should not be performed in patients with toxic megacolon. The risk of perforation in barium enema has been reported at 1:2,500 to 1:12,500.[3,8] The mortality rate of barium has been reported at 1:50,000.[3,8]

Single-contrast barium enema is performed after the rectal placement of a catheter and the infusion of low-weight per volume barium. Intravenous glucagon can be administered to help prevent spasm during the examination. Adequate distention of the colon with contrast followed by careful compression of the entire colon are extremely important technical considerations. Spot radiographs are taken during the examination of all suspicious findings. Postevacuation films are performed to detect lesions that may have been obscured by overlying barium. Postevacuation films are also helpful in the detection of extravasated contrast.

Double-contrast barium enema is performed after the administration of viscous barium. Air or carbon dioxide is then administered to coat the walls of the colon with a thin, even coat of barium. Patients are maneuvered in multiple positions on the fluoroscopic table to maximize the technique. Spot views are obtained of suspicious findings.

Polyps typically appear as small filling defects on barium enema (Figure 7–1). Polyps have a variety of shapes and appearances, including circular, oval, or pedunculated.[9] The size of the stalk of a polyp is important to evaluate. Stalks longer than 2 cm are not usually associated with malignant invasion into the adjacent wall.[10] Polyps measuring between 0.6 and 1 cm should proceed to biopsy.[11]

Colorectal neoplasm has a variety of morphologic appearances. Lesions typically appear as annular regions of poor distensibility and have been likened to the appearance of an apple core (Figure 7–2). These lesions have a sharp transition point to a more normal-appearing colon. Sharp shouldering usually demarcates the lesion. Lesions can also have a semiannular or saddle appearance. Scirrhous neoplasms may produce marked bowel wall thickening. Extravasation of contrast producing the double-tract sign has also been reported with colonic neoplasm.[12]

Barium enema and colonoscopy should be considered complementary examinations. Barium enema and colonoscopy have a similar sensitivity rate for detecting lesions within the colon.[13,14] Colonoscopy carries a greater risk of perforation, with rates reported between 1:200 and 1:5,000.[15] Colonoscopy is approximately 3 to 5 times more expensive than barium enema. Although experienced colonoscopists reach the cecum in 95 percent of patients, rates of less experienced operators can be highly variable. Barium studies are rarely unsuccessful in reaching the cecum. Colonoscopy, however, has the added advantage of a lower false-positive error rate since this technique easily differentiates polyps from stool. Biopsy and polypectomy are tremendous advantages of colonoscopy. By optimizing the combination of

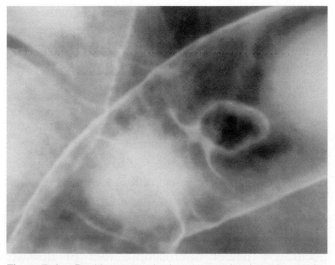

Figure 7–1. Double-contrast barium enema showing a 2-cm polyp in the sigmoid colon arising from a small stalk. Image courtesy of Dr. Deborah Hall.

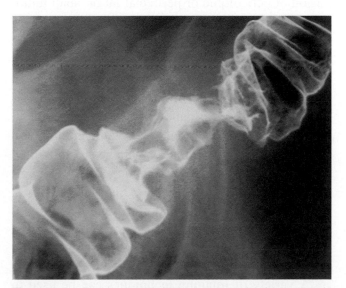

Figure 7–2. Double-contrast barium enema showing an "apple core" lesion involving the sigmoid colon.

examinations to the individual patient, the accuracy of colorectal carcinoma detection can be achieved with maximum benefit to the patient.

COMPUTED TOMOGRAPHY

Computed tomography scanning has become the workhorse diagnostic imaging modality in detecting, staging, and following patients with cancer of the lower gastrointestinal tract. It is an efficient means of obtaining a global assessment of the entire abdomen and pelvis. In addition, CT scanning can determine the thickness of the colonic wall involved with tumor and depict the relationship of the neoplasm with surrounding structures. Metastases to adjacent structures, adrenal glands, lymph nodes, liver, bony structures, and musculature can be ascertained.

Studies consistently indicate that CT is an excellent means of initially staging primary or secondary colorectal tumor. The sensitivity of detecting hepatic metastases has been well documented in the literature, with rates ranging from 85 to 90 percent.[16] Accuracy rates have been reported around 70 percent for determining local tumor extension.[17] CT scanning is particularly useful in staging patients with Dukes stage D lesions, which may lead to changes in surgical planning or preoperative management. Positive predictive value rates have been reported at 100 percent for CT staging of Dukes D lesions.[18] Frequently, however, CT may understage patients with microinvasion of pericolonic or perirectal fat or small tumor foci in normal-sized nodes. Lymph node sensitivity detection has been reported as low as 25.9 percent.[19]

Advances in CT technology have enabled scanners to obtain images in less than 1 second per slice. Helical CT scanning produces continuous three-dimensional CT information by allowing the table to move continuously through a rotating radiograph producing gantry. Information can then be formatted in variable slice thickenesses since a helix, or volume of information, is obtained. Shorter scan times, reduction in patient organ motion, and the ability to acquire images rapidly after intravenous contrast enhancement are advantages of the newer generation CT scanners.[20]

A variety of imaging techniques can be used to enhance images obtained by CT. Intravenous contrast is extremely important in achieving differences in conspicuity between normal and abnormal tissue. Two types of intravenous contrast media are typically available: ionic and nonionic. Nonionic contrast is generally preferred because of its lower incidence of adverse allergic reactions. Adequate opacification of the alimentary tract is required for assessment of mucosal detail in the colon. Adequate distention of the colon can usually be achieved when the patient receives approximately 700 cc of contrast orally. The administration of rectal contrast has also proven helpful in detection and staging of colorectal neoplasm.

The normal distended colonic wall usually measures less than or equal to 3 mm. Wall measurements greater than 6 mm in diameter are considered abnormal[20] (Figure 7–3). Extracolonic tumor spread is suggested by loss of the normal black-appearing pericolonic fat. Streaky, irregular strands of soft tissue density may be seen invading the pericolonic fat by tumor. Tumor may manifest as a large irregular mass, and extracolonic spread can be definitive if invasion into adjacent muscles, bone, or organs is seen (Figure 7–4). Areas of low density within a mass may indicate tumor necrosis. Calcifications within the tumor may suggest a mucinous adenocarcinoma. Abnormal air density in surrounding structures may represent an associated fistulous tract with the tumor. Liver metastases manifest as foci of low density on nonintravenous contrast images and will exhibit fairly uniform enhancement after the administration of intravenous contrast (Figure 7–5). Peritoneal carcinomatosis appears as irregular, soft tissue density masses within the omentum and enhancement of the peritoneal lining after the administration of intravenous contrast.

Computed tomography scanning is a cost effective means of evaluating the entire abdomen and pelvis. The average cost of an abdominal and pelvic CT scan ranges from US $300 to US $1,000. The ease of performing and scheduling a CT has resulted in a 75 percent increase in the volume of examinations over the past 5 years at our institution. As previously mentioned, CT is inadequate in its ability to accurately detect microscopic foci of disease. Images from CT scans can be degraded by artifacts. For example, beam-hardening artifact from a hip prosthesis can markedly impair evaluation of the pelvis. CT scanning, however, continues to be the preferred imaging modality at our institution for staging colorectal neoplasm.

VIRTUAL COLONOSCOPY

Simulated endoscopic visualization of the colon is a new imaging technique used to evaluate the hollow organ viscous. Virtual colonoscopy makes use of specific computer algorithms of helical CT data sets to acquire images that can be viewed two-dimensionally or three-dimensionally. The radiologist can view the colon as if perceiving motion similar to conventional endoscopy (Figures 7–6 to 7–9).

The technique of virtual colonoscopy requires adequate bowel cleansing and the insufflation of air through a rectal enema tube. Intravenous glucagon is usually administered to relieve spasm and reduce motion artifact. Images of the abdomen and pelvis are usually obtained in a single breathhold, with a scan slice thickness of 5 mm that can be reconstructed at 2-mm intervals. The CT data can then be

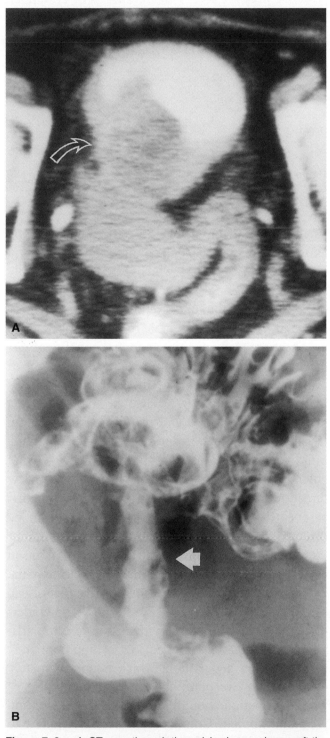

Figure 7–3. *A,* CT scan through the pelvis shows a large soft tissue attenuation lesion involving the distal sigmoid colon. *B,* Barium enema of the same apple core appearing lesion involving the distal sigmoid colon.

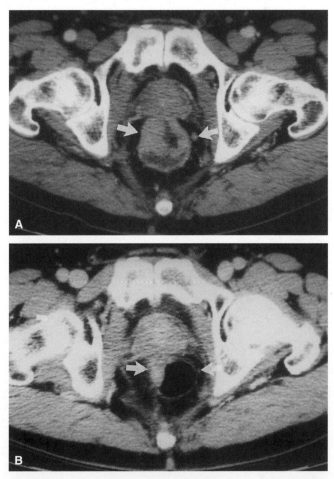

Figure 7–4. *A,* CT scan of the pelvis showing a rectal carcinoma with an associated pericolonic lymph node before radiation and chemotherapy. *B,* CT scan shows interval reduction in size of the rectal tumor and lymph node following radiation and chemotherapy.

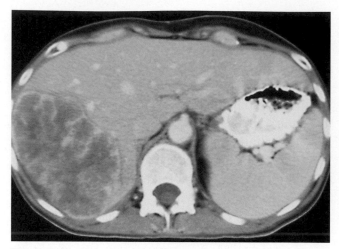

Figure 7–5. CT scan of the abdomen performed after the intravenous adminstration of contrast shows a large metastatic lesion involving the right lobe of the liver with a central area of low density representing necrosis.

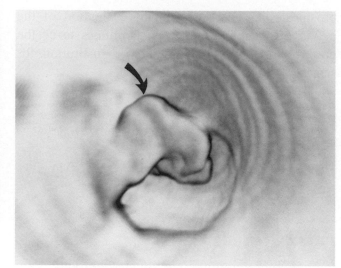

Figure 7–7. Virtual colonoscopy image of a 4.5-cm splenic flexure carcinoma. Image courtesy of Dr. Helen Fenlon.

downloaded to computer workstations equipped with software capable of producing volume rendering analysis.

Initial studies regarding the accuracy, sensitivity, and specificity of virtual colonoscopy have been encouraging.[21] A recent study was able to prospectively identify and localize 100 percent of cancers in the evaluation of 38 patients.[21] All polyps greater than 6 mm in diameter were also identified in this study. Other studies using CT colonographic techniques detected 100 percent of all polyps greater than 1 cm in diameter, 71 percent of polyps between 0.5 and 0.9 cm, and up to 28 percent of polyps

smaller than 0.5 cm in size.[22–24] Virtual colonoscopy allows for adequate visualization of the entire colon in 92 percent of cases, which compares favorably with conventional endoscopy.[20] Polyps were detected proximal to constricting carcinomas in segments of bowel not accessible to endoscopy.

There are many exciting potential benefits of virtual colonoscopy. The test is a noninvasive means of evaluating the entire colon. The risk of perforation is low, approximately 0.075 percent.[25] No anesthesia or sedation is required and scan time is possible in less than 60 seconds. Lesions can be detected on the blind side of haustral folds because virtual colonoscopy does not have the limitation of view direction. The entire colon can be evaluated and disease extent beyond the mucosa of bowel can be detected from the conventional helical CT data set.

Virtual colonoscopy is an imaging technique in evolution. There are limitations to performing the examination in its current form. Retained stool can often mimic and disguise bowel pathology. Under- or overdistention of bowel with air can result in artifacts. The radiation dose is low at approximately 0.44 rems per acquisition, which is approximately equivalent to two plain abdominal radiographs.[24,26] The examination should be avoided in children and pregnant women. Colonoscopy is still required to confirm findings and for biopsy.

As computer software technology capable of producing surface rendering improves, CT virtual

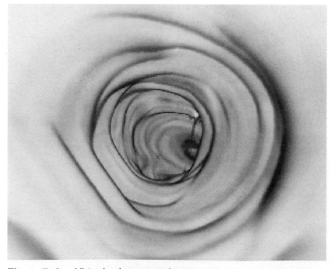

Figure 7–6. Virtual colonoscopy image of the normal colon. Image courtesy of Dr. Helen Fenlon.

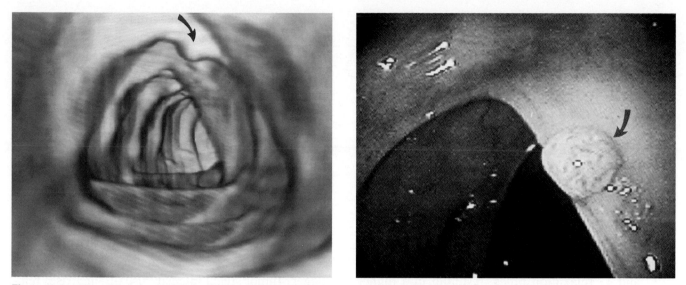

Figure 7–8. Virtual and conventional colonoscopy images of a 6-mm transverse colon polyp. Images courtesy of Dr. Helen Fenlon.

colonoscopy may indeed become a routine screening devise for colorectal disease. Large-scale, prospective, multicenter trials are needed to determine the true accuracy of this imaging method. Until that time, CT virtual colonoscopy is an imaging technique in its infancy with great promise for screening the colon in a timely, cost-effective, and noninvasive manner.

MAGNETIC RESONANCE IMAGING

Magnetic resonance imaging is becoming increasingly popular in the diagnosis and staging of colorectal cancer. The advent of new imaging techniques, such as superior phased array pelvic and endorectal coils, as well as the administration of rectal contrast agents, has improved image quality. The multiplanar imaging capabilities of MRI offer a special advantage of this modality.

Images produced by MRI are based on the interactions between protons in tissues within an alternating magnetic field. Hydrogen protons become excited when a specific radio frequency (RF) is applied. These protons subsequently return to equilibrium (relaxation), resulting in a release of RF energy called an echo. The relaxation of hydrogen protons to equilibrium has been designated T_1 and T_2.

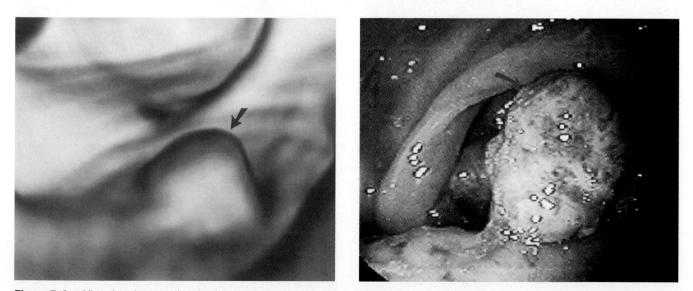

Figure 7–9. Virtual and conventional colonoscopy images of a 15-mm dysplatic cecal polyp. Images courtesy of Dr. Helen Fenlon.

MRI images can be varied by changing the interval between RF pulses (T_R) and the time between the RF pulse and the signal reception (T_E). T_1-weighted images are formed by keeping the T_R and T_E shorter; T_2-weighted images are produced by keeping T_R and T_E longer. Different biologic tissues have characteristic MRI appearances. Free water, such as seen in edema, have a long T_1 and T_2 relaxation and will appear low in signal intensity on T_1-weighted images and high in signal intensity on T_2-weighted images. Fat behaves differently and demonstrates short T_1 relaxation times. Fat therefore appears high in signal intensity on T_1-weighted images. Gadolinium is a paramagnetic contrast agent that causes a reduction in T_1 and T_2 relaxation times, resulting in a higher signal on T_1-weighted images.

Studies have shown MRI to be equally effective in staging colorectal tumors when compared to CT.[27] Overall staging accuracies have been reported at 74 to 82 percent.[27–30] Although only a few studies with small patient populations have been reported using endorectal coils for staging colorectal cancer, initial results have been encouraging, with sensitivities reported at 92 percent for the assessment of local tumor extension[31] (Figure 7–10). MRI has proven particularly useful in the search for hepatic metastases when CT results are technically unsatisfactory or when clinical evaluation is in conflict with good-quality CT results.[32] Favorable results have been reported in staging patients with recurrent colorectal neoplasm, with accuracies reported in the 95 percent range.[33] MRI, like CT, has difficulty in diagnosing metastatic local lymph node involvement, with accuracies of correctly diagnosing lymph nodes reported around 60 percent.[34] Perirectal fat infiltration is also difficult to diagnosis, with reported accuracies of only 71 percent for T3 tumors.[35]

Colorectal neoplasms typically appear as areas of wall thickening, with signal intensity equal to or slightly higher than skeletal muscle on T_1-weighted images (Figures 7–11 and 7–12). Gadolinium enhancement results in better definition of the tumor resulting in higher signal intensity on T_1-weighted images. Tumor signal intensity usually increases relative to skeletal muscle on spin echo T_2-weighted images. T_2-weighted images are typically not as useful in detecting extracolonic tumor extension because of the relatively long T_2 relaxation times of perirectal fat and tumor resulting in poor contrast differences. For rectal cancer, MRI performed in the coronal plane can be helpful in determining whether tumor involves the sphincter near the anal verge. Metastatic liver lesions enhance with gadolinum and usually appear of high signal intensity on T_1-weighted images. On T_2-weighted images, metastases to liver from colorectal neoplasm appear of high signal intensity. Bone metastases are usually easily detected with MRI and are depicted as a loss of normal marrow signal.

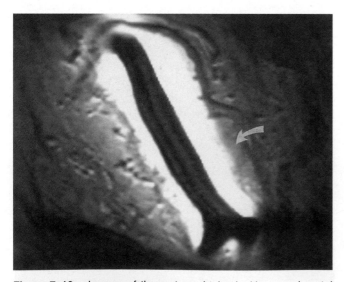

Figure 7–10. Images of the rectum obtained with an endorectal coil in place demonstrating marked thickening of the rectum representing a large adenocarcinoma.

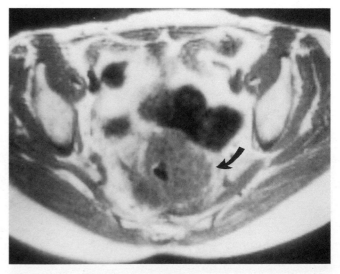

Figure 7–11. Axial images through the pelvis show a large irregular mass involving the rectum, with disruption of the perirectal fat planes.

MRI and CT should be considered complementary in the work-up of colorectal neoplasms. MRI is usually not used as a first-step imaging modality. As previously mentioned, MRI is particularly helpful when there is a high clinical suspicion of hepatic metastases despite a high-quality negative CT scan. MRI and CT are helpful in determining whether a patient will benefit from preoperative radiation or if a sphincter-saving procedure can be performed in rectal carcinoma.[20] CT and MRI are also helpful in designing radiation ports of patients. As accessibility and imaging techniques continue to improve, MRI will undoubtedly play a greater role in the future evaluation of colorectal neoplasm.

ULTRASONOGRAPHY

Transrectal ultrasonography (TRUS) has recently become popular in staging colonic malignancy. TRUS allows visualization of the layers of the colonic wall; therefore, the depth of tumor extension can be ascertained. Pericolonic nodes and extension beyond the serosa can often be diagnosed with TRUS.

Sensitivities ranging from 67 to 96 percent for detection of tumor spread beyond the rectal wall have been reported.[19,36,37] Detection of local adenopathy has been reported at 50 to 75 percent.[19,36,37] Although perirectal infiltration of tumor is usually detected with sensitivities as high as 97 percent, the specificity of examining the perirectal region is low, with numbers reported at 24 percent.[38] Advanced neoplasms are often difficult to evaluate with TRUS and are generally better assessed with CT or MRI.

Images produced from TRUS appear as rings radiating from a transducer that is placed within the colonic lumen. The transducer is covered with a balloon filled with water that appears hypoechoic (black).[20] The various layers of the colonic wall produce different levels of echogenicity. The innermost ring appears as a hyperechoic band (white) and represents the interface of the balloon with mucosa.[20] The second layer seen appears relatively hypoechoic and represents the muscularis mucosa.[20] The third layer is hyperechoic and represents the submucosa.[20] The fourth ring seen is hypoechoic and represents the muscularis propria.[20] The fifth layer is hyperechoic and represents the interface between pericolonic fat and the serosa of the colon.[20]

Colorectal neoplasms often appear as hypoechoic nodules within the wall of the colon. Extent of tumor within the colon is depicted by disruption of the various ultrasonographic layers as previously described (Figures 7–13 and 7–14). Although it is often difficult to distinguish malignant and benign nodes by TRUS, malignant nodes may appear hypoechoic surrounded by the more echogenic fat.

TRUS combined with endoscopy provides a unique method of assessing colonic neoplasm. Lesions can be detected, staged for local extension invasion, and biopsied in one setting. The presence or absence of pericolonic nodes is often possible. CT or MRI is, however, required for assessment of distant metastases.

Recently a new ultrasonographic technique, hydrocolonic sonography, has been described; it uses water instillation into the colon. The abdomen is then scanned with a traditional transabdominal

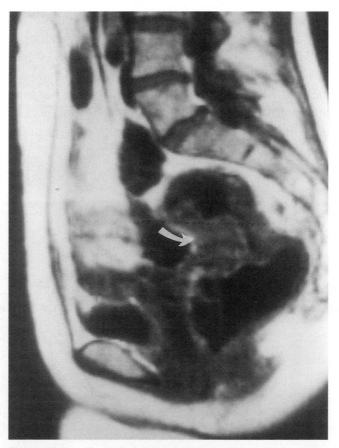

Figure 7–12. T_1 sagittal images demonstrate a large annular lesion involving the distal sigmoid colon.

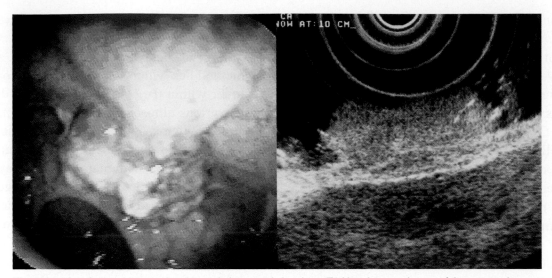

Figure 7–13.   Colonoscopy and endorectal ultrasound showing a T2 N0 adenocarcinoma of the rectum. Images courtesy of Drs. Richard Erickson and Andrejs Avots-Avotins, Scott and White Clinic, Temple, TX.

technique. This examination is usually well tolerated by the patient and has been reported to adequately examine the entire extent of the colon in 97 percent of patients in a prospective trial of 300 patients.[38] Hydrocolonic sonography was able to diagnosis 97 percent of colorectal carcinoma and detect 91 percent of polyps greater than 7 mm in this trial.[38] A detailed evaluation of the colonic wall was also possible. Detection of distant metastases was possible because the examination was performed transabdominally. Although this technique is not widely used in the United States, its role as a primary screening technique has great potential.

POSITRON EMISSION TOMOGRAPHY (PET)

Fluorine-18-fluoro-2-deoxyglucose (FDG) positron emission tomography (PET) has emerged as a useful modality in oncologic imaging in gauging patient treatment responses. PET body cameras have recently been developed, allowing for new applications outside of its more traditional role in the central nervous system.

FDG is a positron emitting radiopharmaceutical that is effective in body tumor imaging. FDG is a glucose analog that competes with glucose at glucose transport sites on the cell membrane. FDG and glu-

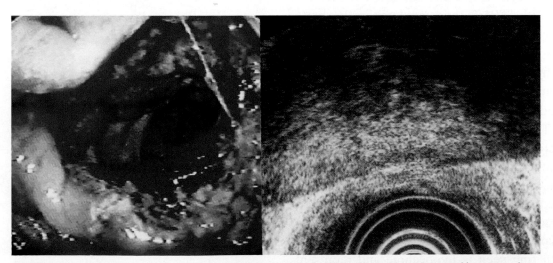

Figure 7–14.   Colonoscopy and endorectal ultrasonography showing a T4 rectal carcinoma with prostate invasion. Images courtesy of Drs. Richard Erickson and Andrejs Avots-Avotins, Scott and White Clinic, Temple, TX.

cose undergo phosphorylation by the enzyme hexokinase, which is used to trap charged species within the cell. Increased hexokinase activity correlates with a variety of neoplastic lesions in body tumor imaging. Tumor conspicuity is therefore increased with PET imaging after the administration of FDG.

PET images are obtained after injecting 5 to 10 mCi of FDG. Obtaining contiguous 9.7-cm segments is generally considered sufficient in the detection to liver neoplasm. Imaging is acquired in 10-minute sequential intervals over a period of 60 to 80 minutes. Hepatic metastases show maximum conspicuity after approximately 60 minutes.[39]

PET imaging is highly effective in identifying liver metastases in patients with colorectal neoplasms.[40] Studies have shown lesion conspicuity to exceed CT in detecting liver metastases.[41] Morphologic features of metastases have been well characterized, including the characteristic ring configuration of hepatic metastases (Figures 7–15 and 7–16). PET imaging has been advocated as a means of evaluating presacral abnormalities in patients with col-

orectal neoplasms. PET is helpful in distinguishing postoperative change and postirradiation change from tumor recurrence.

Although PET remains largely an imaging tool of large academic centers, its clinical usefulness in following patients after receiving complex treatment regimens such as chemoembolization and antibody-directed tumor agents has shown promise. Further improvements with cameras capable of increased spatial resolution could eventually promote PET as a mainstream colorectal imaging tool.

CONCLUSION

A variety of radiologic imaging studies are available in the diagnosis of colorectal neoplasms. The selection of the appropriate study should be tailored to the individual patient. The institutional availability and expertise largely governs which modality should be used. Presently, no one imaging modality adequately detects and stages colorectal neoplasms. Studies should be considered complementary and institutional algorithms should be created for maximum patient benefit.

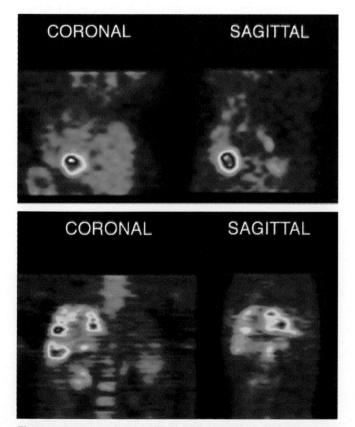

Figures 7–15 and 7–16. FDG PET images showing abnormal uptake of tracer within the liver from colonic metastases.

REFERENCES

1. Morson B. The polyp-cancer sequence in the large bowel. Proc R Soc Med 1974;67:451–457.
2. Muto T, Bussey HJR, Morson BC. The evaluation of cancer of the colon and rectum. Cancer 1975;36: 2251–70.
3. Gelfand DW, Ott DJ. Cost-effective screening for colorectal cancer: the radiologist's view. Primary Care and Cancer 1992;12:11–3.
4. Kelvin FN, Maglinte DDT, Stephens BA. Colorectal carcinoma detected initially with barium enema examination: site distribution and implications. Radiology 1988;169:649–51.
5. Laufer I. The double-contrast enema: myths and misconceptions. Gastrointest Radiol 1976;1:19–31.
6. Gelfand DW, Chen YM, Ott DJ. Radiologic detection of colonic neoplasms: benefits of a system-analysis approach. AJR Am J Roentgenol 1991;156:303–6.
7. MacCarty RL. Colorectal cancer: the case for barium enema. Mayo Clin Proc 1992;67:253–7.
8. Stevenson GW. Normal anatomy and technique of examination of the colon: barium, CT, and MRI. In: Freeney PC, Stevenson GW, editors. Margulis and Burhenne's alimentary tract radiology, ed 5, vol 1. St. Louis: Mosby and Company;1994, p. 692.

9. Smith C. Colorectal cancer radiologic diagnosis. Radiol Clin North Am 1997;35:439–56.

10. Ott DJ, Gelfand DW, Wu WC, et al. Colon polyp morphology on double-contrast barium enema: its pathologic predictive value. AJR Am J Roentgenol 1983; 141:965–70.

11. Kelvin FM, Gardiner R. Techniques of imaging and interpretation. In Kelvin FM, Gardiner R, editors. Clinical imaging of the colon and rectum. New York: Raven Press, 1987, p. 27.

12. Ferrucci JT, Ragsdale BD, Barrett PJ, et al. Double tracking in the sigmoid colon. Radiology 1976;120: 307–12.

13. Fork FT. Double contrast enema and colonoscopy in polyp detection. Gut 1981;22:971–7.

14. Ott DJ, Gelfand DW, Chen YM, et al. Colonoscopy and the barium enema: a radiologic viewpoint. South Med J 1985;78:1033–5.

15. Eddy DM. Screening for colorectal cancer. Ann Intern Med 1990;113:373–84.

16. Berland LL, Lewison TL, Foley WD, et al. Comparison of pre- and post-contrast CT in hepatic metastases. AJR Am J Roentgenol 1982;138:852–8.

17. Thompson WM, Halvorsen RA, Foster WL, et al. Preoperative and postoperative CT staging of rectosigmoid carcinoma. AJR Am J Roentgenol 1986;146:703–10.

18. Bathazar EJ, Megibow AJ, Hulnick D, et al. Carcinoma of the colon: detection and preoperative staging by CT. AJR Am J Roentgenol 1988;150:301–6.

19. Freeney PC, Marks WM, Ryan JA, et al. Colorectal carcinoma evaluation with CT: preoperative staging and detection of postoperative recurrence. Radiology 1986;158:347–53.

20. Thoeni RF. Colorectal cancer radiologic staging. Radiol Clin North Am 1997;35:457–83.

21. Fenlon HM, Nunes DP, Clarke PD, et al. Colorectal neoplasm detection using virtual colonscopy: a feasibility study. Gut 1998;43:806–11.

22. Hara AK, Johnson CD, Reed JE, et al. Colorectal polyp detection with CT colography: two- versus three-dimensional techniques. Radiology 1996;200:49–54.

23. Hara AK, Johnson CD, Reed JE, et al. Detection of colorectal polyps by computed tomographic colography: feasibility of a novel technique. Gastroenterology 1996;110:284–90.

24. Hara AK, Johnson CD, Reed JE, et al. Reducing data size and radiation dose for CT colonography. AJR Am J Roentgenol 1997;168:1181–4.

25. Farley DR, Bannon MP, Zietlow SP, et al. Management of colonoscopic perforations. Mayo Clin Proc 1997; 72:729–33.

26. Fenlon HM, Ferrucci JT. Virtual colonoscopy—what will the issues be? AJR Am J Roentgenol 1997; 169:453–8.

27. Butch RJ, Stark DD, Wittenberg J, et al. Staging rectal cancer by MR and CT. AJR Am J Roentgenol 1986; 146:1155–60.

28. de Lange EE, Gechner RE, Edge SB, et al. Preoperative staging of rectal carcinoma with MR imaging: surgical and histopathologic correlation. Radiology 1990; 176:623–8.

29. Guinet C, Buy JN, Ghossain MA, et al. Comparison of magnetic resonance imaging and computed tomography in the preoperative staging of rectal cancer. Arch Surg 1990;125:385–8.

30. Guinet C, Buy JN, Sezeur A, et al. Preoperative assessment of the extension of rectal carcinoma: correlation of the MR, surgical, and histopathologic findings. J Comput Assist Tomogr 1988;12:209–14.

31. Chan TW, Kressel HY, Milestone B, et al. Rectal carcinoma: staging at MR imaging with endorectal surface coil. Work in progress. Radiology 1991;181:461–7.

32. Demas BE, Hricak J, Goldberg HI, et al. Magnetic resonance imaging diagnosis of hepatic metastases in the presence of negative CT studies. J Clin Gastroenterol 1985;7:553–60.

33. Pema PJ, Bennett WF, Bova JG, et al. CT vs MRI in diagnosis of recurrent rectosigmoid carcinoma. J Comput Assist Tomogr 1994;18:256–61.

34. Thaler W, Watzka S, Martin F, et al. Preoperative staging of rectal cancer by endoluminal ultrasound vs. magnetic resonance imaging. Preliminary results of a prospective, comparative study. Dis Colon Rectum 1994;37:1189–93.

35. Onodera J, Maetani S, Nishikawa T, et al. The reappraisal of prognostic classifications for colorectal cancer. Dis Colon Recum 1989;32:609–14.

36. Ebner F, Kressel HY, Mintz MC, et al. Tumor recurrence versus fibrosis in the female pelvis: differentiation with MR imaging at 1.5T. Radiology 1988; 166:333–40.

37. De Lange EE, Fechner RE, Wanebo HJ. Suspected recurrent rectosigmoid carcinoma after abdominoperineal resection: MR imaging and histopathologic findings. Radiology 1989;170:323–8.

38. Limberg B. Diagnosis and staging of colonic tumors by conventional abdominal sonography as compared with hydrocolonic sonography. N Engl J Med 1992; 327:65–9.

39. Okazumi S, Isono K, Enomoto K, et al. Evaluation of liver tumors using fluorine-18-fluorodeoxyglucose PET: characterization of tumor and assessment of effect of treatment. J Nucl Med 1992;33:333–9.

40. Nagata Y, Yamamoto K, Hiraoka M, et al. Monitoring liver tumor therapy with (18F) FDG positron emission tomography. J Comput Assist Tomogr 1990;14:370–4.

41. Goldberg MA, Lee MJ, Fischman AJ, et al. Fluorodeoxyglucose PET of abdominal and pelvic neoplasms: potential role in oncologic imaging. Radiographics 1993;13:1047–62.

8

Surgery of Primary Colon and Rectal Cancer

MARK J. OTT, MD

JEAN-PIERRE E.N. PIERIE, MD, PhD

The surgical treatment of colorectal cancer has multiple facets. Historically, surgery has been and continues to be the best method of effecting cure in this disease. Along with this primary role, surgery is often required for diagnosis and staging of disease, along with the palliation of symptoms. The purpose of this chapter is to outline and illustrate each of these key components of surgical care in the treatment of these cancers of the lower gastrointestinal tract. An understanding of the appropriate application of surgery in this disease is essential for both surgeons and physicians involved in the treatment of colorectal cancer. Only then can surgery be put to its best use, which is to bring about a cure and/or improve the quality and length of life for patients with cancers of the colon and rectum.

SURGERY AS A DIAGNOSTIC TOOL

With the advent of radiologic and endoscopic methods, the need for surgical exploration to obtain diagnostic tissue has decreased considerably. Whereas preoperative tissue diagnosis was not used in the majority of colorectal tumors three decades ago, the vast majority of patients today have histology prior to definitive surgery. Since greater than 98 percent of colon and rectal cancers are adenocarcinomas arising from the mucosa and thus endoluminal, a thorough lower endoscopy can determine the diagnosis prior to any surgical exploration in the vast majority of cases. In the 5 to 10 percent of cases where the colonoscope

is not able to reach the tumor due to technical reasons (tortuous colon, poor preparation, etc.), a double-contrast barium enema can provide a radiologic diagnosis. It should be emphasized that in the case of colon carcinoma, an actual tissue diagnosis is often not necessary prior to surgery. As long as the location and appearance of the tumor, either endoscopic or radiologic, are adequately obtained, the information necessary to proceed with surgery is in hand. In the case of rectal carcinoma, diagnostic tissue and tumor depth and location are usually essential in planning the appropriate definitive treatment.

For the more rare tumors of the colon and rectum, such as carcinoids, lymphomas, and gastrointestinal stromal tumors that are submucosal or extraluminal, standard endoscopic methods may not make the diagnosis. In these situations, endoscopic ultrasonography can often visualize and biopsy these lesions. When this is not successful, ultrasonography or computed tomography (CT)-guided biopsy techniques can often obtain diagnostic tissue. However, with carcinoids, lymphomas, and gastrointestinal stromal tumors, it is common for the true diagnosis to be made at surgical exploration. Figure 8–1 demonstrates a large gastrointestinal stromal tumor of the sigmoid colon. This patient had normal bowel activity and a normal colonoscopy. The CT scan demonstrates the large primary tumor arising from the sigmoid colon.

Surgery may also be necessary to obtain diagnostic tissue in the case of recurrent disease. A rea-

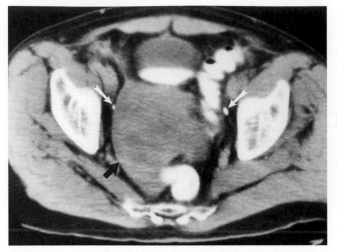

Figure 8–1. A high-grade gastrointestinal stromal tumor arising from the sigmoid colon. The tumor (*black arrow*) fills most of the pelvis. Ureters (*white arrows*) are in close proximity to the tumor.

sonably common scenario is that of a rising carcinoembryonic antigen (CEA) level and a CT scan showing extraluminal thickened tissue in the area of prior surgery. Endoscopic ultrasonography or radiologic-guided biopsies often return nondiagnostic inflammatory or fibrous tissue. When distant disease is ruled out, these patients warrant re-exploration for diagnosis and possible resection. These patients can still be cured through a combination of surgery, radiation therapy, and chemotherapy, but a firm diagnosis needs to be established.

SURGERY AS A CURATIVE AND STAGING TECHNIQUE

The goal of resection for both colonic and rectal cancers is threefold: first, a complete resection of the involved bowel segment with negative proximal, distal, and radial margins; second, a wide lymphadenectomy to encompass all draining lymph nodes for that segment of bowel; and third, restoration of bowel continuity when possible. The restoration of bowel continuity is an important goal, but the bowel resection and lymphadenectomy should never be compromised to avoid an ostomy. All of these goals should be achieved in conjunction with a thorough exploration and a minimal amount of complications (ie, infection, hemorrhage, and sexual or urinary dysfunction). The actual methods of resection vary according to location and will be discussed separately.

Both the colon and especially the rectum normally carry high bacterial counts (ie, *Bacteroides fragilis* and *Escherichia coli* 10^{10} and 10^7/g of wet feces, respectively[1]) and are thus considered contaminated cases. In order to reduce infectious complications from an expected rate of 70 percent down to less than 10 percent, preoperative decontamination of the bowel is indicated. There are many methods of decontamination but most involve a mechanical washout to evacuate the colon followed by an antibiotic sterilization of residual anaerobic and gram negative bacteria. Patients who undergo a colorectal resection with primary anastomosis in an unprepared situation are more likely to have wound infections, anastomotic breakdown, and leakage. This has traditionally prompted most surgeons to perform a diverting colostomy in this situation. However, surgery on the unprepared right or transverse colon, which has a lower bacterial count and liquid stool, can still be safely performed with either a right colectomy or extended right colectomy and primary ileocolonic anastomosis. When faced with a colorectal cancer that cannot undergo proper decontamination prior to surgery (ie, obstruction, severe hemorrhage, or perforation and infection), the surgeon must weigh these risks and benefits in deciding between a resection with colostomy or an anastomosis. In the case of a colostomy, it is useful for the surgeon to identify the distal bowel stump with a colored nonabsorbable suture at the time of the first surgery to facilitate its identification at a subsequent surgery to restore bowel continuity.

COLONIC RESECTIONS

Figures 8–2 and 8–3 demonstrate the classic anatomy and vascular supply of the colon. While variations exist, the lymphatic drainage parallels the vascular supply. Thus, by excising the appropriate segment of colon with its accompanying vascular arcades back to their respective origins from either the superior mesenteric or inferior mesenteric artery, a wide lymphadenectomy will be achieved. There is no oncologic benefit to high ligation of the inferior mesenteric artery flush with the aorta. A ligation below the origin of the left colic is equally curative.[2] In terms of the actual tumor and bowel wall resec-

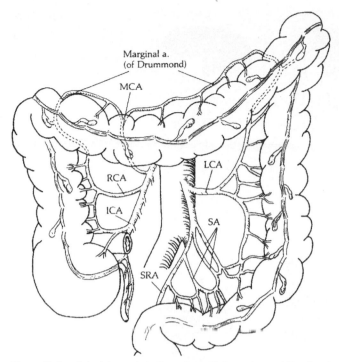

Figure 8–2. Arterial supply to the colon with the colon mobilized and displaced downward (below the marginal artery of Drummond). ICA = ileocolic artery; LCA = left colic artery; RCA = right colic artery; SA = sigmoid arteries; SRA = superior rectal artery. From Nyhus LM, Baker RJ, eds. Mastery of surgery, 2nd ed. Boston: Little, Brown, 1992.

tion, it would be sufficient to resect the involved segment of colon with a 1- to 2-cm margin of normal bowel. This would resect all gross and microscopic disease within the bowel wall. However, this type of resection would not achieve a sufficient lymphadenectomy, and thus wider resections are generally performed. These resections follow the vascular distributions of the colon (Figure 8–4). These hemicolectomies resect the associated lymphatics and minimize the chance of an ischemic anastomosis that can happen with segmental resections in patients with atherosclerotic vessels.

Tumor location and lymphovascular supply determine the appropriate resection. Lesions located in the cecum should be resected to include a segment of terminal ileum and its mesentery. The right colon is resected up to the right of the middle colic vessels. Tumors located in the ascending colon are resected with a standard right hemicolectomy. Lesions at the hepatic flexure may require resection by an extended right hemicolectomy (Figure 8–5). Obviously, the surgeon's judgment is critical in determining the appropriate operation as there are

anatomic variations and other patient issues that must be considered. Tumors in the mid-transverse colon are often resected from the hepatic flexure to the splenic flexure. This includes resection of the contiguous mesentery of the middle colic vessels. When transecting a vessel from the superior or inferior mesenteric artery, there is no curative benefit to a flush transection. A 1-cm cuff of vessel to ligate will give the same lymphadenectomy with less risk of hemorrhage.

The attached segment of omentum should also be resected with the specimen. This is done by transecting the omentum on the colonic side of the gastroepiploic vessels. The omentum also contains lymph nodes, which may be involved with tumor metastases. During right colonic resections, care must be taken to visualize and protect the duodenum, right ureter, and right gonadal vessels. All three of these structures are at risk as the right colon is mobilized out of the retroperitoneum.

Figure 8–6 demonstrates the ligation of the inferior mesenteric artery in order to mobilize the colon during a left hemicolectomy. As stated earlier, ligation of the inferior mesenteric artery does not add to cure rate, but it does remove the inferior mesenteric

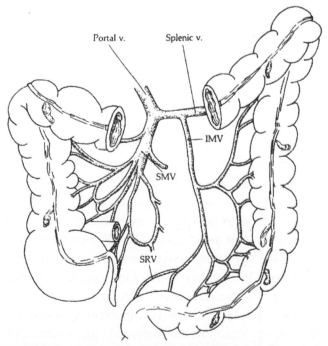

Figure 8–3. Venous drainage of colon. IMV = inferior mesenteric vein; SMV = superior mesenteric vein; SRV = superior rectal vein. From Nyhus LM, Baker RJ, eds. Mastery of surgery, 2nd ed. Boston: Little, Brown, 1992.

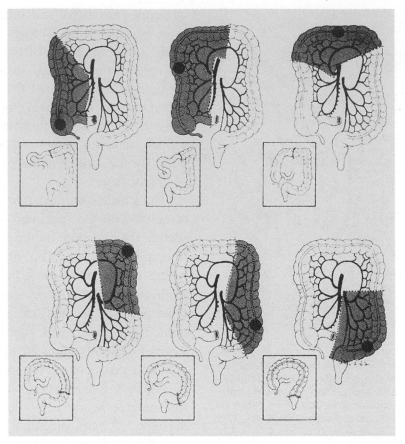

Figure 8–4. Extent of surgical resection for cancer at various sites. A black disk represents the cancer. Anastomosis of the bowel remaining after resection is shown in the small insets. The extent of resection is determined by the distribution of the regional lymph nodes along the blood supply. From Shrock TR. Large intestine. In: Way LW, ed. Current surgical diagnosis and treatment, 7th ed. Los Altos, CA: Lange Medical Publications, 1985.

artery as a point of fixation. This in turn allows for better mobilization of the remaining colon and a tension-free anastomosis. For more proximal lesions, the superior rectal artery can often be preserved with no compromise in cure rates. There is no curative or staging benefit to a para-aortic lymphadenectomy.

During the resection of left colon lesions, the splenocolic and renocolic ligaments will often need to be incised to adequately mobilize the colon for resection and or anastomosis. Small tears in the capsule of the spleen are easily created by too vigorous retraction. Prevention is far more successful than treatment. However, when bleeding occurs from splenic capsular tears, it is important to incise the remaining attachments between the colon and spleen. This releases the tension on the capsule. It is then more likely that topical hemostatic agents, cautery, and direct pressure will be successful in

achieving hemostasis. Other structures that are easily damaged during mobilization of the left colon from the retroperitoneum include the left ureter, left gonadal vessels, and tail of the pancreas. The tail of the pancreas can be inadvertently injured during mobilization of the splenic flexure of the colon. This can lead to either postoperative pancreatitis or a pancreatic fistula. Visualization of these structures will help prevent their injury.

The surgeon's judgment in determining the extent of the resection is critical. A large premalignant polyp not amenable to endoscopic removal can be removed via a colotomy and polypectomy or via a segmental resection, without lymphadenectomy. Large bulky lesions that invade through the bowel wall into adjacent organs should be resected with a negative margin of the adjacent organ (ie, bladder, small bowel, abdominal wall, etc.). Stage for stage,

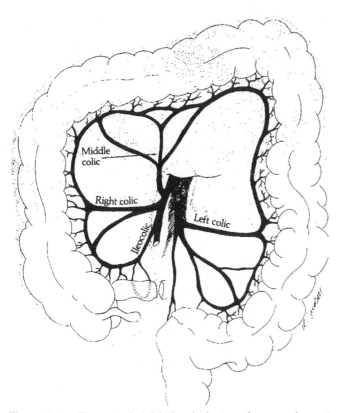

Figure 8–5. The extended right hemicolectomy for a neoplasm at the hepatic flexure side of the transverse colon. Includes a subtotal colectomy with resection of the cecum and the ascending, transverse, and a portion of the descending colon with its mesentery to the level of the left colic vessels. From Nyhus LM, Baker RJ, eds. Mastery of surgery, 2nd ed. Boston: Little Brown, 1992.

tumor. There certainly is evidence that manipulation of the tumor during the operation leads to increased tumor shedding of detectable tumor cells into the blood supply.[7] Turnbull's initial series demonstrated improvement in survival in patients resected with this technique. However, subsequent controlled studies have failed to demonstrate any clinical benefit in decreased local recurrence or increased survival.[8] At the present time it cannot be considered standard of care.

There is great variability in the frequency of postoperative bowel movement following a hemicolectomy. Most patients will have a minimal increase in frequency, but some patients will initially have an increase of two to four movements per day. These patients can have their frequency decreased through the addition of fiber to the diet and, when necessary, an antimotility agent. The remaining colon will often adapt over a 4- to 6-month period to return a patient to a more normal-for-them pattern.

these T4 lesions have no increase in complications and an equal cure rate with en bloc surgical resection.[3] The plane of invasion between the colonic tumor and the invaded organ should not be fractured. Disruption of this plane, even with subsequent surgical resection, decreases the cure rate by greater than 50 percent.[4,5] In the case of invasion into the abdominal wall or retroperitoneum, the area of resection should be marked with metal clips for subsequent radiation therapy to help minimize the risk of a local recurrence. When possible, the area should also be covered by omentum to help exclude as much bowel as possible from the subsequent radiation field.

The No-Touch technique, as popularized by Turnbull and colleagues,[6] involves the early division and ligation of the vascular supply and occlusion of the proximal and distal bowel lumen around the area of the tumor. This is done to limit the shedding of tumor cells into the blood and lymphatic systems and into the bowel lumen during manipulation of the

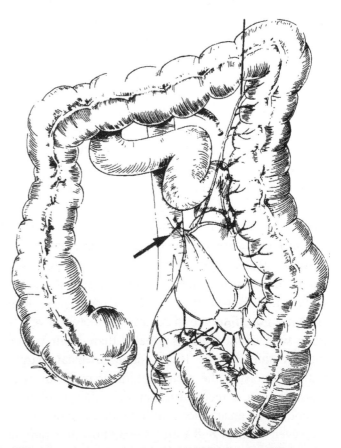

Figure 8–6. Location of division of the inferior mesenteric artery (*arrow*) 1 cm from the aorta during a left hemicolectomy. From Nyhus LM, Baker RJ, eds. Mastery of surgery, 2nd ed. Boston: Little, Brown, 1992.

RECTAL RESECTIONS

There is a wide array of treatment choices facing the clinician managing rectal cancer. Surgical treatment options can vary from transabdominal operations to local excision. Newer techniques are being applied to reduce the necessity for permanent colostomy, improve functional results, and reduce local recurrence. Radiation therapy with chemotherapy, especially in the preoperative setting, has a much more prominent role in the treatment of rectal cancer than in colon cancer. The roles of adjuvant and neoadjuvant therapy are discussed in subsequent chapters in this text.

Low Anterior and Abdominoperineal Resection

The gold standard for removal of a rectal cancer is via a transabdominal low anterior resection (LAR) or a combined abdominoperineal resection (APR). Both of these operations remove the involved bowel segment and the associated lymphatic tissue. There is no curative benefit of the complete rectal resection and permanent colostomy accomplished by an APR versus the LAR if the surgeon is able to obtain adequate proximal and distal margins in combination with a wide resection of the draining mesorectal lymphatic tissue. Best was the first to demonstrate that mucosal involvement 2 cm or more below the distal edge of the lesion was found in less than 1 percent of cases.[9] Others confirmed this finding in several retrospective studies that demonstrated that there was no benefit in local control or metastatic disease for bowel margins greater than 2 cm.[10,11] The question was finally laid to rest by the National Surgical Adjuvant Breast and Bowel Project (NSABP) [R-01] trial showing no difference in recurrence between resections with distal margins greater than 3 cm versus those within 2 cm.[12] If an adequate distal margin without excising the rectal sphincter mechanism is possible, then a reconstruction via either a coloanal or colorectal anastomosis is indicated (Figure 8–7). However, Figures 8–8A and 8–8B show an example of a specimen of a T3N0M0 rectal tumor that was situated too low to be eligible for a sphincter-saving procedure. Consequently, an APR was performed.

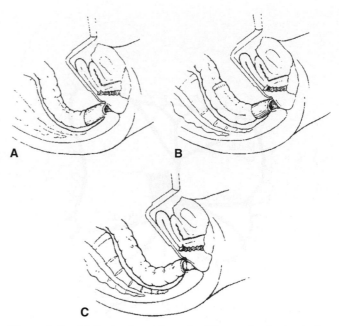

Figure 8–7.   Methods of anastomosis of the proximal colon to the rectum or anus after a low anterior resection: *A,* end-to-end colorectal anastomosis; *B,* end-to-side colorectal anastomosis with J-pouch; *C,* end-to-end coloanal anastomosis. From Enker WE. Total mesorectal excision with sphincter and autonomic-nerve preservation in the treatment of rectal cancer. In: Condon RE, ed. Current techniques in general surgery. New York: Lawrence DellaCorte, 1996.

The proximal extent of lymphatic resection has likewise been contested but never answered in a prospective study. However, several nonrandomized studies would support a dissection to include the nodal tissue up to the bifurcation of the left colic from the inferior mesenteric artery. Division of the artery just distal to this bifurcation preserves the left colic blood supply and has not shown any survival disadvantage relative to a more extensive proximal lymphadenectomy of para-aortic nodes with ligation of the inferior mesenteric artery at its origin. In a retrospective study from St. Mark's Hospital of 784 patients with ligation distal to the left colic versus 586 patients with resection of the inferior mesenteric artery and accompanying nodal tissue, there were no differences in 5-year survival for any Dukes A, B, or C patients.[13] Similarly, in a series by Hojo and colleagues, there was only 1 survivor among 15 patients who had extensive proximal lymphadenectomies when there were pathologically positive nodes along the inferior mesenteric artery.[14] These studies support the practice of resecting proximal nodal tissue up to and including the origin of the superior rectal artery and preserving the inferior mesenteric and left colic artery.

The concept of a sharp total mesorectal excision (TME) has increased the surgical awareness of the importance of obtaining a wide radial margin by encompassing the mesorectum as a defined packet. In 1982, Heald and colleagues published his initial description of the surgical techniques involved in TME[15] (Figure 8–9). He also emphasized the importance of identifying and preserving the sympathetic and parasympathetic nerves to retain postoperative bowel, bladder, and sexual function, the autonomic nerve preservation (TME-ANP) (Figure 8–10). The dissection is continued down to the levator ani muscles to achieve full mobilization of the rectum and mesorectum (Figures 8–11, A and B). Incomplete circumferential mobilization of the rectum limits dis-

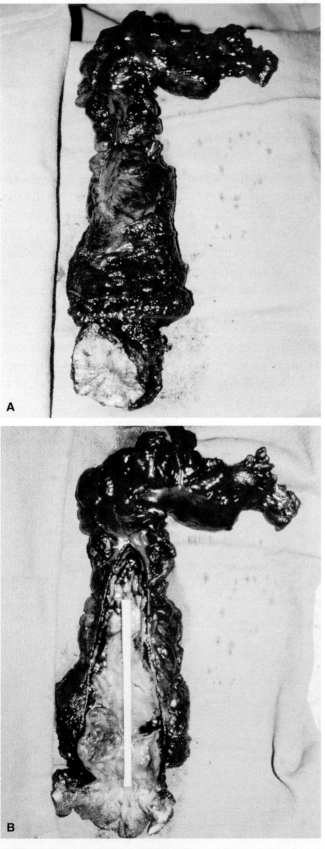

Figure 8–8. *A,* Specimen after an APR and *B,* opened to show a T3N0M0 rectal cancer just above the anal sphincter. It is situated too low to be eligible for a sphincter-saving LAR.

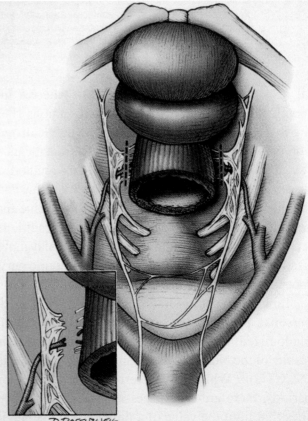

Figure 8–9. Schematic of the critical pelvic structures encountered during a sharp total mesorectal excision. The autonomic nerves and rectal vessels are divided sharply and individually to preserve the autonomic innervation necessary for bladder and sexual function. From Enker WE. Total mesorectal excision with sphincter and autonomic-nerve preservation in the treatment of rectal cancer. In: Condon RE, ed. Current techniques in general surgery. New York: Lawrence DellaCorte, 1996.

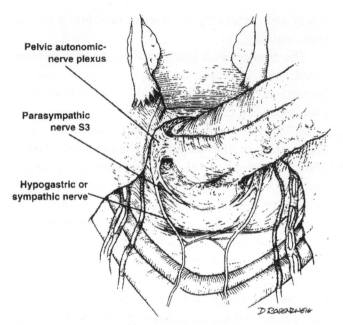

Figure 8–10. Mobilization of the rectum during a sharp mesorectal dissection demonstrating identification and preservation of autonomic nerve structures critical for bladder and sexual function. From Enker WE. Total mesorectal excision with sphincter and autonomic-nerve preservation in the treatment of rectal cancer. In: Condon RE, ed. Current techniques in general surgery. New York: Lawrence DellaCorte, 1996.

tal resection margins (Figure 8–11D), whereas full mobilization will allow more distal resections (Figure 8–11C). Traditionally, much of the pelvic dissection below the peritoneal reflection for rectal cancer was performed in a blunt fashion. This method of dissection was rapid and identified lateral tissue containing vascular, lymphatic, and nervous tissue that was then divided between clamps. The traditional technique will also allow for adequate distal mobilization but is more likely to injure autonomic nerve roots and disrupt the mesorectal lymphatic packet.

Table 8–1 demonstrates the results of Heald's personal, prospectively collected, consecutive, non-randomized series of patients[16] compared to the results of the North Central Cancer Treatment Group (NCCTG).[17] While the two series cover similar time periods, there are differences in patient tumor profiles that limit the value of a direct comparison. His excellent results with local recurrence rates of less than 5 percent and overall recurrence at 10 years of 22 percent in curatively operated patients have provoked intense discussions about the true merit of this more time- and labor-intensive technique. This study covers a 13-year period from 1978 to 1991,

with mean follow-up of 7.5 years. Of the 290 patients, 135 high-risk patients who were most likely to recur after curative resection constituted the group for analysis. There were 126 low anterior resections and 9 abdominoperineal resections in this group. High risk was defined according to the definition from the NCCTG. These investigators excluded Dukes A (Astler Coller A + B1) lesions, those more than 12 cm from the anal verge, and those considered not curative by the surgeon. The operation was considered curative when, at the end of the procedure, the surgeon believed that all grossly detectable cancer had been removed. None of these patients received adjuvant therapy, which reflects a long-term opinion of Heald's that improved survival and local control can be achieved by optimal surgery alone. This is an obvious divergence from the recommendations of the 1990 National Institutes of Health (NIH) consensus conference where the combination of radiation therapy and chemotherapy was recommended as standard of care for stage 2 and 3 disease.[18]

There is a cost for this apparent decrease in local and distal recurrence. Operative times are increased

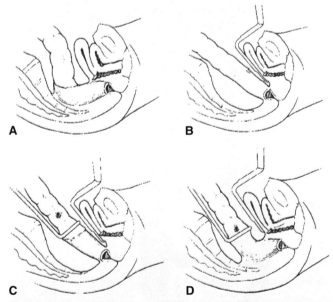

Figure 8–11. Mobilization of the rectum below the peritoneal reflection: *A,* the rectum prior to mobilization; *B,* full mobilization of the rectum to the level of the levator ani muscles; *C,* full mobilization of the rectum allows distal transection of the rectum with a generous distal margin; *D,* incomplete mobilization of the rectum compromises the distal margin of transection. From Enker WE. Total mesorectal excision with sphincter and autonomic-nerve preservation in the treatment of rectal cancer. In: Condon RE, ed. Current techniques in general surgery. New York: Lawrence DellaCorte, 1996.

Table 8–1. LOCAL AND TOTAL RECURRENCE RATES FOR TOTAL MESORECTAL EXCISION AND NCCTG DATA		
Treatment Group	Local Recurrence (%)	Overall Recurrence (%)
TME	5	22
Conventional surgery + radiation	25	62.7
Conventional surgery + radiation + chemotherapy	13.5	41.5

Data from MacFarlane JK, Ryall RDH, Heald RJ. Mesorectal excision for rectal cancer. Lancet 1993; 341:457–60.

by 2.5 hours, and there are increased blood transfusion requirements. There is an 11 percent clinical and an additional 6.4 percent radiologic leak rate with TME. Heald and many others now routinely use a temporary diverting colostomy. Due to complications, 5 percent of these colostomies were never reversed. A similar series of 350 patients in Norway undergoing TME had an anastomotic leak rate greater than 20 percent, leading to emergency surgery, morbidity, and two deaths.[19]

While TME is touted as improving autonomic nerve function postoperatively, no good randomized studies exist to document this fact. The standard blunt dissection technique with clamping of the lateral pedicles undoubtedly has resulted in numerous unintended injuries to the pelvic autonomic nerve plexus. It would seem reasonable that a more meticulous dissection with preservation of the defined nerve roots would lead to better function.[20]

All of the preceding discussion serves to emphasize the point that surgical technique does make a difference in patient outcome. Hermanck and colleagues surveyed rectal cancer outcomes in seven major German cities and found that local recurrence rates varied among individual surgeons from less than 10 percent to more than 50 percent.[21,22] Quirke and colleagues demonstrated the importance of radial margin clearance.[23] In this prospective series of 52 patients with rectal adenocarcinoma, careful whole-mount sectioning of APR specimens revealed spread to the lateral margins in 14 patients (27%). Twelve of these patients (85%) developed local recurrence whereas only 1 of 38 patients (3%) with negative radial margins developed a local recurrence. Sharp dissection employed in TME to excise

the entire mesorectum reproducibly provides a maximal intact lateral resection margin and may explain the beneficial effects on local control.

Local Excision of Rectal Carcinoma and Sphincter-Sparing Techniques

The best operation in the treatment of rectal cancer is one that achieves a curative resection with the least morbidity and mortality. As the incidence of large bowel cancer increases with each decade of life, many patients diagnosed with cancer of the rectum are older than 70 years of age with coexistent medical problems. An advantage of local excision is that it is usually associated with a mortality rate near zero and similar low morbidity rates.[24,25] The avoidance of a permanent stoma is another great advantage to the patient if the cure of cancer is not jeopardized. Approximately 10 to 15 percent of all patients with rectal carcinoma have tumors confined to the rectal wall and might be eligible for local excision after proper patient selection. The approach may be transanal, transcoccygeal, or trans-sphincteric as described in more detail later in this chapter.[26–28] However, regardless of the surgical approach, the resection must achieve a negative margin and a full-thickness excision; otherwise, therapy is inadequate and further surgical therapy is indicated.

The most important criterion for local excision is accessibility, which will influence surgical treatment.[29] To maximize the chance of a good oncologic procedure, several surgical groups have reported criteria for local excision, mostly in single institution, retrospective studies.[25,27] Ideal rectal tumors for this approach are situated below the peritoneal reflection, are less than 4 cm in diameter, take up less than 40 percent of the rectal circumference, have no palpable or radiologically visible perirectal nodes, are mobile on digital examination, and have a well-differentiated histology without lymphatic or vascular invasion.[30,31] All of these factors identify tumors that have a low likelihood of nodal metastases. Since local resections generally do not remove draining lymph nodes, these unresected lymph nodes can lead to local and distant recurrence if they in fact contain tumor. This is supported by the finding that local recurrence rates after local resection and the frequency of lymph node metastases found at APR are closely matched for similar stage diseases.[29] Therefore, local excision with curative intent is only appropriate when the risk of nodal metastases is as near zero as possible. The methods presently available to determine the depth of tumor invasion of the rectal wall (the T status) and to document regional lymph nodes (N status) are limited. A good digital rectal examination in experienced hands can predict invasion of the rectal wall in up to 80 percent of cases but is less useful for detecting regional tumor-positive lymph nodes.[32] CT scan and MRI are useful for identification of intra-abdominal metastases and can accurately identify locally advanced tumors that have invaded adjacent pelvic structures, but the negative predictive value for regional lymph nodes is only 50 to 70 percent. Endoluminal ultrasonography has been reported to be a more accurate diagnostic instrument for assessment of penetration of the rectal wall by carcinoma. It has a negative predictive value of 70 to 95 percent in experienced centers. The same expert groups report a negative predicted value of 80 to 90 percent for detection of regional lymph nodes by ultrasonography.[33,34] The caveats are that an expert sonographist is needed for a reliable intraluminal sonographic examination and, even then, not all lymph nodes containing tumor are enlarged in colon and rectal carcinoma.[35,36] Therefore, despite the best preoperative staging presently available, the status of lymphatic involvement is often still uncertain. This has important implications, as lymph node involvement has the single greatest impact on survival and is present in 40 to 60 percent of all rectal cancer patients treated by surgery alone.[37,38] When deciding whether to perform a local resection where lymph nodes are generally not removed versus transabdominal resections where lymph nodes are resected, there is always some uncertainty. When a patient is a candidate for a local resection (tumor confined to mucosa, submucosa, or muscularis propria), tumor biopsy information in terms of tumor grade and evidence of lymphatic or vascular invasion can be very important. Patients with poorly differentiated tumors and evidence of lymphatic or vascular invasion on biopsy have a 36 to 53 percent rate of local recurrence after local resections alone versus a 12 to 15 percent rate of local recurrence after transabdominal resection.[39] Because rectal cancer

histology can affect the type of operation, most rectal cancers require a tissue diagnosis and thorough staging prior to definitive surgical treatment.

Steele and his co-workers have recently published the only multi-institutional prospective controlled trial of sphincter-sparing treatment for distal rectal carcinoma in the literature, conducted by the CALGB (Cancer and Leukemia Group B).[24] Their inclusion criteria for local excision of a rectal tumor match the criteria mentioned earlier in this chapter, although no effort was made to differentiate between high-grade (including a histology of vascular and lymphatic invasion) and low-grade tumors. After local excision, patients with T1 tumors received no further treatment and were followed for recurrence and survival. Patients with T2 tumors were given adjuvant radiation and chemotherapy. Any patient with a local recurrence was salvaged with a formal APR. Only patients who underwent excision with negative margins were included. After 6 years of follow-up, survival and failure-free survival rates of the eligible patients are 85 and 78 percent, respectively, with no difference between the T1 and T2 (plus adjuvant treatment) groups. Comparing these results to historical control patients who received a formal APR, the authors conclude no significant therapeutic disadvantage in the sphincter-sparing approach thus far, when the strict selection criteria are applied. The efficacy of surgical salvage after local recurrence remains uncertain because too few patients were salvaged and the follow-up was relatively short. The results concerning salvage surgery following local recurrence (mostly a formal APR) are of utmost importance, since disappointing results from retrospective studies have been reported until now.[29]

After local resection, postoperative radiation and chemotherapy are usually given for lesions penetrating the rectal wall. The two prospective series that have looked at this form of therapy indicate a local recurrence rate of 6.5 to 8 percent and a survival rate of 90 percent, which is equal to the expected results of an abdominoperineal resection.[40,41] Rectal function is reported as good or satisfactory in greater than 80 percent of the patients.

Although local excision of rectal carcinoma can be accomplished through a transsacral or trans-sphincteric approach, transanal exposure is the technique chosen most frequently. The prone jackknife position is used for lesions in the anterior and lateral locations. For lesions of the posterior rectum, the lithotomy position is preferred.[42] The preoperative bowel preparation is the same as in other large bowel procedures. In the operating room, the rectum is irrigated with an antiseptic solution to minimize contamination during the procedure. Exposure is achieved by an anal speculum and/or retractor. The procedure requires full-thickness excision, with an in vivo margin of 1 cm beyond the edge of the tumor (Figure 8–12, A and B). The positioning of traction sutures

helps in removal of the tumor and orients the specimen for the pathologist (Figure 8–13, A and B). To minimize operative bleeding, electrocautery should be used. Primary closure of the resulting defect shortens the time required for healing, but this aspect is not a strict requirement as long as the defect lies caudad to the peritoneal reflection (Figure 8–14, A and B). Proctoscopic examination should be performed at the completion of the procedure to ensure that an adequate lumen has been preserved. Figure 8–15 gives an endoscopic view of the rectal wound 1 year after local excision.

For very low rectal tumors, at or near the anorec-

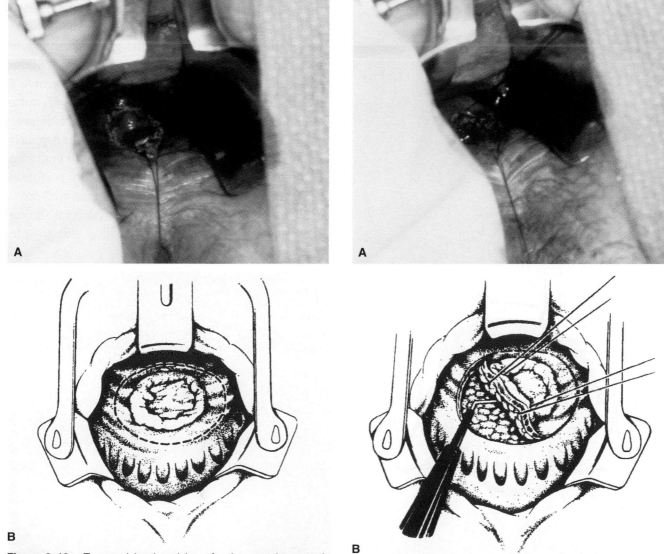

Figure 8–12. Transanal local excision of a low rectal tumor: *A,* exposure of a posterior wall rectal carcinoma with Parks anal retractor and *B,* diagram of the same stage of the operation. The 1-cm margin is marked. From Bailey HR, Huval WV, Max E, et al.[27]

Figure 8–13. *A,* Full-thickness excision of the tumor using traction sutures for presentation of the specimen, and *B,* diagram of the same stage of the operation. From Bailey HR, Huval WV, Max E, et al.[27]

tal junction, an intersphincteric resection with partial excision of the internal anal sphincter might be possible[28] (Figure 8–16). In a small prospective study, 5-year survival rates of 75 percent were reported after this procedure for T2 and T3 tumors plus adjuvant therapy in very low tumors between 2.5 cm and 4.5 cm from the anal verge. Continence was normal in half of the patients and half of the patients suffered from occasional minor leaks.

Kraske was the first to describe a transsacral approach for midrectal cancers in 1885.[26] Others have modified this technique, but the principles are the same.[43] Tumors situated on the anterior side of the midrectum are suitable for this approach. Post-

operative fistulae are the most frequent postoperative complications after this procedure and occur in approximately 15 percent of cases. The technique can be ideal for midrectal tumors and should be a part of the surgeon's armamentarium.

In conclusion, local excision as a sphincter-saving procedure is possible in 10 to 15 percent of patients with rectal cancers. Strict selection minimizes the chance of regional lymph node metastases and is the key to a good outcome.

PALLIATIVE COLORECTAL SURGERY

Not all colorectal surgery is performed with curative intent. Patients presenting with truly unresectable primary tumors or patients with metastatic disease constitute this group. In the case of patients with unresectable primary tumors, the goal of surgery is usually to relieve obstruction. For distal tumors of the rectum and sigmoid colon, this will usually involve a diverting colostomy and probably a mucous fistula. Patients with distal obstruction who are unresectable should not have an end colostomy and blind pouch proximal to the obstruction. The colon will continue to secrete mucus and can potentially freely perforate or fistulize into an adjacent organ from internal pressure. Patients with more proximal unresectable colon cancers can usually be bypassed with a side-to-side

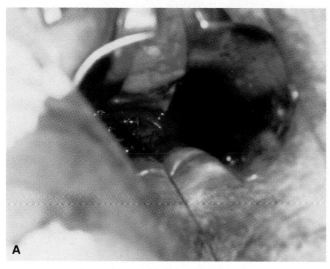

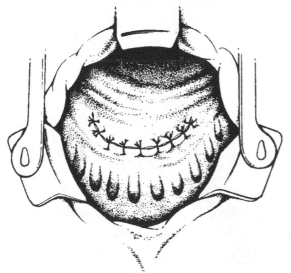

Figure 8–14. *A,* Primary longitudinal closure of the defect with absorbable sutures, without narrowing of the lumen; and *B,* diagram of the same stage of the operation, although a transverse closure is depicted. From Bailey HR, Huval WV, Max E, et al.[27]

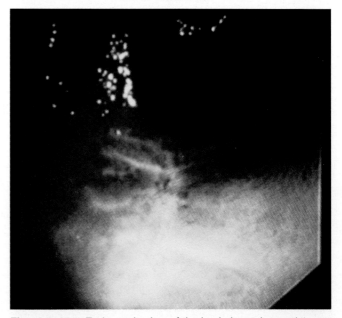

Figure 8–15. Endoscopic view of the healed rectal wound 1 year after local excision of a rectal cancer.

anastomosis between bowel proximal and distal to the obstruction. This will circumvent the obstruction and allow internal decompression of the potentially obstructed segments while keeping the patient free of a colostomy. A side-to-side anastomosis between the cecum and sigmoid colon is usually easily performed and causes only a minimal increase in the number of bowel movements per day.

Patients with unresectable primary tumors and bleeding from the tumor present a more difficult situation. These patients will often have a resolution or decrease in bleeding with colonic diversion or bypass. The continued presence of the fecal stream contributes to the bleeding process. When this fails to control the bleeding, external beam radiation will often be successful.

Patients who present with distant metastases and resectable primary colorectal tumors should generally have their primary tumor resected. Possible exceptions to this include widespread carcinomatosis with expected survival of less than 6 months or multiple medical problems that make the patient a high-risk surgical candidate or that preclude any systemic chemotherapy. Due to difference in tumor biology, almost every surgical series has about a 5 percent, 5-year survival rate for these patients.[44]

LAPAROSCOPIC TECHNIQUES IN COLORECTAL CANCER SURGERY

Laparoscopy has been used in colorectal surgery for several decades.[45] The initial clinical reports of laparoscopic colorectal surgery (LCR) suggested many advantages in comparison to conventional (open) techniques, including reduced postoperative pain, earlier recovery of bowel function, shorter length of hospital stay, and earlier return to normal activities.[46] More recent studies have not been as favorable.[47] To date, there at least appear to be no significant differences in perioperative complications or mortality between laparoscopic and open colorectal surgery, and short-term outcomes seem equivalent. Despite a trend toward a reduced length of stay, the overall costs of laparoscopic resections have historically been higher. This in part has been related to both a longer operative time and higher equipment costs. Many of the expenses would be expected to decline,

as advances in both laparoscopic equipment design and surgical technique reduce the surgeon's operative time and costs. Some of the specific complications related to laparoscopic technique include port-site herniation, inadvertent organ injury, complications of pneumoperitoneum (respiratory acidosis), and resection of the wrong segment of bowel.[48]

Another aspect is the learning curve. There are major differences in surgical technique between LCR and other more common laparoscopic procedures like laparoscopic cholecystectomy. These differences include working in multiple anatomic regions, the need to divide multiple mesenteric vessels, removal of a fairly large specimen, and the performance of a safe anastomosis. The number of supervised laparoscopic colorectal resections needed to comfortably learn the procedure is not well documented but is estimated to be more than 40 completed cases, partly depending on the laparoscopic experience of the surgeon.[49,50] This implies that a second qualified surgeon and a high-volume setting are needed to overcome this problem. Furthermore, if conversion from LCR to an open procedure is needed, one gets the worst of both methods: higher cost and operative time combined with a larger incision and an increased incidence of postoperative complications.[51]

There are three potential uses of laparoscopy in colorectal cancer. The first is an occasional need for

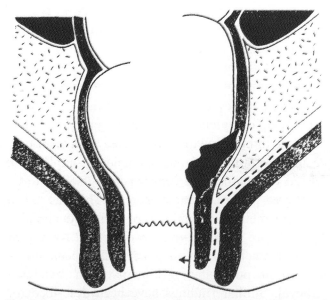

Figure 8–16. Intersphincteric resection of a very low rectal cancer at the anorectal junction, with partial excision of the internal anal sphincter. From Rullier E, Zerbib F, Laurent C, et al.[28]

diagnostic or staging information prior to definitive treatment. Given the success of endoscopic and radiologic studies, this is an extremely rare event. Nevertheless, laparoscopy allows inspection of the entire abdominal cavity and permits biopsy of serosal lesions. Furthermore, intraoperative laparoscopic ultrasonography is especially useful for diagnosing occult, small intraparenchymal liver metastasis from colorectal cancer.

The second possible role is in palliative colorectal surgery. In cases where advanced colorectal carcinoma is diagnosed preoperatively, laparoscopic surgery permits a variety of palliative measures, such as resection of the primary tumor, intestinal bypass, and stomal diversion without the need for a large incision. Alternative procedures, including laparoscopically assisted feeding jejunostomies and cathether placement for intraperitoneal chemotherapy, can be performed in the same setting. As compared to open surgery, LCR is generally believed to have a more rapid return of bowel function, decreases length of hospitalization, and results in less postoperative pain, although there are also studies that refute these claims.[52] Given the specific disadvantages of LCR as outlined earlier, the surgeon has to decide whether the potential benefits outweigh these problems.

The role LCR in curative cancer surgery is still to be defined and is presently being evaluated. Although similar 5-year survival rates after LCR and open procedures have been reported in a comparative prospective trial, there is still considerable debate whether there will be a compromise in cure rate.[47,53] This question is currently being investigated in multiple randomized prospective studies, conducted in several countries.[50,54] There is some experimental evidence that laparoscopic procedures decrease tumor growth as compared with open procedures.[55] On the other hand, a unique complication related to laparoscopic cancer surgery seems to be an altered pattern of tumor spread. This has led to port-site metastases and is not well understood.[56] Not only are such recurrences present at the site of tumor extraction, but they have also been documented at port sites not involved in specimen removal. Similar findings have been described for other intra-abdominal malignancies, including pancreatic, ovarian, and gallbladder cancer. It is not

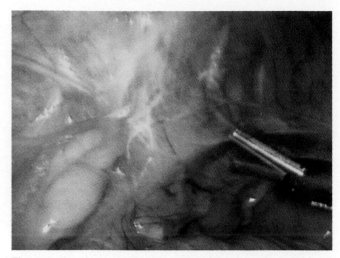

Figure 8–17. Laparoscopic view of intra-abdominal dissection with a harmonic scalpel.

clear whether these types of recurrences are an inevitable consequence of minimally invasive techniques or perhaps related to a learning experience. Current ongoing studies indicate that the incidence of trocar site recurrence seems to be decreasing, suggesting that the learning curve may have influenced this adverse outcome.[50]

As stated earlier, there are specific techniques and equipment for the laparoscopic procedure. Dissection is primarily performed using a laparoscopic harmonic scalpel (Figure 8–17), and vascular struc-

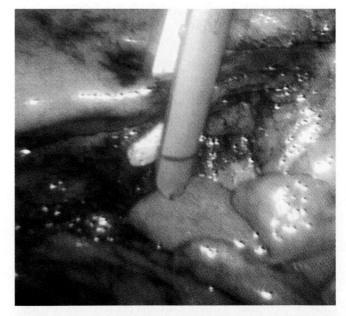

Figure 8–18. Laparoscopic view of transsection of a vascular structure in the mesentery of the colon using the laparoscopic vascular stapler device.

tures are preferably divided by a laparoscopic vascular stapler (Figure 8–18). The bowel is transsected with the help of a laparoscopic roticulating gastrointestinal stapler (Figure 8–19). After the bowel is dissected out and transsected distally (Figure 8–20), the specimen is taken out of the abdominal cavity through a 4- to 5-cm incision (Figure 8–21). Although the anastomosis can be performed intracorporally, the easier and therefore safer extracorporal technique is chosen by many surgeons, including the

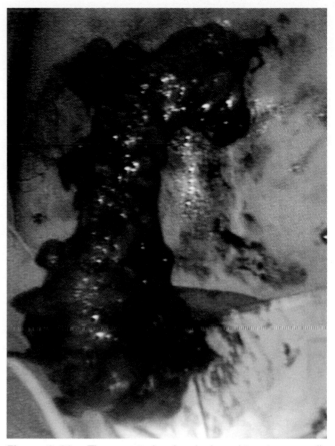

Figure 8–21. The resected colon is brought extracorporally through the 4-cm abdominal incision.

authors, in case of a right-sided or transverse colectomy. However, when the anastomosis is to be performed between the distal left colon and rectum, a stapled anastomosis can be carried out intracorporally using a circular stapling device.

Laparoscopy will certainly have an important role in colorectal surgery, but until such time as more prospective trials become conclusive, only patients enrolled in one of these studies should be offered a laparoscopic resection for cancer with curative intent.

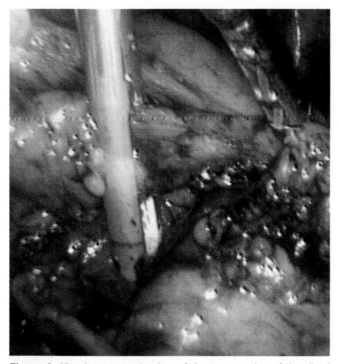

Figure 8–19. Laparoscopic view of the transsection of the distal colon using a laparoscopic roticulating gastrointestinal stapler device.

REFERENCES

1. Mackowiak PA. The normal microbial flora. N Engl J Med 1982;307:83–93.
2. Grinnell RS. Results of ligation of inferior mesenteric artery at the aorta in resections of carcinoma of the descending and sigmoid colon and rectum. Surg Gynecol Obstet 1965;120:1031–6.
3. Gebhardt C. Multi-visceral resection in colorectal carcinoma. Langenbecks Arch Chir Suppl Kongressbd 1998;115:327–30.

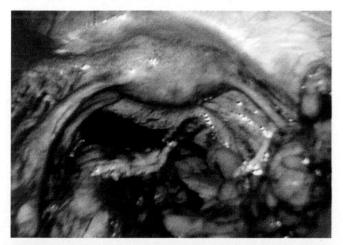

Figure 8–20. Laparoscopic view of the pelvic cavity showing the transsected distal colon and the uterus anterior of that.

4. Gall FP, Tonak J, Altendorf A. Multivisceral resections in colorectal cancer. Dis Colon Rectum 1987;30: 337–41.

5. Hunter JA, Ryan JA Jr, Schultz P. En block resection of colon cancer adherent to other organs. Am J Surg 1987;154:67–71.

6. Turnbull RB, Kyle K, Watson FR, Spratt J. Cancer of the colon: the influence of the no-touch isolation technique on survival rates. Ann Surg 1967;166: 420–5.

7. Hayashi N, Egami H, Kai M, et al. No-touch isolation technique reduces intraoperative shedding of tumor cells into the portal vein during resection of colorectal cancer. Surgery 1999;125:369–74.

8. Wiggers T, Jeekel J, Arends JW, et al. No touch isolation technique in colon cancer: a controlled prospective trial. Br J Surg 1988;75:873–8.

9. Best RR. Rectosigmoidectomy with anastomosis in carcinoma of rectum and rectosigmoid. J Int Coll Surgeons 1950;13:203–8.

10. Hojo K. Anastomotic recurrence after sphincter-saving resection for rectal cancer: length of distal clearance of the bowel. Dis Colon Rectum 1986;29:11–4.

11. Pollett WG, Nicholls RJ. The relationship between the extent of distal clearance and survival and local recurrence rates after curative anterior resection for carcinoma of the rectum. Ann Surg 1983;198:159–63.

12. Wolmark N, Fischer B. An analysis of survival and treatment failure following abdominoperineal and sphincter-saving resection in Dukes' B and C rectal carcinoma. Ann Surg 1986;204:480–9.

13. Pezim ME, Nicholls RJ. Survival after high or low ligation of the inferior mesenteric artery during curative surgery for rectal cancer. Ann Surg 1984;200:729–33.

14. Hojo K, Koyama Y, Moriya Y. Lymphatic spread and its prognostic value in patients with rectal cancer. Am J Surg 1982;144:350–4.

15. Heald RJ, Husband EM, Ryall RDH. The mesorectum in rectal cancer surgery – the clue to pelvic recurrence? Br J Surg 1982;69:613–6.

16. MacFarlane JK, Ryall RDH, Heald RJ. Mesorectal excision for rectal cancer. Lancet 1993;341:457–60.

17. Krook JE, Moertel CG, Gunderson LL, et al. Effective surgical adjuvant therapy for high-risk rectal carcinoma. N Engl J Med 1991;324:709–15.

18. NIH consensus conference. Adjuvant therapy for patients with colon and rectal cancer. JAMA 1990; 264:1444–50.

19. Heald RJ. Rectal cancer: the surgical options. Eur J Cancer 1995;31A:1189–92.

20. Havenga K, Enker WE, McDermot K, et al. Male and female sexual and urinary function after autonomic nerve preservation for carcinoma of the rectum. J Am Coll Surg 1996;182:495–502.

21. Hermanek P, Wiebelt H, Staimmer D, Riedl S. Prognostic factors of rectum carcinoma—experience of the German multicenter study SGCRC. German study group colo-rectal carcinoma. Tumori 1995;81:60–4.

22. Hermanek P, Hohenberger W. The importance of volume in colorectal cancer surgery. Eur J Surg Oncol 1996;22:213–5.

23. Quirke P, Durdey P, Dixon MF, Williams NS. Local recurrence of rectal adenocarcinoma due to inadequate surgical resection. Lancet 1986;Nov:996–8.

24. Steele GD, Herndon JE, Bleday R, et al. Sphincter-sparing treatment for distal rectal adenocarcinoma. Ann Surg Oncol 1999;6:433–41.

25. Murray JJ, Stahl TJ. Sphincter-saving alternatives for treatment of adenocarcinoma involving distal rectum. Surg Clin North Am 1993;73:131–144.

26. Kraske P. Zur extirpation hochsitzender masdarmkrebs. Verh Dtsch Ges Chir 1885;14:464.

27. Bailey HR, Huval WV, Max E, et al. Local excision of carcinoma of the rectum for cure. Surgery 1992;111: 555–61.

28. Rullier E, Zerbib F, Laurent C, et al. Intersphincteric resection with excision of internal anal sphincter for conservative treatment of very low rectal cancer. Dis Colon Rectum 1999;42:1168–75.

29. Killingback M. Local excision of carcinoma of the rectum: indications. World J Surg 1992;16:437–46.

30. Breen E, Bleday R. Preservation of the anus in the therapy of distal rectal cancers. Surg Clin North Am 1997;77:71–83.

31. Tanaka S, Yokota T, Saito D, et al. Clinicopathologic features of early rectal carcinoma and indications for endoscopic treatment. Dis Colon Rectum 1995;38: 959–63.

32. Nicholls RJ, Galloway DJ, Mason AY, et al. Clinical local staging of rectal cancer. J Surg 1985;72(Suppl): S51–2.

33. Rifkin MD, Ehrlich SM, Marks G. Staging of rectal carcinoma: prospective comparison of endorectal US and CT. Radiology 1989;170:319–22.

34. Saitoh N, Okui K, Sarashina H, et al. Evaluation of echographic diagnosis of rectal cancer using intrarectal ultrasonic examination. Dis Colon Rectum 1986;29:234–42.

35. Nicholls RJ, Mason AY, Morson BC, et al. The clinical staging of rectal cancer. Br J Surg 1982;69:404–9.

36. Herrera-Ornelas L, Justiniano J, Castillo N, et al. Metastases in small lymph nodes from colon cancer. Arch Surg 1987;122:1253–6.

37. Dukes C, Bussey H. The spread of rectal cancer and its effect on prognosis. Br J Cancer 1958;12:309–20.

38. Gabriel W, Dukes C, Bussey H. Lymphatic spread in cancer of the rectum. Br J Surg 1935;23:395–413.

39. Willett C, Compton C, Shellito P, Efird J. Selection fac-

tors for local excision or abdominoperineal resection of early stage rectal cancer. Cancer 1994;73:2716–20.

40. Bleday R, Breen E, Jessup JM, et al. Prospective evaluation of local excision for small rectal cancers. Dis Colon Rectum 1997;40:388–92.

41. Ota D, Skibber J, Rich T. M.D. Anderson cancer center experience with local excision and multimodality therapy for rectal cancer. Surg Oncol Clin N Am 1992;1:147–52.

42. Nivatvongs S, Wolff BG. Technique of per anal excision for carcinoma of the low rectum. World J Surg 1992; 16:447–50.

43. Hargrove WC, Gertner MH, Fitts WT. The Kraske operation for carcinoma of the rectum. Surg Gynecol Obstet 1979;148:931–3.

44. Knoch M, Hohenberger W. Long-term survival after noncurative therapy of colorectal carcinomas. Langenbecks Arch Chir Suppl Kongressbd 1996;113:133–5.

45. Monson JRT, Hill AD, Dapzi A. Laparoscopic colonic surgery. Br J Surg 1995;82:150–7.

46. Phillips EH, Franklin M, Carroll BJ, et al. Laparoscopic colectomy. Ann Surg 1992;216:703–7.

47. Franklin ME, Rosenthal D, Abrego-Medina D, et al. Prospective comparison of open versus laparoscopic colon surgery for carcinoma: five year results. Dis Colon Rectum. 1996;39:S35–46.

48. Wexner SD, Cohen SM, Ulrich, et al. Laparoscopic colorectal surgery: are we being honest with our patients? Dis Colon Rectum 1995;38:723–7.

49. Agachan F, Joo JS, Weiss EG, Wexner SD. Intra-operative laparoscopic complications. Are we getting better? Dis Colon Rectum 1996;39:S14–9.

50. Stocchi L, Nelson H. Laparoscopic colectomy for colon cancer: trial update. J Surg Oncol 1998;68:255–67.

51. Slim K, Pezet D, Riff Y, et al. High morbidity rate after converted laparoscopic colorectal surgery. Br J Surg 1995;82:1406–8.

52. Ortiz H, Armendariz P, Yarnoz C. Early postoperative feeding after elective colorectal surgery is not a benefit unique to laparoscopy assisted procedures. Int J Colorectal Dis 1996;11:246–9.

53. Wexner SD, Cohen SM. Port site metastases after laparoscopic colorectal surgery for cure of malignancy. Br J Surg 1995;82:295–8.

54. COST Study Group. Early results of laparoscopic surgery for colorectal cancer. Dis Colon Rectum 1996;39:S53–8.

55. Bouvy ND, Marquet RL, Jeekel J, Bonjer HJ. Laparoscopic surgery is associated with less tumour growth stimulation than conventional surgery: an experimental study. Br J Surg 1997;84:358–61.

56. Tomita H, Marcello PW, Jeffrey MD, Milsom MD. Laparoscopic surgery of the colon and rectum. World J Surg 1999;23:397–405.

9

Radiation Therapy in Colon and Rectal Cancer

CHRISTOPHER G. WILLETT, MD

COLON CANCER

Recent prospective randomized trials have established the value of adjuvant chemotherapy for patients with resected high-risk colon cancer. Patients with stage III colon cancer receiving 1 year of 5-fluorouracil (5-FU) and levamisole or 6 months of 5-FU and leucovorin have had statistically significant improvements in survival compared to patients receiving no adjuvant therapy or levamisole alone.[1-3] Currently, there is active investigation in defining the optimal sequence, administration, and modulation of 5-FU-based chemotherapy. Because of the documented efficacy of adjuvant chemotherapy and the perception among many oncologists that colonic carcinoma (as opposed to rectal cancer) is much more likely to recur systemically than locally, there has been little systematic examination of the value of postoperative irradiation with chemotherapy.

The potential indications for postoperative irradiation in patients with colon cancer stem from examinations of the patterns of failure after resection.[4,5] For rectal carcinoma, the most important predictor of local failure is tumor stage, but for colonic carcinoma, both stage and location are important. For lesions in the ascending and descending colon (anatomically immobile bowel), invasion into the retroperitoneum may limit a wide surgical resection. Compromised radial resection margins invite local failure. Unless there is invasion into an adjacent organ, local failure is rare for tumors in the sigmoid and transverse colon (mobile bowel), since a wide resection margin is usually achievable regardless of the extent of invasion into the mesentery. For tumors that arise in the cecum, flexures, or proximal and distal ends of the sigmoid colon, the risk of local failure may be variable depending on the amount of mesentery and the ability to obtain a satisfactory circumferential margin. For any colon tumor that adheres to adjacent structures (with and without lymph node involvement), local failure rates exceed 30 percent. In summary, local failure is an important consideration for large bowel tumors, where there are anatomic constraints on radial resection margins and for tumors invading adjacent structures. Figure 9–1 illustrates a representative case of a patient with a cecal cancer invading the anterior abdominal wall and psoas muscle posteriorly. Because of the improved survival seen in patients with node-positive colon carcinoma who receive 5-FU and levamisole or 5-FU and leucovorin, adjuvant radiation therapy for these patients with resected high-risk colon cancer will need to be combined with systemic chemotherapy.

Adjuvant Therapy

Published reports on the use of adjuvant postoperative radiation therapy to the tumor bed with and without chemotherapy for colonic carcinoma are limited to single-institution retrospective analysis.[6-9] These studies suggest that failure rates in the operative bed are reduced in patients receiving radiation therapy compared with historical controls. Since 1976, patients at the Massachusetts General Hospital (MGH) with completely resected but high-risk

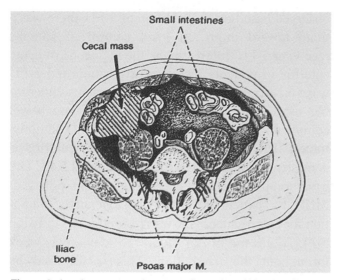

Figure 9–1. A representative case of a patient with a cecal cancer invading the anterior abdominal wall and psoas muscle posteriorly.

colonic carcinoma have been considered for postoperative radiation therapy to the tumor bed.[6,7] These high-risk groups included patients with stage B3 and C3 disease, patients with stage C2 disease except middle sigmoid and transverse colon cancer, and selected patients with stage B2 disease with tight margins. In all, 171 patients (1976–1989) have received postoperative radiation therapy via a high-energy linear accelerator by parallel opposed fields or multifield techniques to irradiate the tumor bed with approximately a 3- to 5-cm margin to a total dose of 45 Gy in 1.8 Gy fractions. This was followed by a shrinking field technique, sparing the small bowel, to 50.4 Gy. Additional treatment above 50.4 Gy was attempted in patients with stage B3 and C3 disease only if the small bowel could be displaced from the field. Of 171 patients, 53 were treated with adjuvant chemotherapy, usually 5-FU as IV bolus for 3 consecutive days (500 mg/m²/d) during the first and last weeks of radiation therapy. These 171 patients receiving postoperative radiation therapy were compared with 395 patients in the MGH series with stage B2, B3, and C3 tumors who underwent surgery only during the period from 1970 to 1977.[4,6] Table 9–1 shows by stage the 5-year actuarial local control and recurrence-free survival rates for patients undergoing postoperative radiation therapy and patients having only surgery. Local control and recurrence-free survival was statistically improved for patients with stage B3 and C3 tumors

receiving postoperative radiation therapy compared with similarly matched surgical patients. Local control rates for irradiated patients with stage B3 and C3 tumors were 93 and 72 percent, whereas the figures were 69 and 47 percent for stage B3 and C3 in patients having only surgery. Patients with stage B3 and C3 disease receiving postoperative radiotherapy experienced a 16 and 15 percentage point increase in disease-free survival, respectively, compared with the group that had surgery only. In contrast, local control and recurrence-free survival was not improved for B2 and C2 patients receiving postoperative radiation therapy compared with surgery alone. It should be noted, however, that for irradiated patients with stage B2 and C2 lesions, these comparisons may be unfavorably biased against irradiation, since most were referred because of concerns about the adequacy of local control with surgery alone. In this context, to have achieved similar local control and recurrence-free survival in the high-risk irradiated B2 and C2 patients may actually represent a positive gain.

In a recent updated analysis of the MGH experience, the 10-year actuarial rates of local control and recurrence-free survival were 88 and 58 percent, respectively, for patients treated with adjuvant irradiation for T4N0 or T4N+ cancer with one lymph node metastasis.[7] Results were less satisfactory for patients with more extensive nodal involvement.

Other studies have demonstrated improved local control in irradiated patients with high-risk colon cancer.[8,9] The results of postoperative radiotherapy at the Mayo Clinic for patients with locally advanced colon cancers were recently analyzed.[8] More than 90 percent of these had modified Astler-Coller

	TABLE 9–1. FIVE-YEAR ACTUARIAL LOCAL CONTROL AND RECURRENCE-FREE SURVIVAL AFTER SURGERY; POSTOPERATIVE RADIOTHERAPY VERSUS SURGERY ALONE ACCORDING TO STAGE (MGH EXPERIENCE)					
	Surgery Plus Radiation			**Surgery Alone**		
Stage	**No. of Patients**	**LC (%)**	**RFS (%)**	**No. of Patients**	**LC (%)**	**RFS (%)**
B2	23	91	72	163	90	78
B3	54	93	79	83	69	63
C2	55	70	47	100	64	48
C3	39	72	53	49	47	38

LC = local control; RFS = recurrence-free survival.

(MAC) stage B3 and C3 lesions. The 5-year actuarial local failure rate was 10 percent for patients with no residual disease, 54 percent for patients with microscopic residual disease and 79 percent for patients with gross residual disease ($p < .0001$).

A recent report summarized the results of postoperative radiotherapy at the University of Florida for patients with locally advanced but completely resected colon cancers.[9] This study reported a local control rate of 88 percent, which was quite similar to the 90 percent reported at the Mayo Clinic in patients who had completely resected tumors. In addition, a significant relationship between the radiation dose delivered and the rate of local control was found. The 5-year rate of local control was 96 percent for those who received 50 to 55 Gy as compared with 76 percent for those who received < 50 Gy ($p = .0095$).

To assess the merits of postoperative radiation therapy for selected patients with colonic cancer, a randomized prospective intergroup trial combining postoperative irradiation plus 5-FU and levamisole versus 5-FU and levamisole alone was initiated in 1993 under the auspices of the North Central Cancer Treatment Group and the Radiation Therapy Oncology Group. Eligible patients included those with stage B3 and C3 lesions and C2 tumors arising in the ascending and descending colon. Unfortunately, this trial was closed prematurely because of poor patient accrual. An analysis of the 222 patients entered in this trial in May 1999 showed no difference in survival between treatment arms.[10] A higher rate of grade 3 hematologic toxicity was observed in the patients receiving chemotherapy and radiation combined compared to chemotherapy only. However, these data are preliminary and must be interpreted cautiously in light of the small patient numbers in this study.

There are few data evaluating the combined effect of 5-FU and irradiation in colon cancer. In the MGH adjuvant series, 53 patients received bolus 5-FU (500 mg/m^2/day) for 3 consecutive days during the first and last weeks of irradiation. Local control and recurrence-free survival rates for the adjuvantly treated patients based on 5-FU administration during radiation therapy are listed in Table 9–2. Although no statistically significant differences in local control or recurrence-free survival were

observed based on the addition of 5-FU, there was a trend toward improved local control in patients receiving 5-FU. Interestingly, the incidence of acute enteritis in patients receiving irradiation and 5-FU was 16 percent versus 4 percent in patients undergoing irradiation only. No difference in late bowel complications have been observed by 5-FU administration. This higher incidence of acute enteritis is consistent with other reports of combined 5-FU and irradiation in rectal cancer. Our current policy at MGH for patients receiving postoperative irradiation for colon cancer is to utilize continuous infusion 5-FU (225 mg/m^2/24 hours) 5 days per week throughout the irradiation. This is followed by 6 months of maintenance 5-FU and leucovorin.

Because of the high incidence of hepatic metastases and peritoneal failures developing in patients with advanced-stage colonic carcinoma, there have been clinical investigations of the efficacy of adjuvant hepatic irradiation as well as whole abdominal radiation therapy. There has only been one randomized prospective trial.[11] The Gastrointestinal Tumor Study Group reported the results of a phase III trial of adjuvant hepatic irradiation.[11] In this study, 300 patients with completely resected transmural or node-positive colon carcinoma were randomized between two treatment arms: (1) observation or (2) 5-FU and 21 Gy to the liver (1.5 Gy per fraction for 14 treatments). The 5-FU was given as an intravenous bolus during the first 3 days of radiation therapy as well as maintenance treatment. No statistical differences in survival, recurrence-free survival, or liver recurrence were seen between the control patients and the treated patients.

Several investigators have reported the results and toxicity of whole abdominal irradiation as an adjuvant

	Without 5-FU			With 5-FU		
Stage	No. of Patients	LC (%)	RFS (%)	No. of Patients	LC (%)	RFS (%)
B2	16	91	87	7	100	80
B3	37	93	94	16	100	83
C2	41	70	69	14	70	43
C3	24	72	67	15	79	52

TABLE 9–2. FIVE-YEAR ACTUARIAL LOCAL CONTROL AND RECURRENCE-FREE SURVIVAL OF ADJUVANTLY IRRADIATED PATIENTS BASED ON 5-FU ADMINISTRATION

LC = local control; RFS = recurrence-free survival.

treatment for patients at risk for hepatic and peritoneal failure.[12-14] None of these studies had concurrent controls. Wang and colleagues reported the experience at Princess Margaret Hospital of 30 patients receiving whole abdominal irradiation of 14 to 25 Gy over 3 to 5 weeks with or without local tumor boost.[12] The 5-year actuarial survival was 55 percent. For patients without regional nodal involvement survival was 72 percent compared with 41 percent for patients with nodal involvement. After treatment, 4 patients had failure in the peritoneum and 12 had hepatic and extra-abdominal failure. Brenner and colleagues described 21 patients with Dukes C colonic cancer who received whole abdominal radiation therapy of 20 to 30 Gy in 3 weeks to areas at high risk and concurrent weekly 350-mg/m² doses of 5-FU given intravenously[13] The patients who underwent radiation therapy were compared with a matched control group of patients who underwent surgery alone, and a statistically significant improvement in the disease-free survival was noted (55% vs 12%, respectively).

In 1995, the results of a phase I/II Southwestern Oncology Group Study (SWOG 8572) utilizing 30 Gy of whole abdominal irradiation and an additional 16 Gy tumor boost with continuous infusional 5-FU (200 mg/m²/24 hr) for 41 patients with T3N1-2 colon cancer were described.[14] In view of the early intolerance, the protocol was amended to insert a 1-week break from external beam irradiation and 5-FU. The 5-year actuarial disease-free and overall survival for all 41 patients was 58 and 67 percent, respectively. For the 19 patients with four or fewer positive nodes, the 5-year overall survival and disease-free survival rates were both 61 percent. For the 20 patients with more than four involved nodes, the 5-year actuarial disease-free and overall survival rates with chemoirradiation were 55 and 74 percent, respectively. This is higher than the disease-free and overall survival results of 35 and 39 percent reported in the 5-FU and levamisole intergroup trial. Based on these results, these investigators propose that this regimen be evaluated against 5-FU and levamisole in a phase III trial.

Estes and colleagues compared patterns of relapse for MAC C2 patients in SWOG 8591 (arms of surgery alone or surgery plus 5-FU/levamisole), SWOG 8572 (whole abdominal irradiation plus tumor bed irradiation and infusion 5-FU), and the surgery alone arm from the MGH analysis.[15] In SWOG 8591, although lung relapse was decreased from 34 to 21 percent with the addition of 5-FU/levamisole to surgical resection, the chemotherapy adjuvant had no impact on the rate of local-regional relapse (surgery alone, 20%; 5-FU/levamisole, 27%), which was equivalent to the 32 percent incidence alone in the MGH analysis. Patients who received chemoirradiation (whole abdominal irradiation and tumor bed irradiation with infusion 5-FU) in SWOG 8572 had only a 12 percent tumor bed nodal relapse rate along with a reduction in liver and peritoneal relapse rates (liver relapse rate of 22% with chemoirradiation vs 54% and 57% in the two arms of SWOG 8591; peritoneal relapse rates of 15% in SWOG 8572 vs 37% and 40% in SWOG 8591).

Techniques of Irradiation of Colon Cancer

As is true in the treatment of rectal carcinoma, great care must be taken in the postoperative treatment of adenocarcinoma of the colon. The field arrangement will vary to a great degree depending on the exact site of the primary tumor and the areas thought to be at high risk for local recurrence. Although recommendations on specific fields cannot be made, some general suggestions can be made.

One should try to treat the primary tumor site with a 4- to 5-cm margin proximally and distally and a 3- to 4-cm margin medially and laterally so as to provide adequate coverage of the local tumor spread. Figure 9–2 shows a standard simulation film of a patient receiving postoperative irradiation of a cecal cancer. Clips placed at resection delineated the tumor bed, thus aiding in the design of the radiation portal and necessitating less irradiation of small bowel. Generally, the lymph nodes in the mesentery beyond the margins of the surgical resection are not treated. At times one may wish to treat lymph nodes draining from adjacent structures that are involved by tumor, such as the para-aortic nodes with deep retroperitoneal involvement. The surgeon can usually obtain good mesenteric nodal margins with standard lymph node dissections.

We have often found it helpful to treat patients in the right or left decubitis position. When patients are treated with one side up, often much of the small bowel will fall by gravity away from the radiation field. A special small bowel series must be obtained in the treatment position and compared to the standard supine position to confirm movement of small bowel and define the exact amount of small bowel in the field. The total radiation dose needs to be adjusted by the amount of small bowel included.

One often finds that part or all of one kidney needs to be irradiated. We have generally accepted the finding that irradiation of a large portion of one kidney results in long-term lack of function in that kidney. We have, however, been willing to treat these patients if their other kidney functions well and their blood-urea nitrogen (BUN) and creatinine values are within normal limits. An evaluation of the long-term effects of renal irradiation has been performed at the MGH and has shown minimal long-term clinical sequelae from unilateral renal irradiation.[16]

For colon carcinomas, a dose of 45 Gy is delivered through large fields 1.8 Gy per fraction as described earlier. At this point, an attempt is made to design a boost that will exclude as much small bowel as possible from the radiation field. The exact dose delivered to the boost area will vary according to the stage of tumor and the location of normal tissue. For a B3 or C3 tumor, we try to treat with 55 to 60 Gy if this is thought to be safe, given the position of the small intestine. Often two-field reductions will be required, one at 45 Gy and one at 50 Gy. The first field reduction may include a small portion of small bowel but, beyond 50 Gy, small bowel should be completely excluded. Although data are not available at present, the use of intraoperative radiation therapy in certain stage B3 and C3 patients such as those with uncertain margins may also be appropriate.

Summary

Selected subsets of patients with colon cancer have local recurrence risks equivalent to those seen with rectal cancer if surgery alone is used. In view of the positive results seen with combined irradiation and chemotherapy in the adjuvant treatment of rectal cancer, encouraging pilot study results with postoperative irradiation with or without 5-FU for resected high-risk colon cancers at MGH, and the positive

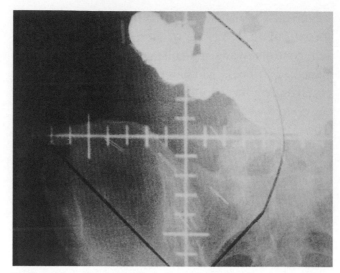

Figure 9–2. Simulation film of a patient receiving postoperative irradiation of a cecal cancer.

results of 5-FU and levamisole in high-risk adjuvant colon cancer, an intergroup randomized trial was conducted comparing 5-FU and levamisole with 5-FU and levamisole and tumor bed irradiation in patients at high risk for local recurrence following surgical resection (modified Astler-Coller B3, C3, and retroperitoneal C2 lesions; TNM T4bN0 or T4bN1,2; T3,4aN1,2). This protocol did not reach planned accrual objectives as 6 months of adjuvant 5-FU/leucovorin were shown to be equivalent to 12 months of adjuvant 5-FU/levamisole. Preliminary analysis shows no difference in survival rates between treatment arms but, given the small sample size, these data must be interpreted cautiously. Until a trial with adequate patient accrual determines the exact role of radiation therapy in colon cancer, including the proper administration of radiation-sensitizing chemotherapy, one must treat each case individually and examine relevant pathologic, clinical, and radiographic data when deciding the optimal approach to adjuvant local treatment of this disease.

RECTAL CANCER

Carcinoma of the rectum is a heterogeneous disease. At one end of the clinical spectrum, a small number of patients who present with superficially invasive favorable cancers are well served by limited procedures, such as local excision or endocavitary irradiation. The great majority of patients with rectal cancer, however, have mobile but more deeply invasive tumors that require low anterior or abdominoperineal resection. At the other and less favorable end of the clinical spectrum, a subset of patients present with locally advanced tumors that are adherent or fixed to adjoining structures such as the sacrum, pelvic side-walls, prostate, or bladder. The surgical and oncologic management of these patients varies greatly depending on stage. The following sections will review relevant clinical issues in these three presentations: favorable, mobile, and locally advanced rectal cancer.

Favorable Rectal Cancer

Approximately 34,700 patients will have developed carcinoma of the rectum in the United States in 1999.[17] Since the introduction of the abdominoperineal resection by Miles, a surgical approach to removal of this tumor and its adjacent tissues, has offered a high probability of local control and survival. Despite its merits, the abdominoperineal resection has profound drawbacks: loss of anorectal function with a permanent colostomy and a high incidence of sexual and genitourinary dysfunction. To overcome these limitations, there has been the development of an array of surgical procedures ranging from simple excision to complex resections with reconstruction. In appropriately staged patients, these operations appear to offer not only comparable rates of local control as the abdominoperineal resection but importantly preserve sphincter integrity. With continued experience, selection criteria and the role of radiation therapy and chemotherapy have become more clearly defined.

One obvious consideration in the selection of patients for sphincter preservation is tumor location within the rectum. Patients with tumors in the upper rectum have long been well managed by a sphincter-preserving anastomosis. With the advent of the end-to-end anastomotic stapling instrument, tumors of the mid-rectum, even in a narrow pelvis, become amenable to treatment by low anterior resection and preservation of the anal sphincter. Although with the lower anastomoses there is a real incidence of sexual dysfunction and less than perfect anorectal function, the avoidance of a permanent colostomy is perceived by the patient as an extremely fortunate situation. In contrast to tumors of the upper and middle rectum,

management of distal rectal cancer continues to pose a major challenge to the surgeon and oncologist. Clearly, an important consideration in treatment selection of patients with low rectal cancer is the local extent of the primary tumor.

For small tumors in the distal rectum, there has been increasing interest in local excision procedures as an alternative to the abdominoperineal resection. These operations involve an excision of the primary tumor through the anus (per-anal excision), by division of the anal sphincter (transanal, transphincteric, or Park's resection) or using a parasacral approach (Kraske). The latter two procedures are somewhat more extensive than a simple per-anal excision and have a greater degree of associated morbidity. Clearly, this technique is limited to tumors that can be excised and the excision site closed without significant narrowing of the rectal lumen.

Clinical and Radiologic Evaluation

The usual criteria for rectal cancers suitable for local excision are as follows: tumor size less than 4 cm, location 8 cm or less from the anal verge, well or moderately well-differentiated histology, mobile, not ulcerated, and no suspicion of perirectal or presacral nodes.[18] One is attempting to select patients with tumors confined to the rectal wall where there is a low probability of lymph node metastases. Local excision procedures are most suitable for these patients.

Although impressive advances have been made in the radiologic imaging of rectal cancer, digital examination by an experienced practitioner is one of the most reliable (and inexpensive!) methods of determining the depth of penetration of the primary tumor. The accuracy rates of staging the primary tumor by digital examination have been reported to be approximately 80 percent.[19] Because lymph node metastases are seen only microscopically in a high percentage of cases, it is not surprising that digital examination is insensitive at identifying metastatic perirectal nodal involvement.

In addition to digital examination, endoscopic ultrasound staging (EUS) has been used in assessing loc tumor extent as well as lymph node involvement.[19,20] Correlation of ultrasound T stage to pathologic T stage ranges from 70 to greater than 90 percent in most series.[21] To achieve high accuracy rates

(90% or greater), this examination must be performed by experienced operators. In a study from the University of Minnesota, the accuracy rates rose from 59 percent during the early phase of the study to 88 percent in the latter phase of the study.[22] Because ultrasonography and other imaging modalities can only visualize macroscopic changes, these techniques are inherently limited in their ability to discriminate lesser degrees of invasion between tumors. In one study, 30 percent of 24 patients believed to have T2 lesions based on EUS in fact had transmural invasion pathologically.[23] In assessing parirectal nodal involvement, EUS has been less helpful, with reported accuracy rates ranging from 50 to 80 percent.[20] With these caveats, EUS is generally acknowleged to be complementary to digital examination in staging and more accurate than axial CT and MRI scans.

Although CT and MRI may be inferior to EUS in staging rectal cancer, there are potential advantages of these studies. These imaging modalities offer a larger field of view than EUS and may be less operator and technique dependent and allow study of stenotic tumors.[19,20] It is our policy to obtain a CT scan as well as EUS to aid in the selection of patients for local excision. Patients with convincing evidence of transmural penetration or perirectal lymph node involvement are probably best managed by radical surgical resection because of the risk of tumor cut-through and inadequate lymph node removal by local excision procedures.

Surgery and Pathologic Evaluation

The selection of the local excision technique is important. Surgical procedures such as per-anal and transphincteric (York-Mason) excision and excision via midline posterior proctotomy (Kraske) procedure are advocated as these operations permit removal of the tumor and adjoining rectum in one piece without fragmentation of the tumor and allow assessment of inked margins, histologic differentiation, vessel involvement, and depth of penetration through the bowel wall. The pathologist should carefully define the narrowest margin in fresh tissues and on slides using an ink margin. Fulguration or electrocoagulation are not recommended as these

procedures are associated with a high likelihood of residual disease after the procedure and inadequate pathologic analysis.

A critical limitation of local excision procedures is the inability to sample or resect perirectal and mesenteric lymphatics. The incidence of perirectal lymph node metastases progressively rises as the tumor penetrates from submucosa through muscularis propria to fat.[24–26] In a collective series, lymph node metastases were observed in 12, 35, and 44 percent of lesions involving the submucosa, muscularis propria, and perirectal fat, respectively.[18] In addition to T stage, histologic grade and vascular involvement are independent predictors of lymph node metastasis. One analysis reported a 29 to 50 percent risk of perirectal nodal metastasis for patients with T1 and T2 tumors, respectively, showing poorly differentiated histology or lymphatic/blood vessel involvement.[25] Table 9–3 summarizes the incidence of perirectal nodal metastases by T stage and histologic features of the primary tumor.

Because many patients with pathologically high-risk T1 and T2 tumors have perirectal lymph metastases, local excision procedures alone would be inadequate treatment. Studies examining the outcome of patients undergoing local excision only show a clear association of local failure rate to the risk of perirectal nodal metastases as assessed by primary tumor histopathology. In a study from Erlangen, Germany, patients with low-risk tumors had less than 10 percent local failure whereas patients with high-risk tumors had greater than 30 percent local failure.[26] To improve the outcome of these patients, treatment programs of postoperative pelvic irradiation with concurrent 5-FU after local excision of "high-risk" tumors are being

Table 9–3. RISK OF PERIRECTAL LYMPH NODES BY PRIMARY TUMOR HISTOPATHOLOGY		
Low Risk: Less Than 10%	Intermediate Risk: 10% to 20%	High Risk: Greater Than 30%
Well-differentiated histology	Moderately differentiated histology	Poorly differentiated histology
Submucosa or inner muscularis propria invasion	Muscularis propria invasion	Muscularis propria or perirectal fat invasion Lymphatic or venous vessel invasion

investigated at many centers in the United States.[27–35] The results of several studies are summarized in Table 9–4.

Treatment Recommendations and Results

Treatment recommendations should be guided by the surgical and pathologic findings of the local excision. For patients with small tumors invading the mucosa and submucosa, local excision alone probably suffices. Studies from several centers have shown that the results of local excision only for patients with T1 lesions with favorable histology are excellent, with local control and recurrence-free survival rates of 90 percent or greater. Postoperative irradiation is usually not advised for patients with locally excised T1 tumors unless the margins are compromised or the primary tumor exhibits poorly differentiated histology or lymphatic/venous invasion.

In tumors that are somewhat larger or in which there is deeper invasion of the tumor into the rectal wall, more aggressive techniques of combined local excision and radiation therapy and chemotherapy have been employed. Because of the risk of perirectal nodal metastases and reported local failure rates of 20 percent or greater after local excision only, postoperative pelvic irradiation with 5-FU-based chemotherapy is advised for all patients with T2 lesions. Single-institution studies reporting on the results of postoperative irradiation for these patients indicate excellent local control and survival rates. In a report from the MD Anderson Hospital, the local control rate of 15 patients with T2 tumors treated by local excision with postoperative irradiation and 5-FU-based chemotherapy was 93 percent.[30] Similar results were reported by MGH where the 5-year actuarial local control of 33 patients with T2 tumors treated by local excision and adjuvant irradiation with and without 5-FU was reported at 85 percent.[29]

The results from single-institution studies of local excision of T1 and T2 rectal cancer with appropriate selection of postoperative irradiation appears to be supported by results of the CALGB Intergroup Phase II study.[35] In this study, 59 patients underwent local excision of T1 tumors without further therapy whereas 51 patients with T2 tumors received postoperative irradiation with 5-FU after local excision.

Overall, 13 of the 110 (12%) patients have had tumor recurrence. Four of the 59 patients with T1 tumors failed; two underwent APR for local recurrence only, and both were reported without evidence of disease at the time of last visit. Nine of 51 patients with T2 primaries failed. Three had distant recurrence and died without evidence of salvage attempted. Six underwent APR for local recurrence. Two had local and distant disease and subsequently died. Four had initial recurrence limited to the local site; three of these four were reported free of disease at the time of last visit; the remaining patient failed at distant sites but was disease free locally at the time of death. Thus, five of six potentially curable patients after APR were reported without disease at the time of last visit and one of six had died of distant disease despite local tumor control.

For patients with tumors invading the perirectal fat (T3), radical surgical resection is recommended (if feasible) because of the risk of tumor cut-through and inadequate lymph node removal by local excision procedures. The experience of local excision with postoperative irradiation and chemotherapy is limited and the available data suggest higher local failure rates. Three of 15 patients (20%) with T3 tumors from the MD Anderson report have experienced local failure following local excision and postoperative irradiation with 5-FU.[30] In a study from MGH, three of four patients (75%) with T3 tumors suffered a local recurrence after local excision and postoperative irradiation.[28] Unless there is a medical contraindication or patient refusal, we would not advise a treatment program of local excision and postoperative irradiation and chemotherapy for patients with T3 tumors.

Table 9–4. OUTCOME FOLLOWING LOCAL EXCISION AND POSTOPERATIVE IRRADIATION

Study	Local Control (%)	Survival (%)
Princess Margaret Hospital[32]	76	80 (6-year median)
Fox Chase Cancer Center[33]	81	75 (5-year DFS)
Memorial Sloan Kettering Cancer Center[34]	73	70 (Overall)
CALGB Intergroup[35]	90	74 (Crude figures)
MGH/Emory University[29]	90	74

Radiation Therapy Techniques and 5-Fluorouracil Administration

At the time of surgery, radiopaque markers are placed at the perimeter of the excision, identifying the high-risk region to aid in treatment planning. For patients with disease limited to the submucosa and muscularis propria, pelvic irradiation to 45 Gy in 25 fractions by a four-field technique is given followed by the first-field reduction with lateral fields to 50.4 Gy and a second-field reduction (if appropriate) with lateral fields to 54.0 Gy. During the 5.5- to 6-week course of irradiation, our patients receive continuous infusion 5-FU (225 mg/m^2/24 hrs) 5 days per week. Chemotherapy alternatives could include bolus 5-FU with leucovorin during the first and last weeks of irradiation.

Patients are treated in the prone position. For the initial fields (45 Gy), the superior border should be 1.5 cm above the level of the sacral promontory and the lower border of the field 4 to 5 cm below the defined tumor bed (Figures 9–3 and 9–4). Laterally, the posteroanterior-anteroposterior (PA-AP) fields extend 1 to 1.5 cm beyond the true bony pelvis. To treat the entire presacral space with adequate margins and full dose, the lateral fields are designed so that the posterior border encompasses the entire sacrum with a 1-cm margin posterior to the sacrum. Anteriorly, the fields are designed to encompass the previous tumor bed, including the posterior wall of the vagina for females and a large portion of the prostate for males. The radiopaque markers placed at surgery are helpful in designing the field reductions (Figure 9–5). After 45 Gy, lateral fields with an approximately 3-cm margin around the marked tumor bed are typically used for three fractions to 50.4 Gy, followed by a further field reduction with a 2-cm margin around the marked tumor bed to 54 Gy. A small bowel series must be performed to ensure

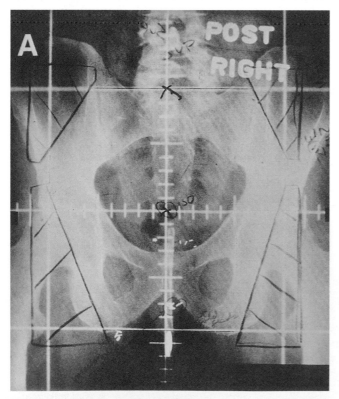

Figure 9–3. Anteroposterior simulation film of a patient with rectal cancer that has been locally excised.

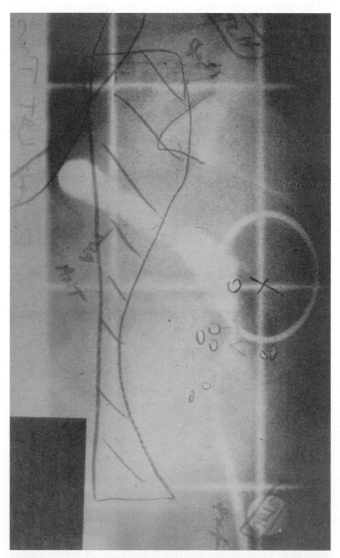

Figure 9–4. Lateral simulation film of a patient with rectal cancer that has been locally excised.

that no small bowel is within these lateral boost fields. For patients with positive or tight resection margins or poor prognostic features suggesting a higher risk of local recurrence, additional irradiation to 55 Gy to 65 Gy may be appropriate. Specialized techniques, such as interstitial implant, split beams with rectal dilatation, or perineal proton beam irradiation, allow homogeneous irradiation of high-risk regions in the rectum and adjacent perirectal fat with sparing of uninvolved rectum, perineum, and pelvic viscera. These techniques may allow a substantial number of patients to obtain local control with good preservation of anorectal function.

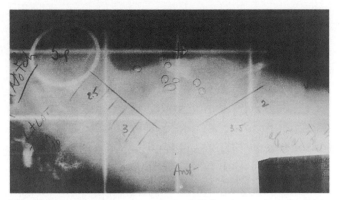

Figure 9–5. Radiopaque markers outlining tumor bed to aid in designing field reductions.

Summary

The combination of local excision with postoperative irradiation and chemotherapy appears to offer not only satisfactory local control and survival but, importantly, sphincter preservation for selected patients with distal rectal cancer. For patients with favorable histology T1 rectal cancer, local excision alone suffices. Postoperative irradiation and chemotherapy should follow local excision procedures for patients with unfavorable histology T1 and all T2 tumors. The data for T3 tumors with this approach are limited; however, results from single-institution studies suggest unacceptably high local failure rates. Radical resection is advised.

Mobile Rectal Cancer

Adjuvant Therapy

The efficacy of postoperative irradiation and 5-FU-based chemotherapy as adjuvant therapy for resected high-risk rectal cancer (stage II or III disease) was established by a series of prospective randomized trials during the 1980s and 1990s.[36–40] These studies examined the role of postoperative irradiation and chemotherapy for rectal carcinoma. The Gastrointestinal Tumor Study Group (GITSG) randomized patients with Dukes B2 and C rectal carcinomas to one of four arms: observation, postoperative irradiation only (40 or 48 Gy), chemotherapy only (semustine [methyl-CCNU] and 5-FU), and postoperative irradiation (40 or 44 Gy) with concurrent 5-FU and maintenance chemotherapy with 5-FU and methyl-CCNU.[36] This study demonstrated improved local control and survival for patients receiving combined irradiation and chemotherapy compared with surgery alone. The National Surgical Adjuvant Breast and Bowel Project (NSABP) randomized patients with Dukes B and C rectal cancers to one of three arms: observation only, adjuvant chemotherapy only (methyl-CCNU, vincristine, and 5-FU), or postoperative irradiation only (46 to 47 Gy).[37] There was a reduction in local recurrence in patients receiving postoperative irradiation but no improvement in survival compared with surgery alone. Male patients receiving chemotherapy had improved survival compared with control patients. The Mayo/North Central Cancer Treatment Group (NCCTG) study compared postoperative irradiation only (50.4 Gy), postoperative irradiation (50.4 Gy) with concurrent 5-FU, and pre- and postirradiation chemotherapy (5-FU and methyl-CCNU).[38] This study showed improved local control and survival in patients who received combined modality treatment versus postoperative irradiation only. Most investigators have interpreted these data to show that combined pelvic irradiation with concurrent and maintenance 5-FU-based chemotherapy results in both improved pelvic control and survival compared with surgery alone for patients with rectal tumors extending through the bowel wall or with nodal involvement.

All of these chemotherapy regimens contain methyl-CCNU, a known risk factor for acute non-lymphocytic leukemia. The estimated risk of delayed acute leukemia in patients receiving multiple doses of methyl-CCNU over 12 to 18 months is

2.3 cases per 1,000 persons per year (14 cases of leukemia in 2,067 patients given methyl-CCNU; 6-year cumulative risk of developing leukemia is 4%). Importantly, two subsequent randomized postoperative trials from the GITSG and the NCCTG have demonstrated that methyl-CCNU does not produce an additive benefit to irradiation plus 5-FU.[39,40] Thus, methyl-CCNU is no longer utilized in the adjuvant chemotherapy regimens in colorectal cancer.

A major issue at present in the adjuvant therapy of rectal cancer is how best to optimize the proven combination of radiation and 5-FU. If there is a combined modality effect of radiation therapy and 5-FU, it is logical to try to use both modalities optimally. Both the use of 5-FU as a long-term continuous infusion (225 mg/m²/d) and 5-FU combined with leucovorin have been shown to produce higher response rates in patients with metastatic disease than doses of conventional bolus 5-FU. The GI Intergroup has run a study testing the value of continuous infusion 5-FU given with radiation therapy compared with bolus 5-FU during radiation therapy.[40] Both groups of patients also received pre- and postirradiation 5-FU. Although there was a reduction in distant metastases and improved recurrence-free and overall survival in patients receiving PVI 5-FU compared to bolus 5-FU, there was no difference in local control rates by 5-FU administration ($p = .11$) (Table 9–5). A study has also been recently completed testing the value of pelvic irradiation with combinations of 5-FU; 5-FU and leucovorin; and 5-FU, leucovorin, and levamisole in the adjuvant therapy of rectal cancer.[41] Preliminary analysis indicates that the three-drug regimen is more toxic and no more efficacious than the one- or two-drug regimen. Additional studies will continue to be run to attempt to determine the optimal mode of administration as well as modulation of 5-FU. In a nonstudy setting, we have utilized continuous infusion schedules of 5-FU (225 mg/m²/24 hrs) throughout the 5- to 6-week course of pelvic irradiation.

Although improvements in local control and survival have been achieved by adjuvant therapy, acute and late treatment-related morbidity have also been observed. In a recent intergroup trial, 24

Table 9–5. RANDOMIZED POSTOPERATIVE RADIATION/ CHEMOTHERAPY TRIALS OF RECTAL CANCER

	Local Failure (%)	Distant Failure (%)	Overall Survival (%)
GITSG[36]			
RT + ChT	11	26	57
RT	20	30	43
ChT	27	27	43
Control	24	34	28
NSABP[37]			
RT	16	31	50
ChT	21	24	58
Control	25	26	48
NCCTG/Mayo[38]			
RT - ChT	14	29	53
RT	25	46	38
GI Intergroup[40]			
RT - PVI 5-FU	NS	31	70
RT - Bolus 5-FU	NS	40	60

NS = not stated; PVI = peripheral venous infuson.

percent of patients receiving concurrent pelvic irradiation and 5-FU by peripheral venous infusion experienced severe or life-threatening diarrhea.[40] In addition to acute toxicity, there may be significant late effects as well. In an analysis of 306 rectal cancer patients treated with postoperative irradiation at the Mayo Clinic from 1981 to 1990, the 10-year probability of developing chronic bowel injury was 25%.[42] Besides the standard endpoints of acute and late bowel injury, there is also increasing awareness of changes in quality of life induced by adjuvant therapy. Kollmorgen and colleagues[43] from the Mayo Clinic reported major long-term detrimental effects on the bowel function (frequency, incontinence, pad requirements, etc.) of patients undergoing low anterior resection and postoperative chemoirradiation compared to patients undergoing low anterior resection alone.

Preoperative Irradiation

In the United States, the principal focus of clinical research of rectal cancer has been directed at studies examining combinations of postoperative irradiation and chemotherapy. In contrast, European investigators have conducted a series of trials evaluating different schedules of preoperative irradiation with surgery compared to surgery only for patients with rectal cancer.[44-47] Table 9–6 summarizes the results of these studies according to the dose intensity of preoperative irradiation (low dose, moderate dose, and Swedish style). As Table 9–6 shows, there is no improvement in local control or survival for patients undergoing low-dose preoperative irradiation compared to patients undergoing surgery alone. For patients undergoing moderate-dose preoperative irradiation, local failure rates have been decreased by this schedule but no improvements in survival were seen. The most recent of the Swedish studies evaluating the schedule of 25 Gy in 5 fractions[47] has shown statistical improvements in local control and survival compared to patients undergoing surgery alone. This Swedish approach of preoperative irradiation has been adopted by many European oncologists but has not been widely accepted in the United States principally because of concerns of late treatment related morbidity with this rapid and high-dose fractionation schedule as well as the desire to integrate chemotherapy concurrently with preoperative irradiation.

Neoadjuvant Therapy

Because of the success of combined modality treatment in the postoperative setting, there has been intense interest in utilizing this approach neoadjuvantly. Numerous phase II studies[48-52] have demonstrated the safety of this program and preliminary analyses indicate satisfactory local control and survival rates. These studies have also shown higher rates of complete pathologic response following chemoirradiation compared to irradiation only. Complete pathologic responses occur in only 6 to 12 percent of patients following moderate- to high-dose (45–50 Gy) preoperative irradiation (Table 9–7).

In some studies, continuous infusion 5-FU programs or various 5-FU-based regimens with irradiation have increased these complete pathologic response rates to 20 to 29 percent (see Table 9–7). The significance of increased pathologic responses in terms of local control and survival will require further maturation of these and other studies.

Although the techniques and dose of irradiation are similar in these chemoirradiation studies (45 to 50.4 Gy in 25 to 28 fractions to the pelvis with a three- or four-field arrangement), there is marked variability in modes of 5-FU administration. Some studies employ a schedule of 5-FU given as a bolus for 3 or 4 consecutive days during the first and last weeks of irradiation whereas other investigators have utilized a continuous infusion approach throughout irradiation. Additionally, several investigators have incorporated other agents such as leucovorin and cisplatin in combination with 5-FU. Because of the intergroup trial showing a survival advantage for patients treated with continuous infusion 5-FU throughout irradiation compared to patients treated with bolus 5-FU in the postoperative setting, it would seem appropriate that this approach should be adopted for preoperative irradiation programs in rectal cancer. The value of additional agents such as leucovorin, levamisole, and cisplatin in combination with 5-FU is under active investigation. It is becoming clear from the adjuvant rectal trials that more chemotherapy with irradiation is not necessarily a better situation. As previously discussed, the three-drug combination of 5-FU, levamisole, and leucovorin is more toxic and no more effective than the one- or two-drug regimen.[41] At present, we are using a 5-FU schedule of 225 mg/m^2/24 hours for 5 days per week throughout the 5.5-week course of preoperative irradiation (45 Gy to the pelvis followed by a tumor boost of 5.4 Gy in 28 1.8 Gy fractions). In our experience, this 5-FU schedule has been well tolerated.

For larger and more invasive tumors of the distal rectum where local excision is inappropriate, preoperative irradiation and more recently preoperative

Table 9–6. SELECTED RANDOMIZED TRIALS OF PREOPERATIVE IRRADIATION AND SURGERY VERSUS SURGERY ONLY				
		% LC		5-Year Survival
Study	Dosage	C	TX	C	TX
Low Dose					
Princess Margaret[44]	5 Gy	—	—	35	40
Medical Research Council[45]	5 Gy/20 Gy	—	—	39	40
Moderate Dose					
EORTC[46]	34.5 Gy	70	85	59	69
Swedish Style					
Swedish Rectal Cancer Trial[47]	25 Gy	73	89	48	58

Table 9–7. CORRELATION OF PATHOLOGIC RESPONSE TO NEOADJUVANT REGIMEN

Study	Patients	Preoperative EBRT Dose (Gy)	Chemotherapy	Complete Pathologic Response Rate (%)
U. Florida[48]	132	30–50	None	11
Jewish H.[49]	208	40-50	None	6
MDAH[50]	77	45	5-FU Inf.	29
Duke[51]	43	45	5-FU & CDDP	27
MSKCC[52]	20	50.4	5 FU & leucovorin	20

chemoirradiation have been utilized to promote tumor regression, thus facilitating a resection sparing the sphincter and employing the left colon in a coloanal anastomosis. The sphincter is disturbed by this surgery, and many patients experience initial difficulty with control, a sense of urgency, and stool frequency, although most patients eventually have acceptable functional results. Table 9–8 summarizes the results of three studies[53–55] utilizing this approach of preoperative irradiation and resection with coloanal anastomosis. The data demonstrate that approximately 80 percent of patients with low rectal cancers can undergo a resection with a coloanal anastomosis as an alternative to abdominoperineal resection. Analyses of local control, survival, and bowel function are encouraging.

There is much debate regarding the relative merits and disadvantages of adjuvant versus neoadjuvant combined modality therapy in the treatment of patients with rectal carcinoma. Currently, there is one active randomized trial (NSABP R-03) in the United States assessing the merits of neoadjuvant therapy (5-FU and leucovorin, pelvic irradiation) versus adjuvant therapy (5-FU, leucovorin, pelvic irradiation). In a preliminary analysis of 116 patients, preoperative chemotherapy and irradiation appeared as safe and tolerable as postoperative therapy.[56] There appeared to be a trend to tumor downstaging and sphincter preservation in the preoperative arm. Final determination of survival benefit and long-term toxicity awaits completion of this study.

Technical Aspects of Postoperative or Preoperative Radiation Therapy

In treatment of abdominopelvic tumors, careful attention must be paid to radiation therapy technique. It is generally inappropriate to treat rectal tumors with PA-AP fields alone where the anterior structures, not substantially at risk for local failure, are treated to a high dose. This invariably leads to increased toxicity from the treatment, with minimal gain in terms of improved local control. At the MGH, patients are generally treated with a four-field box technique, although a three-field technique, with right and left lateral fields and a posterior field, is also reasonable (Figures 9–6 and 9–7). The use of lateral fields allows a portion of the bladder and some anteriorly placed small bowel to be spared.

The PA-AP fields extend from approximately the lower level of the L5 vertebral body to 4 to 5 cm below the anastomosis (or below the tumor when treating preoperatively) in patients who had a low anterior resection. For patients with an abdominoperineal resection, the fields always extend to include the perineum. There are a substantial number of local recurrences in the perineum and this area needs to be in the high-dose volume. Laterally, the fields extend approximately 1.0 to 1.5 cm beyond the bony pelvis so that the lateral pelvic soft tissue receives the full radiation dose. The lateral fields have the same cephalad and caudad extent as the PA-AP fields. Patients are treated prone. The posterior

Table 9–8. PRELIMINARY RESULTS OF PREOPERATIVE IRRADIATION AND RESECTION WITH COLOANAL ANASTOMOSIS

Study	Patients (n)	Preoperative EBRT Dose (Gy)	Patients Undergoing Sphincter-Preserving	Local Control (%)	Actuarial Survival (%)	Bowel Function (%)
Minsky et al[53]	30	50.4	24 (80)	83 (4 y)	75 (4 y)	75% good to excellent
Rouanet[54]	27	60	21 (78)	93 (crude)	83 (2 y)	NA
Mohiuddin et al[55]	52	45–60	NA	86 (crude)	85 (5 y)	90% acceptable

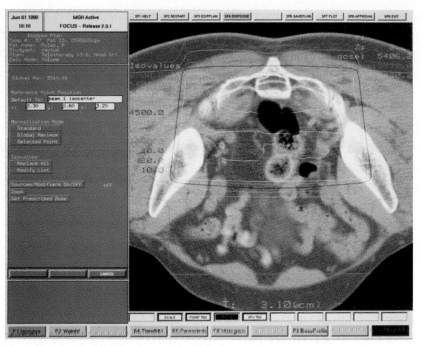

Figure 9–6.   CT treatment plan showing isodose distribution of a three-field arrangement (posterior and right and left laterals). Patient is in prone position.

border of the lateral field extends beyond the bony sacrum so that the full dose is delivered to the presacral space, a common site of local failure. Anteriorly, the fields extend to cover adequately the original tumor with at least a 2-cm margin. Blocks can often be used to spare a portion of the femoral neck on the lateral fields.

Patients are treated with a full bladder so as to push some of the small intestine out of the radiation field. When the perineum needs to be treated, a bolus

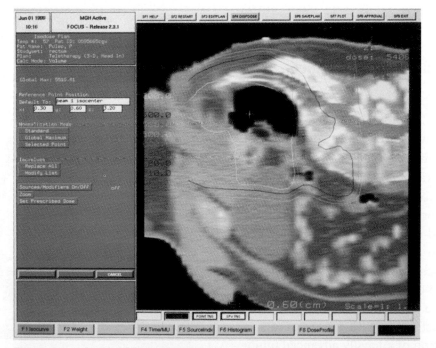

Figure 9–7.   Sagittal CT plan showing isodose distribution of a three-field arrangement (posterior and right and left laterals).

is placed on it so that a full dose will be delivered to the scar in this region. If the reaction becomes marked, the bolus can be removed. Generally, perineal reactions have not produced major symptoms.

Patients are treated at 1.8 Gy, five fractions per week, to a total dose of 45 Gy to these fields. The field size is then reduced and a boost dose is delivered to the tumor bed. Prior to designing the boost field, a special small bowel radiographic series is obtained so as to define the exact location of the small bowel with respect to the boost area. Only by defining the exact bowel position can one design the radiation fields so as to eliminate excess irradiation of the small intestine. Great effort is made to avoid doses greater than 45 Gy to any small bowel that is fixed in the pelvis. In this regard, it is helpful to have the surgeon (at the time of the initial surgical procedure) try to mobilize small intestine from the pelvis. This can best be accomplished by reperitonealizing the pelvic floor. When this is not possible it is helpful to have a loop of omentum mobilized to cover the pelvic floor or to have the uterus retroverted to accomplish the same purpose. Some centers have investigated the use of prostheses or artifical mesh, but these are still being investigated. This is most important in treating patients after an abdominoperineal resection, as after a low anterior resection the remaining rectum and colon prevent some small bowel from being immobilized deep in the pelvis.

Locally Advanced Rectal Cancer

Within this group of patients categorized as having locally advanced rectal cancer, there is also variability in disease extent with no uniform definition of resectability. Depending on the series, a locally advanced lesion can range from a tethered or marginally resectable tumor to a fixed cancer with direct invasion of adjacent organs or structures. The definition will also depend on whether the assessment of resectability is made clinically or at the time of surgery. In some cases, tumors thought to be unresectable at the time of clinical or radiographic examination may be more mobile when the patient is examined under anesthesia. With these caveats, a good working definition of a locally advanced tumor is a tumor that cannot be resected without leaving microscopic or gross residual disease in the local site because of tumor adherence or fixation to that site.

Figure 9–8 shows the CT scan of a patient with locally advanced rectal cancer involving the posterior and left pelvic side walls. At surgery the tumor was adherent to the side walls and pathologic review of the resection specimen showed that this radial soft-tissue margin was positive for carcinoma.

Since these patients do poorly with surgery alone, treatment programs of irradiation, chemotherapy, and surgery have evolved to improve the outcome of these patients.

External Beam Irradiation

In the past, the management of locally advanced rectal cancer has been variable. Some patients have had incomplete surgical resections alone, while others have had radiation alone or surgery combined with post- or preoperative irradiation. The results of high-dose external beam irradiation as a primary curative treatment have been unsatisfactory, with local failure rates of at least 90 percent or greater and 5-year survivals of less than 10 percent. Wang and Schulz reported that of 58 patients with recurrent, inoperable, or residual rectosigmoid carcinoma treated with 35 to 50 Gy in 4 to 5 weeks, six patients survived 5 years disease free.[57] O'Connell and colleagues noted that 37 of 44 patients with locally unresectable or recurrent rectal carcinoma treated with 50 Gy in a split-course fashion over 7 weeks with and without adjuvant immunotherapy had progression of disease.[58] Of 31 patients assessable for sites of initial

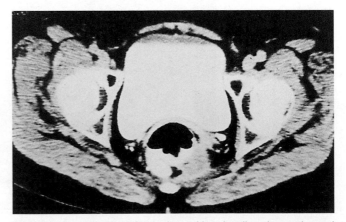

Figure 9–8. CT scan of a patient with a locally advanced rectal cancer involving the posterior and left pelvic side wall.

tumor progression, 17 had local progression only, 11 had concurrent local progression and distant metastases only, and 3 developed only distant metastases. Brierley and colleagues reported that of 77 patients with clinically fixed tumors who were treated with 50 Gy in 20 fractions over 4 years, local control was 3 percent and survival was 4 percent.[59] Unless the patient is not a candidate for surgery, external beam irradiation has no role as definitive treatment.

External Beam Irradiation and Surgery

Combinations of external beam irradiation and surgical resection have been used to improve local control and survival. Radiation therapy after subtotal resection gives better local control and survival in patients treated for residual microscopic disease compared to patients treated with gross residual disease. Allee and colleagues reported the results of 31 patients with residual microscopic cancer treated with 45 Gy followed by additional radiation therapy to as much as 60 to 70 Gy if small bowel could be moved from the radiation field.[60] The local control rate and 5-year disease-free survival rates were 70 and 45 percent, respectively. In contrast, these figures were 43 and 11 percent for 25 patients treated for gross residual disease. A possible dose-response correlation was seen in patients with microscopic residual disease; the risk of local failure was 11 percent (1 of 9) with doses of 60 Gy or greater versus 40 percent (8 of 20) if the boost dose was less than 60 Gy. There was no clear dose-response relationship in patients with gross disease. Of 17 patients receiving external beam irradiation after subtotal resection, Schild and colleagues observed that local control was achieved in 3 of 10 patients (30%) with microscopic residual cancer and 1 of 7 patients (14%) with gross remaining cancer.[61] Four of the 17 patients (24%) have remained disease-free for more than 5 years. Ghossein and colleagues treated patients with 46 Gy in 1.8 Gy fractions followed by a field reduction to the area of persistent disease and received 60 Gy.[62] The incidence of local failure and survival for patients treated with microscopic disease was 16 and 84 percent, whereas for patients with gross disease these figures were 50 and 39 percent, respectively.

For patients presenting with locally advanced disease (unresectable for cure because of tumor fixation), high-dose preoperative irradiation (45 to 50 Gy) has been used to reduce tumor size and facilitate resection. Emami and colleagues reported that the rate of resectability of 28 patients after full-dose preoperative irradiation was 50 percent.[63] Dosoretz and colleagues reported on 25 patients with unresectable tumors in the rectum or rectosigmoid treated with 40 to 52 Gy preoperative radiation therapy.[64] Of the 25 patients, 16 underwent potentially curative resection and the 6-year survival was 26 percent (with three postoperative deaths). Total pelvic failure after curative resection was 39 percent (5 of 13 patients). Mendenhall and colleagues reviewed 23 patients with locally advanced carcinoma who received 35 to 60 Gy of preoperative irradiation.[65] Eleven patients were able to undergo complete resection with a 5-year absolute survival of 18 percent and local failure of 55 percent. As reported by Stevens and Fletcher, 28 of 72 patients (39%) with locally advanced carcinoma of the rectum or rectosigmoid received 50 to 72 Gy preoperatively and were resectable.[66] However, tumor recurred locally in 9 of 28 (32%) of these patients and the 5-year survival was 10 percent. Of 20 patients with unresectable rectal cancer undergoing 43 to 55.8 Gy preoperative irradiation reported by Whiting and colleagues, 13 patients (65%) underwent resection with curative intent.[67] Three of 13 (23%) subsequently developed a local failure; the 5-year survival was 40 percent.

There has been one randomized prospective study examining the merits of preoperative irradiation in patients with locally advanced rectal cancer. Under the auspices of the Northwest Rectal Cancer Group (Manchester, United Kingdom), 284 patients with tethered or fixed rectal cancer were entered into a prospective randomized trial between 1982 and 1986 assessing the effects of preoperative irradiation given 1 week before surgery.[68] A group of 141 patients was allocated to undergo surgical treatment alone and 143 were allocated to receive 20 Gy in four fractions. This study showed a highly significant reduction in local recurrences in the irradiated group (12.8%) versus the surgery alone group (36.5%). Although there was no significant difference in either overall survival or cancer-related mortality between the two treatment groups, subset analysis of the patients who underwent curative surgery alone reveals an overall mortality of 53.3 percent for patients allocated to surgery alone and 44.9 percent for patients allocated to preoperative radiotherapy. This was a significant reduction in mortality.

In summary, following full-dose preoperative irradiation, most series report that one-half to two-thirds of patients will be converted to a resectable status. However, despite a complete resection and negative margins, the local failure rate depending on the degree of tumor fixation varies from 23 to 55 percent.

Preoperative External Beam Irradiation with Chemotherapy and Surgery

Because of the efficacy of postoperative irradiation and 5-FU in the adjuvant treatment of rectal cancer, there has been interest in examining this approach preoperatively. These investigations have studied combinations of moderate- to full-dose preoperative irradiation (45 to 50.4 Gy) with 5-FU-based chemotherapy for patients with clinical T3 and T4 rectal cancer. Comments in this section will be limited to analysis of patients with clinical T4 tumors. The endpoints of these studies have included not only resectability, local control, and survival but pathologic downstaging and sphincter preservation rates. One such report recently came from the MD Anderson Hospital.[69] Patients with locally advanced rectal cancer who received 45 Gy of preoperative irradiation with continuous infusion chemotherapy of 5-FU and/or cisplatin and surgery had 3-year survival and local recurrence rates of 82 and 3 percent, respectively. These results were in contrast with 3-year survival and local recurrence rates of 62 and 33 percent for 36 similarly staged patients undergoing preoperative irradiation without chemotherapy. Although there was a higher rate of sphincter-preserving procedures in patients receiving chemoirradiation (35%) versus patients undergoing irradiation only (7%), there were no differences in rates of resectability or pathologic downstaging between these groups of patients receiving chemotherapy versus no chemotherapy. Other investigations, however, have reported higher resectability and pathologic downstaging rates with the use of preoperative

chemoirradiation schedules. In an analysis of 36 patients (30 primary and 6 recurrent) with locally advanced, unresectable disease who were treated with 50.4 Gy of pelvic irradiation and concurrent 5-FU and leucovorin at Memorial Sloan Kettering Cancer Center, the resectability rate with negative margins was 97 percent and the total complete response rate was 25 percent.[70] Similarly, a Swedish study reported an enhanced resectability rate in patients with unresectable rectal cancer who received preoperative irradiation, 5-FU, methotrexate, and leucovorin rescue compared with 38 patients who received radiation alone (71% vs 34%).[71] Investigators from Tom Baker Cancer Centre reported an 89 percent complete resection rate in 46 patients with tethered and fixed rectal cancer treated with 40 Gy and 5-FU infusion and mitomycin-C.[72] Of 31 patients receiving continuous 5-FU infusion throughout irradiation at Thomas Jefferson University, 29 patients (94%) underwent complete resection with negative margins.[73] Enhanced resectability is an important endpoint since patients with initially unresectable rectal cancer who have microscopic or gross residual disease have higher local failure and lower survival rates compared with those patients who undergo a complete resection.

Analyses of local control and survival following treatment programs of preoperative chemoirradiation and surgery for locally advanced rectal cancer are limited by small patient numbers and short follow up. Nevertheless, preliminary results suggest improved outcomes in patients receiving chemoirradiation compared to prior studies evaluating patients undergoing irradiation only[69–74] (Table 9–9). Based on this data, combinations of moderate to high-dose preoperative irradiation with concurrent 5-FU-based chemotherapy result in improved rates of resectability and possibly local control and survival.

Although the dose and techniques of irradiation are similar in these studies (45 to 50.4 Gy in 25 to 28 fractions to the pelvis via a three- or four-field arrangement), there is marked variability in 5-FU administration. Some studies employ a schedule of 5-FU administered as a bolus for 3 consecutive days during weeks 1 and 5 of irradiation whereas other investigators have utilized a continuous infusion approach

Table 9–9. PREOPERATIVE CHEMOTHERAPY, RADIATION THERAPY, AND RESECTION OF LOCALLY ADVANCED RECTAL CANCER

Study	No. of Patients	Drug Program	EBRT Dose	Complete Resection Rate	Local Failure	Survival
MD Anderson[69]	38	5-FU infusion ± CDDP	45 Gy	84%	Crude – 3%	3 Yr – 82%
MSKCC[70]	36	5-FU/leucovorin	50.4 Gy	97%	4 Yr.Act. – 30%	4 Yr – 67%
Tom Baker Cancer Center[72]	46	5-FU / mit-C	40 Gy	89%	2 Yr.Act. – 16%	3 Yr – 31%
Thomas Jefferson[73]	31	C.I. 5-FU	55.8 Gy	94%	Crude – 16%	3 Yr – 68%
Emory[74]	20	5-FU bolus	50 Gy	N.S.	Crude – 10%	3 Yr – 82%

throughout irradiation. Additionally, several investigators have used other agents such as leucovorin, cisplatin, and mitomycin C in combination with 5-FU. Because of the intergroup trial showing a survival advantage for patients treated with continuous infusion 5-FU throughout irradiation compared to patients treated with bolus 5-FU in the postoperative setting,[70] it would seem appropriate that this approach should be adopted for preoperative irradiation programs in rectal cancer. The value of additional agents such as leucovorin, levamisole, cisplatin, and mitomycin-C in combination with 5-FU is under investigation. It is becoming clear from the adjuvant rectal trials that more chemotherapy with irradiation is not necessarily a better option. In the adjuvant postoperative chemoirradiation rectal trials, its appears that the three-drug combination of 5-FU, levamisole, and leucovorin is more toxic and no more efficacious than 5-FU only or the two-drug regimen of 5-FU and leucovorin.[41] At present, we are using a 5-FU schedule of 225 mg/m^2/24 hours for 5 days per week throughout the 5.5-week course of preoperative irradiation (45 Gy to the pelvis followed by a tumor boost of 5.4 Gy in 28 1.8 Gy fractions). In our experience, this 5-FU schedule with pelvic irradiation has been well tolerated.

Intraoperative Electron Beam Irradiation

Despite full-dose preoperative irradiation and complete resection of locally advanced rectal cancer, local failure occurs in at least one-third of patients. These local failure rates are even higher in patients undergoing subtotal resection. At the MGH, Mayo Clinic, and other centers in the United States, Europe, and Asia, intraoperative electron beam radiation therapy (IOERT) has been used in combination with preoperative irradiation (with and without 5-FU) and surgical

resection when there is gross residual cancer, positive resection margins, or simply tumor adherence.

The IOERT program at MGH was started in 1978 and involved transporting the patient from the operating room to the Radiation Oncology department for IOERT. In 1996, a dedicated IOERT suite was opened at the MGH. This suite allows full-time availability of this technology (Figure 9–9). With this system, a cone (which is used to direct the IOERT) is first placed and then secured in the patient by a modified Bookwalter retractor system (Figures 9–10 and 9–11). There is no further movement of the cone in the patient after it has been immobilized. Following this, the patient is positioned under the linear accelerator (Figure 9–12) and geometric alignment of the cone with the gantry head is achieved by a laser alignment system with appropriate couch movement and gantry rotation (Figures 9–13 to 9–15). During the actual treatment, all operating room personnel step out from the operating room to an adjoining room where the patient is monitored by video (Figure 9–16).

At MGH, all patients with locally advanced rectal cancer receive full-dose preoperative irradiation with infusional 5-FU (225 mg/m^2/day 5 days per week throughout irradiation).[75] Following this, surgical exploration is undertaken 4 to 6 weeks later. At surgery, the abdomen is carefully evaluated for liver and peritoneal metastases. If metastases are found, intraoperative irradiation is not performed and treatment ends with surgical resection or external beam radiation therapy alone. If no metastases are found, the patients undergo abdominoperineal resection, low anterior resection, or pelvic exenteration depending on the extent and location of the tumor. Attempts are made to resect as much disease as possible, even if some gross residual disease remains. The surgical specimen and the tumor bed are examined pathologically to define areas of possible residual disease, microscopic positive margins, or gross residual tumor. It is critical to define all high-risk areas accurately so as to determine the optimal position for the IOERT field. If no tumor adherence and adequate soft-tissue radial margins are present (> 1 cm), IOERT is usually not used. Patients with residual cancer or with positive or minimal (< 5 mm) radial soft-tissue margins are evaluated for IOERT.

The areas at highest risk for local tumor recurrence are defined by the surgeon and radiation oncologist. To direct the IOERT, cones are used with internal diameters ranging from 4 to 8 cm (Figure 9–17). Some have beveled ends, enabling good apposition of the cone to sloping surfaces in the pelvis. Cone size is selected to cover fully the high-risk area, generally on the sacrum or pelvic sidewall. These cones allow the geometry of the cone to fit the specific situation of tumor versus normal tissue. The cone must abut the site being treated, which can be difficult if the high-risk area is located in an anatomically confined region such as the pelvis. Further, the angle of the edge of the cone should optimally be placed flat against the body surface so as to maximize dose homogeneity. It is important that the applicator be placed so that the tumor is fully covered, that sensitive normal tissues are not included in the beam, and that there is no fluid build-up in the treatment area. During treatment, suction tubes are positioned to minimize fluid build-up. If necessary, lead sheets can be cut out to block sensitive normal tissues that cannot be removed from the path of the beam: retraction and packing are often necessary to move normal tissues. Most IOERT treatments in rectal cancer are given through the abdomen but a perineal port is occasionally used to treat a very low-lying tumor involving the coccyx, distal pelvic side-wall, or portions of the prostate and bladder when an exenteration is not performed.

Typical doses of radiation delivered intraoperatively are in the range of 10 to 20 Gy, with the lower doses being given for minimal residual disease and the higher doses for gross residual disease after resection. For patients undergoing complete resection with negative margins, the IOERT dose is usually 10 to 12.5 Gy, whereas for patients undergoing subtotal resection with microscopic residual the dose is 12.5 to 15 Gy. For patients with macroscopic tumor after resection, the dose is 17.5 Gy to 20 Gy. Typical electron energies used are 9 to 15 MeV, depending on the thickness of residual tumor. The dose is quoted at the 90 percent isodose.

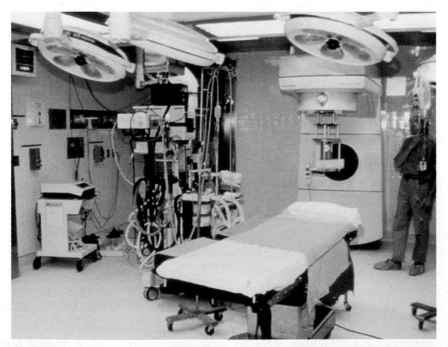

Figure 9–9. MGH dedicated IOERT suite. A wall-mounted linear accelerator is seen on the far wall.

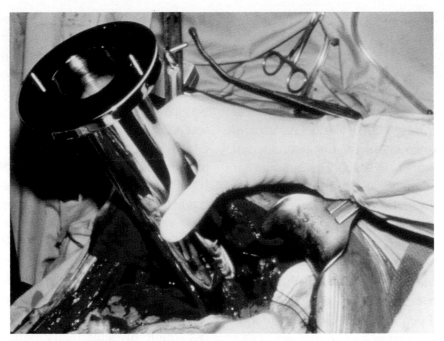

Figure 9–10.   Cone being positioned into the pelvis.

Sixty-four patients with locally advanced rectal cancer have undergone full-dose preoperative irradiation and resection with IOERT. The 5-year actuarial local control and disease-specific survival for 40 patients undergoing complete resection with IOERT were 91 and 63 percent, respectively. For patients undergoing partial resection, local control and disease-specific survival correlated with the extent of residual cancer: 65 and 47 percent, respectively, for microscopic residual disease, and 57 and 14 percent, respectively, for gross residual disease. The 5-year actuarial risk of complications of the 64 patients receiving IOERT was 16 percent. Two patients developed osteoradionecrosis of the sacrum requiring surgical intervention. No deaths were seen as a consequence of these complications.

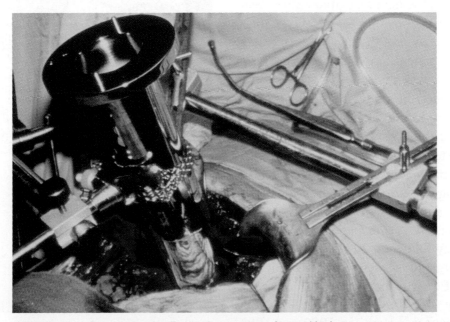

Figure 9–11.   Cone secured to Bookwalter retractor after positioning.

At the Mayo Clinic, the treatment approach of primary locally advanced rectal carcinoma has been similar to MGH, combining external beam irradiation with surgery and IOERT to high-risk regions.[76] From April 1981 through August 1995, 61 patients with primary locally advanced colorectal cancer received an IOERT dose of 10 to 20 Gy, usually combined with 45 to 55 Gy of fractionated external beam radiation therapy (EBRT). The amount of residual disease remaining at IOERT after exploration and maximal resection in the 56 patients was gross in 16, microscopic or less in 39, and unresected in 1. The 5-year survival for the entire group of patients was 46 percent. Patients with microscopic or less residual fared better than those with gross residual, with a 5-year actuarial overall survival of 59 versus 21 percent. Failures within an irradiation field have occurred in 4 of 16 patients (25%) who presented with gross residual after partial resection versus 2 of 39 (5%) with microscopic or less residual after gross total resection. An in-depth analysis of neuropathy following IOERT was also performed. Symptomatic or objective neuropathy was documented in 18 of 56 patients (32%). Ten of 18 (56%) had only Grade 1 toxicity, usually manifesting as mild or intermittent paresthesis and/or pain not requiring narcotics. Of the 7 patients with presumed treatment-related Grade 2 or 3 nerve toxicity, the data suggested a relationship between IOERT dose and the incidence of Grade 2 or 3 neuropathy (< 12.5 Gy–1 of 29 or 3%, > 15 Gy–6 of 26 or 23%, $p = .03$). Because of the high rates of distant metastases in these patients, more routine use of systemic chemotherapy was advised.

In the MD Anderson study, 11 of 38 patients (29%) with primary locally advanced rectal cancer received IOERT to high-risk regions in the pelvis because of persistent tumor adherence or residual tumor following preoperative irradiation and infusional chemotherapy.[69] No local failures were seen in these patients, although 7 of 11 patients developed distant metastases. One patient developed a sensory neuropathy following 20 Gy of IOERT.

The New England Deaconess Hospital has recently analyzed their orthovoltage intraoperative radiation therapy (IORT) experience for locally advanced rectal cancer.[77] Between 1982 and 1993,

33 patients with locally advanced rectal cancer (primary–22 patients and recurrent–11 patients) received preoperative irradiation with 5-FU-based chemotherapy and curative resection. Intraoperative irradiaton through a 300 kVp orthovoltage unit was given to 26 patients. The median dose of IORT was 12.5 Gy (range 8 to 20 Gy). The 5-year actuarial overall survival and local control rates for patients undergoing gross complete resection and IORT were 64 and 75 percent, respectively. The crude local control rate for patients following complete resection with negative margins was 92 percent for patients treated with IORT. IORT was ineffective for gross residual disease with all 4 patients progressing locally despite therapy. Seventeen patients (65%) developed pelvic soft-tissue complications and were treated successfully by posterior thigh myocutaneous flap. The incidence of complications was similar in the patients with primary or recurrent disease.

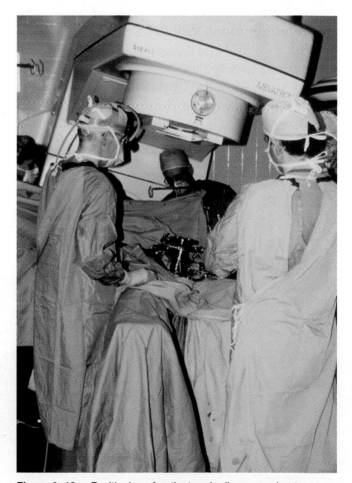

Figure 9–12.   Positioning of patient under linear accelerator.

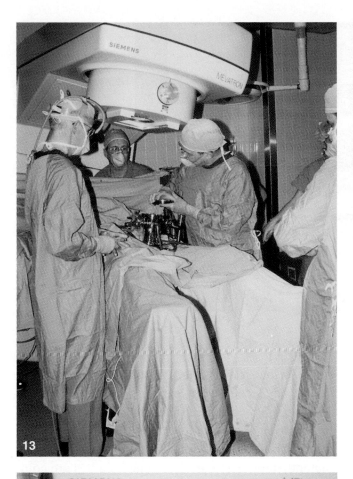

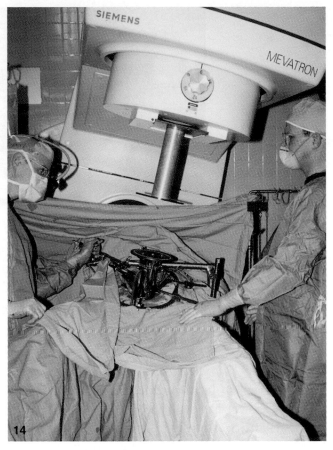

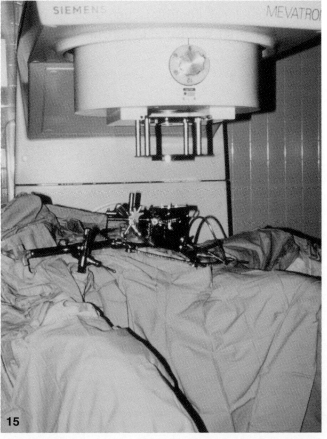

Figure 9–13 to 9–15. Docking of patient. Cone is geometrically aligned to gantry head of linear accelerator by a laser alignment system.

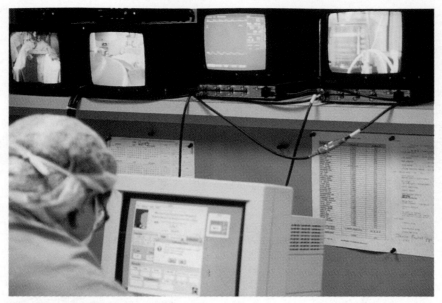

Figure 9–16.   Monitoring of patient during treatment.

Summary

The treatment of locally advanced or clinical stage T4 rectal cancer has evolved over the past 20 years. In the 1980s, treatment programs of moderate- to high-dose irradiation followed by surgery were carried out at several centers in the United States. These studies showed that a complete resection was possible in one-half to two-thirds of patients with locally advanced rectal cancer after full-dose preoperative irradiation. Despite irradiation and complete resection, local failure occurred in at least one-third of these patients. Recent efforts to improve local control have included the administration of concurrent chemotherapy with preoperative irradiation and the use of IOERT at resection.

Because of the efficacy of postoperative irradiation and 5-FU in the adjuvant treatment of rectal cancer, there has been interest in investigating this approach neoadjuvantly. These investigations have studied combinations of moderate- to full-dose preoperative irradiation (45 to 50.4 Gy) with 5-FU-based chemotherapy. Although limited by small patient numbers and short follow-up, the data from these studies show improved rates of resectability and possibly local control and survival. Concurrent 5-FU-based chemotherapy should be utilized with moderate- to high-dose preoperative irradiation programs.

To further improve local control in patients with locally advanced rectal cancer, investigators from the United States and Europe have studied IOERT in combination with treatment programs of external beam irradiation, surgery, and more recently chemotherapy. The data from these studies are compelling that local control is improved in patients receiving IOERT compared to patients not receiving

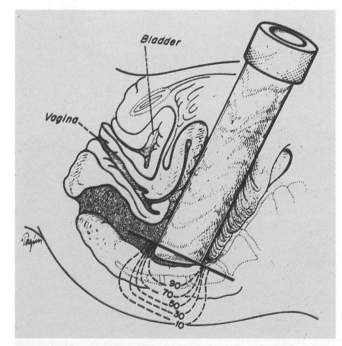

Figure 9–17.   IOERT cone to direct electron beam to irradiate high-risk region in presacral tissues.

this therapy. The result is most beneficial in patients undergoing complete resection versus patients undergoing partial resection. The treatment-related morbidity of IOERT in patients with primary locally advanced rectal cancer has been minimal. In this disease site, IOERT has been integrated successfully into treatment programs utilizing external beam irradiation, chemotherapy, and surgery.

REFERENCES

1. Moertel CG, Fleming TR, Macdonald JS, et al. Levamisole and fluorouracil for adjuvant therapy of resected colon carcinoma. N Engl J Med 1990;322: 352–8.
2. International Multicentre Pooled Analysis of Colon Cancer Trials (IMPACT) investigators: efficacy of adjuvant fluouracil and folinic acid in colon cancer. Lancet 1995;345:939–44.
3. O'Connell MJ, Mailliard JA, Kahn MJ, et al. Controlled trial of 5-FU and low-dose leucovorin given for 6 months as postoperative adjuvant therapy for colon cancer. J Clin Oncol 1997;15:246–50.
4. Willett CG, Tepper JE, Cohen AM, et al. Failure patterns following curative resection of colonic carcinoma. Ann Surg 1984;200:685–90.
5. Gunderson LL, Sosin H, Levitt S. Extrapelvic colon—areas of failure in a reoperation series: implications for adjuvant therapy. Int J Radiat Oncol Biol Phys 1985;11:731–41.
6. Willett CG, Fung CY, Kaufman DS, et al. Postoperative radiation therapy for high-risk colon cancer. J Clin Oncol 1993;11:1112–7.
7. Willett CG, Goldberg S, Shellito PC, et al. Does postoperative irradiation play a role in the adjuvant therapy of stage T4 colon cancer. Cancer J Sci Am 1999; 5:242–7.
8. Schild SE, Gunderson LL, Haddock MW, Nelson H. The treatment of locally advanced colon cancer. Int J Radiat Oncol Biol Phys 1997;37:97.
9. Amos EH, Mendenhall WM, McCarty PJ, et al. Postoperative radiotherapy for locally advanced colon cancer. Ann Surg Oncol 1996;3:431–6.
10. Martenson J, Willett CG, Sargent, et al. A phase III study of adjuvant radiation therapy, 5-fluorouracil and levamisole vs 5-FU and LEV in selected patients with resected, high risk colon cancer. Proc ASCO 1999;18:235a.
11. The Gastrointestinal Tumor Study Group. Adjuvant therapy with hepatic irradiation plus 5-FU in colon carcinoma. Int J Radiat Oncol Biol Phys 1991;21: 1151–6.
12. Wang CS, Harwood AR, Cummings BJ, et al. Total abdominal irradiation for cancer of the colon. Radiother Oncol 1984;2:209–14.
13. Brenner HJ, Bibe C, Chaitchik S. Adjuvant therapy for Dukes' C adenocarcinoma of the colon. Int J Radiat Oncol Biol Phys 1983;9:1789–92.
14. Fabian C, Giri S, Estes N, et al. Adjuvant continuous infusion 5-FU, whole abdominal radiation and tumor bed boost in high-risk stage III colon carcinoma: a Southwest Oncology Group pilot study. Int J Radiat Oncol Biol Phys 1995;32:457–64.
15. Estes NC, Giri S, Fabian C. Patterns of recurrence for advanced colon cancer modified by whole abdominal radiation and chemotherapy. Am Surg 1996; 62:546–50.
16. Willett CG, Tepper JE, Orlow E, et al. Renal complications secondary to radiation treatment of upper abdominal malignancies. Int J Radiat Oncol Biol Phys 1986;12:1601–4.
17. Landis S, Murray T, Bolden S, et al. Cancer statistics, 1999. CA Cancer J Clin 1999;49:8–31.
18. Billingham RP. Conservative treatment of rectal cancer: extending the indication. Cancer 1992;70:1355–63.
19. Nichos RJ, York-Mason AM, Morson BC, et al. The clinical staging of rectal cancer. Br J Surg 1982;69:404–7.
20. Ng A, Recht A, Busse PM. Sphincter preservation therapy for distal rectal cancer—a review. Cancer 1997; 79:671–83.
21. Alexander AA. The effect of endorectal ultrasound scanning on the preoperative staging of rectal cancer. Surg Oncol Clin N Am 1992;1:39–56.
22. Orrom WJ, Wong WD, Rothenberger DA, et al. Endorectal ultrasound in the preoperative staging of rectal tumors: a learning experience. Dis Colon Rectum 1990;33:654–9.
23. Hulsmans FJH, Tio TL, Fockens P, et al. Assessment of tumor infiltration depth in rectal cancer with transrectal sonography: caution is necessary. Radiology 1994;190:715–20.
24. Minsky BD, Rich T, Recht A, et al. Selection criteria for local excision with or without adjuvant radiation therapy for rectal cancer. Cancer 1989;63:1421–9.
25. Brodsky JT, Richard GK, Cohen AM, Minsky BD. Variables correlated with the risk of lymph node metastasis in early rectal cancer. Cancer 1991;69:322–6.
26. Gall FP, Hermanek P. Update of the German experience with local excision of rectal cancer. Surg Oncol Clin N Am 1992;1:99–109.
27. Willett CG, Tepper JE, Donnelly S, et al. Patterns of failure following local excision and local excision and postoperative radiation therapy for invasive rectal cancer. J Clin Oncol 1989;7:1003–8.
28. Wood WC, Willett CG. Update of the Massachusetts General Hospital experience of combined local excision and radiotherapy for rectal cancer. Surg Oncol Clin N Am 1992;1:131–6.

29. Chakravarti A, Compton C, Shellito P, et al. Long-term follow-up of patients with rectal cancer managed by local excision with and without adjuvant irradiation. Ann Surg 1999;230:49–54.

30. Ota DM, Skibber J, Rich TA. MD Anderson Cancer Center experience with local excision and multimodality therapy for rectal cancer. Surg Oncol Clin N Am 1992;1:147–52.

31. Jessup JM, Bothe A, Stone MD, et al. Preservation of sphincter function in rectal carcinoma by a multimodality treatment approach. Surg Oncol Clin N Am 1992;1:137–45.

32. Wong CS, Stern H, Cummings BJ. Local excison and postoperative radiation therapy for rectal carcinoma. Int J Radiat Oncol Biol Phys 1993;25:669–75.

33. Fortunato L, Ahmad NR, Yeung RS, et al. Long-term follow-up of local excision and radiation therapy for invasive rectal cancer. Dis Colon Rectum 1995;38: 1193–9.

34. Wagman R, Minsky B, Cohen A, et al. Conservative management of rectal cancer with local excision and postoperative adjuvant therapy. Int J Radiat Oncol Biol Phys 1999;44:841–6.

35. Steele GD, Tepper J, Herndon JE, Mayer R. Failure salvage after sphincter sparing treatment for distal rectal adenocarcinoma: a CALGB Coordinated Study. Proc ASCO 1999;186:235a.

36. Gastrointestinal Tumor Study Group. Prolongaton of the disease-free interval in surgically treated rectal carcinoma. N Engl J Med 1985;312:1465–72.

37. Fisher B, Wolmark N, Rockette H, et al. Postoperative adjuvant chemotherapy or radiation therapy for rectal cancer: results from NSABP Protocol R-01. J Natl Cancer Inst 1988;80:21–9.

38. Krook JE, Moertel CG, Gunderson LL, et al. Effective surgical adjuvant therapy for high-risk rectal cancer. N Engl J Med 1991;324:709–15.

39. Gastrointestinal Tumor Study Group. Radiation therapy and 5-FU with or without semustine for the treatment of patients with surgical adjuvant adenocarcinoma of the rectum. J Clin Oncol 1992;10:549–57.

40. O'Connell MJ, Martenson JA, Wieand HS, et al. Improving adjuvant therapy for rectal cancer by combining protracted-infusion 5-FU with radiation therapy after curative surgery. N Engl J Med 1995; 331:502–7.

41. Tepper JE, O'Connell M, Petroni G, et al. Adjuvant postoperative fluorouracil-modulated chemotherapy combined with pelvic radiation therapy for rectal cancer. J Clin Oncol 1997;15:2030–9.

42. Miller AR, Martenson J, Nelson H, et al. The incidence and consequences of treatment related bowel injury. Int J Radiat Oncol Biol Phys 1999;43:817–25.

43. Kollmorgen C, Meaghan A, Pemberton JH, et al. The long-term effect of adjuvant postoperative chemora-diotherapy for rectal cancer on bowel function. Am Surg 1999;220:676–82.

44. Rider WD, Palmer JA, Mahoney LJ, et al. Postoperative irradiation in rectal cancer. Can J Surg 1997;20:335–8.

45. Second Report of an MRC Working Party. Evaluation of low-dose preoperative x-ray therapy in the management of rectal cancer. Br J Surg 1989;71:21–5.

46. Gerard A, Buyse M, Wordlinger B, et al. Preoperative radiotherapy as adjuvant treatment in rectal cancer. Ann Surg 1998;208:606–14.

47. Swedish Rectal Cancer Trial. Improved survival with preoperative radiotherapy in resectable rectal cancer. N Engl J Med 1997;336:980–7.

48. Mendenhall WM, Bland KI, Copeland EM, et al. Does preoperative radiation therapy enhance the probability of local control and survival in high-risk distal rectal cancer? Ann Surg 1992;215:696–706.

49. Myerson RJ, Michalsi JM, King ML, et al. Adjuvant radiation therapy for rectal carcinoma: predictors of outcome. Int J Radiat Oncol Biol Phys 1995;32:41–50.

50. Rich TA, Skipper JM, Ajani JA, et al. Preoperative infusional chemoirradiation for stage T3 rectal cancer. Int J Radiat Oncol Biol Phys 1995;32:1025–9.

51. Chan RS, Tyler DS, Anscher MS, et al. Preoperative radiation and chemotherapy in the treatment of adenocarcinoma of the rectum. Ann Surg 1995;221:779–87.

52. Minsky BD, Cohen AM, Kemeny N, et al. Enhancement of radiation-induced downstaging of rectal cancer by 5-FU and high-dose leucovorin chemotherapy. J Clin Oncol 1992;10:79–84.

53. Wagman R, Minsky BD, Cohen AM, Enker WE. Sphincter prevention with preoperative radiation therapy and coloanal anastomosis. Int J Radiat Oncol Biol Phys 1995;553–9.

54. Rouanet P, Fabre JM, Dubois JB, et al. Conservative surgery for low rectal cancer after high dose radiation. Functional and oncologic results. Am Surg 1995;221:67–73.

55. Mohiuddin M, Regine WF, Marks GJ, et al. High-dose preoperative radiation and the challenge of sphincter preservation surgery for cancer of the distal 2 cm of the rectum. Int J Radiat Oncol Biol Phys 1998;40: 569–74.

56. Hyams DM, Mamounas EP, Petrelli N, et al. A clinical trial to evaluate the worth of preoperative multimodality therapy in patients with operable carcinoma of the rectum: a progress report of NSABP R-03. Dis Colon Rectum 1997;40:131–9.

57. Wang CC, Schulz MD. The role of radiation therapy in the management of carcinoma of the sigmoid, rectosigmoid, and rectum. Radiol Soc N Am 1962;79:1–5.

58. O'Connell MJ, Childs DS, Moertel CG, et al. A prospective controlled evaluation of combined pelvic radiotherapy and methanol extraction residue of BCG (MER) for locally unresectable or recurrent

rectal carcinoma. Int J Radiat Oncol Biol Phys 1982; 8:1115–9.

59. Brierley JD, Cummings BJ, Wong CS, et al. Adenocarcinoma of the rectum treated by radical external radiation therapy. Int Radiat Oncol Biol Phys 1995; 31:255–9.

60. Allee PE, Tepper JE, Gunderson LL, et al. Postoperative radiation therapy for incompletely resected colorectal carcinoma. Int J Radiat Oncol Biol Phys 1989; 17:1171–6.

61. Schild SE, Martenson JA, Gunderson LL, et al. Long-term survival and patterns of failure after postoperative radiation therapy for subtotally resected rectal adenocarcinoma. Int J Radiat Oncol Biol Phys 1988; 16:459–63.

62. Ghossein NA, Samala EC, Alpert S, et al. Elective postoperative radiotherapy after incomplete resection of colorectal cancer. Dis Colon Rectum 1981;24:252–6.

63. Emami B, Pilepich M, Willett CG, et al. Effect of preoperative irradiation on resectability of colorectal carcinomas. Int J Radiat Oncol Biol Phys 1982;8:1295–9.

64. Dosoretz DE, Gunderson LL, Hedberg S, et al. Preoperative irradiation for unresectable rectal and rectosigmoid carcinomas. Cancer 1983;52:814–8.

65. Mendenhall WM, Bland KI, Pfaff WW, et al. Initially unresectable rectal adenocarcinoma treated with preoperative irradiation and surgery. Ann Surg 1987; 205:41–4.

66. Stevens KR, Fletcher WS. High dose preoperative pelvic irradiation for unresectable adenocarcinoma of the rectum or sigmoid. Int J Radiat Oncol Biol Phys 1983;9:148.

67. Whiting JF, Howes A, Osteen RT. Preoperative irradiation for unresectable carcinoma of the rectum. Surg Gynecol Obstet 1993;176:203–7.

68. Marsh PJ, James RD, and Scholfield PF. Adjuvant preoperative radiotherapy for locally advanced rectal carcinoma. Dis Colon Rectum 1994;37:1205–14.

69. Weinstein GD, Rich TA, Shumate CR, et al. Preoperative infusional chemoradiation and surgery with or without an electron beam intraoperative boost for advanced primary rectal cancer. Int J Radiat Oncol Biol Phys 1995;32:197–204.

70. Minsky BD, Cohen AM, Enker WE, et al. Preoperative 5-FU, low-dose leucovorin, and radiation therapy for locally advanced and unresectable rectal cancer. Int J Radiat Oncol Biol Phys 1997;37:289–95.

71. Prykolm G, Glimelius B, Pahlman L. Preoperative irradiation with and without chemotherapy (MFL) in the treatment of primary non-resectable adenocarcinoma of the rectum. Results from two consecutive studies. Eur J Cancer Clin Oncol 1989;25:1535–41.

72. Chan A, Wong A, Langevin J, Khoo R. Preoperative concurrent 5-fluorouracil infusion, mitomycin C and pelvic radiation therapy in tethered and fixed rectal carcinoma. Int J Radiat Oncol Biol Phys 1992;25: 791–9.

73. Chen ET-ESU, Mohiuddin M, Brodovsky H, et al. Downstaging of advanced rectal cancer following combined preoperative chemotherapy and high dose radiation. Int J Radiat Oncol Biol Phys 1994;30:169–75.

74. Landry G, Koretz MJ, Wood WC, et al. Preoperative irradiation and fluorouracil chemotherapy for locally advanced rectosigmoid carcinoma: phase I-II study. Radiology 1993;188:423–6.

75. Nakfoor B, Willett CG, Shellito PC. The impact of 5-fluorouracil and intraoperative electron beam irradiation on the outcome of patients with locally advanced rectal cancer. Ann Surg 1998;228:194–200.

76. Gunderson LL, Nelson H, Martenson JA, et al. Locally advanced primary colorectal cancer: intraoperative electron and external beam irradiation ± 5-FU. Int J Radiat Oncol Biol Phys 1997;37:601–14.

77. Kim HK, Jessup M, Beard CJ, et al. Locally advanced rectal carcinoma: pelvic control and morbidity following preoperative radiation therapy, resection and intraoperative radiation therapy. Int J Radiat Oncol Biol Phys 1997;38:777–83.

10

Systemic Therapy Approaches for Colorectal Cancer

JEFF CLARK, MD

There are approximately 130,000 new cases of colorectal adenocarcinoma with an estimated 57,000 deaths each year in the United States, making it the second leading killer among malignancies.[1] Surgery remains the only curative treatment. Although there have been improvements in surgical treatment, including appropriate settings in which resection of metastatic lesions may provide survival benefit, approximately 40 percent of patients still eventually die from the disease. There clearly is a need for continued development and evaluation of novel treatment approaches.

A number of clinical trials are addressing specific questions related to the treatment of patients who have colorectal cancer. These include (1) Will combining currently available chemotherapeutic agents improve survival over that seen with fluorouracil-based therapy in the adjuvant disease settings (as has been seen with the combination of 5-fluorouracil [5-FU] and leucovorin [LV] therapy with irinotecan patients with metastatic disease)? (2) Will new methods of enhancing radiation therapy's effectiveness (eg, new or combined radiation sensitizers; improvements in imaging and treatment planning utilizing technological developments in CT, MRI, and PET scanning; or newer approaches to intraoperative therapy) improve local control of disease and/or survival for patients with rectal cancer? (3) Are there new chemotherapeutic agents or combinations that have greater efficacy than existing ones? and (4) Will new therapeutic approaches (eg, gene therapy, vaccines, antisense oligonucleotides, or monoclonal antibodies against cell-surface antigens such as growth factor receptors [such as the epidermal growth factor receptor (EGFR)], growth factor-fusion toxins, antiangiogenic agents, and small molecules directed against specific proteins), which take advantage of discoveries about the molecular and cell biology of colorectal cancer, have a role in the treatment of this disease?

SYSTEMIC TREATMENT APPROACHES

Chemotherapeutic Agents

5-Fluorouracil

5-FU and related compounds remain an integral component of chemotherapy for treatment of patients in both the adjuvant and metastatic disease setting (Figure 10–1). 5-FU is an analog of the pyrimidine uracil. It has a fluorine in place of hydrogen at the 5-carbon position of the pyrimidine ring (see Figure 10–1A). It is actively and rapidly transported into cells via the uracil transport sys-

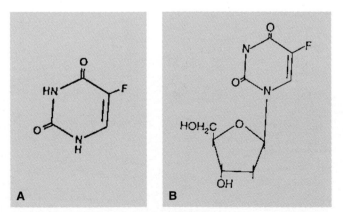

Figure 10–1. *A,* Fluorouracil (5-FU). *B,* Fluorodeoxyuridine (FUDR).

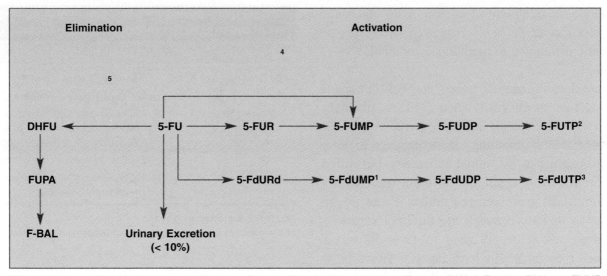

Figure 10–2. 5-FU activation and elimination. 1. Target = Thymidylate synthase 2. Target = RNA 3. Target = DNA 4. 5-FUMP is also a direct metabolite of 5-FU via oratate phosphoribosyltransferase 5. Dihydropyrimidine dehydrogenase (DPD) reduces 5-FU to DHFU and is a rate-limiting step in elimination of 5-FU.

tem. 5-FU must be activated intracellularly for its cytotoxic activity (Figure 10–2). 5-FU has two main mechanisms of action that have been identified, as well as several other potential mechanisms by which it may inhibit cell growth.[2–5] The major mechanism by which it inhibits cell growth involves conversion of 5-FU in vivo to the fluorouridine monophosphate (FdUMP) that directly inhibits the enzyme thymidylate synthase (TS), which is a critical enzyme in the conversion of uridine to thymidine. Its inhibition leads to a decrease in cellular thymidine monophosphate and, as a result, the inhibition of DNA synthesis. The second major mechanism by which it works involves the conversion of 5-FU to the fluorouridine triphosphate (FUTP), which can be incorporated into RNA leading to termination of the RNA strands. This leads to inhibition of protein synthesis. To a lesser extent, the deoxyglucose triphosphates (FdUTP and dUTP) can be incorporated into DNA as fraudulent nucleotides, but it is not certain how significant a role this plays in 5-FU's cytotoxic activity against cancer cells in vivo.

5-FU is rapidly metabolized and has a serum half-life of only approximately 6 to 20 minutes, with considerable interindividual variation.[4] Approximately 90 percent is eliminated by metabolism, especially in the liver, with less than 5 percent being renally excreted in intact form (see Figure 10–2). The major metabolic enzyme for 5-FU is dihydropy-

rimidine dehydrogenase (DPD), which is distributed in tissues throughout the body, including the liver. DPD metabolizes 5-FU to dihydrofluorouracil (DHFU) (see Figure 10–2).

Functional levels of DPD vary in the population,[4] which is probably the major factor contributing to interindividual variations in metabolism and clinical toxicities that are seen. There are a number of polymorphisms in the DPD gene.[5] Ongoing studies are evaluating whether these are associated with significant differences in the functional level of DPD in different individuals. Better understanding of these pharmacogenomic relationships might provide a means for appropriate dosing of 5-FU for each individual.

5-FU can be administered by a number of routes and schedules.[2–4,6–10] The most commonly used of these include once a week bolus; daily × 5 bolus once monthly; a 24-hour infusion once weekly; combined bolus and infusional for 48 hours every 2 weeks; and by continuous infusion (Table 10–1). When it is given by bolus it is usually administered with LV (5-formyltetrahydrofolate). LV enhances 5-FU cytotoxicity by increasing the intracellular pools of 5,10-methylenetetrahydrofolate.[4,11,12] This stabilizes the ternary complex formed between 5-FU, TS, and reduced folate. A meta-analysis has suggested that the response rate is significantly higher when 5-FU is combined with LV (23%) than when 5-FU is used alone for treatment of patients with metastatic colorectal cancer (11%).[13] However, there was no detectable difference in median survival (11.5 vs 11 months).

There does not appear to be a large difference in response rate or survival when 5-FU is given by bolus (with LV) versus infusion (with or without LV).[2,4,7,9,10,14,15] If anything, there appears to be a slight advantage to infusional schedules, but differences are relatively small and have not been statistically significant in randomized studies. There are differences in toxicity between the different schedules and doses, which overall tend to favor infusional schedules (see under Toxicity below). However, at least until oral regimens are fully developed, protracted infusions have the additional morbidity associated with intravenous catheters and wearing pumps.

In addition to using LV, a number of other approaches have been attempted to modulate 5-FU, including combinations with antifolates, DPD inhibitors, other TS inhibitors, and alpha interferon. Sequence-dependent synergy has been seen for the use of antifolates followed by 5-FU + LV in a number of preclinical models.[16] A meta-analysis suggests that the response rate (19% vs 10%) and median survival (10.7 vs 9.1 months) may both be enhanced when the antifolate methotrexate (MTX) is given prior to 5-FU as compared with 5-FU alone for treatment of patients with colorectal cancer.[17] However, the use of LV (to rescue MTX) makes clean interpretation of the value of MTX in these results difficult to interpret. Given the small difference seen in median survival as well as the significant inconvenience of this schedule, the use of sequential MTX with 5-FU and LV in this setting has not been widely pursued.

Trimetrexate (TMTX), a nonclassic antifolate, has several theoretical advantages over MTX. It inhibits dihydrofolate reductase and purine synthesis. This leads to increased intracellular levels of 5-phosphoribosyl-1-pyrophosphate that enhances conversion of 5-FU to 5-FdUMP, which inhibits TS.[18] As opposed to MTX, TMTX does not compete with LV for cellular uptake or polyglutamation. This could provide an advantage for its use (as opposed to MTX) in conjunction with 5-FU combined with LV. The studies evaluating whether pretreatment with TMTX increases the activity of 5-FU + LV for the treatment

Table 10–1. COMMONLY USED 5-FU REGIMENS FOR THE TREATMENT OF COLORECTAL CANCER

LV (mg/m²)	5-FU (mg/m²)
500 Q week × 6 of 8	500*–600 Q week × 6 of 8
20 days 1–5, Q 4–5 weeks	425 days 1–5, Q 4–5 weeks
200 days 1, 2	400 bolus days 1, 2 followed by 600 continuous infusion over 22 hrs days 1, 2 every 2 weeks
0–500	2,600 as 24 hr-infusion once weekly
None	300 continuous infusion days 1–28 every 5 weeks

*500 mg/m² most commonly used.
All chemotherapy doses need to be carefully adjusted for patient factors and toxicity.

of metastatic colorectal cancer are ongoing. A recent update of these results suggests a small advantage of the TMTX arm, although final results are pending.[19]

Combinations of 5-FU (+/- LV) with alpha interferon have not shown any advantage over 5-FU + LV and have been associated with increased toxicity.[20] Similarly, combinations with N-phosphonacetyl-L-aspartate (PALA) or hydroxyurea have not shown either a response or survival advantage over 5-FU alone.[21] Combinations of other TS inhibitors (eg, Tomudcx) with 5-FU are synergistic in the preclinical setting.[22,23] Clinical trials evaluating these combinations are currently being undertaken. Based on the potential enhancement of cellular toxicity by a false thymidine in the setting of 5-FU inhibition of thymidine production, azidothymidine (AZT) has been given in combination with 5-FU and LV.[24,25] Although the results of these phase II studies were potentially encouraging, it is not possible to know whether this improves the therapeutic efficacy of 5-FU + LV in the absence of phase III trials.

Levamisole has been combined with 5-FU for the adjuvant treatment of patients with resected colorectal cancer[26,27]; it does not increase the activity of 5-FU in the metastatic setting. Despite the fact that it still remains unclear what its exact role is in the adjuvant setting, based on the results of randomized clinical trials showing equivalent efficacy to 6 months of 5-FU + LV, 1 year of 5-FU and levamisole therapy still remains one of the accepted treatment options for patients with Dukes C colorectal cancer in the adjuvant setting.

Finally, pilot studies have evaluated whether the addition of sulindac (which inhibits colonic polyp formation) might potentially be beneficial in the adjuvant setting.[28] However, no phase III studies have yet evaluated this combination. Given the potential importance of pathways involved in COX-2 synthesis in proliferation of cells involved in colonic polyp formation, more selective COX-2 inhibitors are being evaluated for their potential role in this setting.[29]

Resistance. The major mechanism of resistance to 5-FU is thought to be elevated TS levels within tumor cells. Although it still has not been established in randomized clinical trials, a number of studies have suggested a direct correlation between high TS levels in colorectal tumors and lack of response to 5-FU treatment.[30,31] In addition, for patients treated with 5-FU-based regimens in the adjuvant setting, those whose tumors had higher TS levels had shorter median disease-free and overall survival than those whose tumors had lower TS levels.

Toxicity. Toxicity due to 5-FU (and related compounds and metabolites) is primarily manifested in rapidly dividing tissues, especially the gastrointestinal tract and bone marrow.[4–10] Although qualitatively similar toxicities are seen with different routes and durations of administration, the severity and frequency of individual toxicities seen are dose and schedule dependent. Diarrhea, stomatitis, and mild to moderate neutropenia are the most frequent serious toxicities seen with 5-FU administration (Table 10–2). Other moderately frequent toxicities include mild nausea and/or vomiting, dermatitis, esophagitis, excessive tearing, and mild alopecia. Protracted-infusion 5-FU is also associated with a higher incidence of hand-foot syndrome, although diarrhea is less frequent than with bolus regimens.

There are two uncommon but potentially serious toxicities that can occur with 5-FU treatment. Neurotoxicity (cerebellar ataxia, somnolence, and upper motor neuron signs) can be seen and is usually reversible. The neurotoxicity has been seen more frequently in patients receiving intracarotid arterial delivery of 5-FU. Myocardial ischemia has also been reported uncommonly, usually in patients with prior history of cardiac disease. This has been more commonly reported for infusional as opposed to bolus delivery of 5-FU.

Table 10–2. TOXICITIES SEEN WITH 5-FU TREATMENT	
Frequent	Diarrhea, stomatitis, mild to moderate neutropenia, mild nausea, excessive tearing, hand-foot syndrome (especially protracted infusion 5-FU)
Uncommon but serious	Neurotoxicity (cerebella ataxia, somnolence, upper motor neuron), myocardial ischemia

All chemotherapy doses need to be carefully adjusted for patient factors and toxicity.

Irinotecan (CPT-11)

Camptothecins are plant alkaloids that inhibit the topoisomerase I enzyme, which plays a role in DNA translation and transcription.[32–35] Topoisomerase I is involved in controlling the structure of DNA and relaxing the supercoiled double-stranded DNA helix (Figure 10–3). During the process of DNA replication, topoisomerase I forms a transient covalent bond with DNA that nicks one of the DNA strands. Subsequently, the DNA strand passes, the break is religated, and the enzyme is then released, allowing unwinding of the DNA helix and relieving tortional stress.

Camptothecins stabilize the topoisomerase I/DNA cleavable complex (see Figure 10–3). Irreparable double-stranded breaks in DNA occur when the protein-DNA complex meets a moving DNA replication fork. The presence of these irreparable double-strand breaks in DNA initiates a process resulting in cell death by apoptosis. There is evidence that the process may be mediated, at least partially, by the interleukin-1 beta converting enzyme pathway. Although topoisomerase I is constitutively expressed, cells must be in the S-phase of the cell cycle for camptothecins to mediate cell death since DNA replication is required.

The camptothecin irinotecan (CPT-11, Camptosar) is a prodrug that must be converted to its active metabolite SN-38 by carboxylesterase enzymes[36] (Figure 10–4A and B). The major source of conversion is in the liver via hepatic carboxylesterases, although carboxylesterases also exist in other organs, including the intestines. At least two known hepatic carboxylesterases are responsible for conversion of irinotecan to SN-38 in humans. SN-38 must be in its

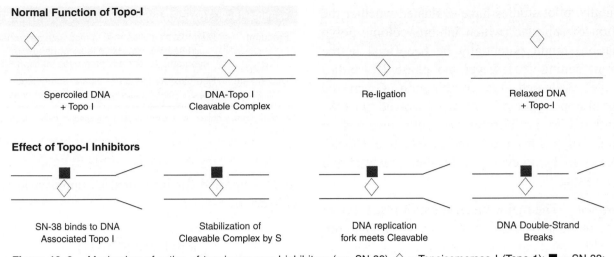

Normal Function of Topo-I

| Spercoiled DNA + Topo I | DNA-Topo I Cleavable Complex | Re-ligation | Relaxed DNA + Topo-I |

Effect of Topo-I Inhibitors

| SN-38 binds to DNA Associated Topo I | Stabilization of Cleavable Complex by S | DNA replication fork meets Cleavable | DNA Double-Strand Breaks |

Figure 10–3. Mechanism of action of topoisomerase I inhibitors (eg, SN-38). ◇ = Topoisomerase I (Topo-1); ■ = SN-38; ▭ = DNA.

lactone form to be active and can be inactivated by pH-dependent hydrolysis of the lactone ring. Inactivation occurs at more alkaline pH.

SN-38 is primarily eliminated through conjugation by hepatic uridine glucoronosyltransferase (UGT1.1), which is the isoform that glucoronidates bilirubin. Patients with an isoform of this enzyme containing an extra TA DNA base sequence in the TATA (an area of DNA to which proteins bind during transcription) box have Gilbert's syndrome. This isoform has an altered ability to glucuronidate bilirubin or SN-38, leading to decreased biliary clearance of SN-38 and susceptibility to severe toxicity when irinotecan is administered.[37] Glucoronidated SN-38 is rapidly secreted into the bile.

Deconjugation, by beta glucuronidase, can occur by bacteria in the intestine leading to enterohepatic recirculation, which may contribute to both local intestinal toxicity as well as systemic redistribution of the drug.[38,39] Since alkalinization leads to hydrolysis of the lactone ring of SN-38, it is thus possible that alkalinization of the gastrointestinal tract could decrease the gastrointestinal toxicity of irinotecan. However, since this might also lead to decreased systemic reabsorption, the overall effect of such an approach on the therapeutic index of irinotecan would have to be evaluated in clinical trials.

Irinotecan has most commonly been given by one of two schedules: either once weekly at a somewhat lower dose as a 90-minute infusion for 4 weeks on followed by 2 weeks off or as a higher dose 90-

minute infusion every 3 weeks[40–42] (Table 10–3A). The results of studies evaluating each of the schedules separately do not suggest a clear difference in response rates. The results of trials that have evaluated the regimens separately suggest that neutropenia, diarrhea, and nausea are somewhat greater for the high-dose, less-frequent schedule. This is somewhat offset by the more convenient schedule and lack of repeated weekly acute toxicity when the

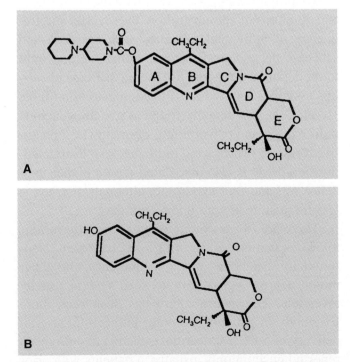

Figure 10–4 *A,* Irinotecan (CPT-11, Camptosar). *B,* SN-38 (active metabolite or irinotecan).

Table 10–3A. DOSE SCHEDULES FOR IRINOTECAN ALONE	
(Mg/m²)/Duration	Schedule
125/over 90 minutes	Once weekly × 4 weeks followed by 2 weeks off
350 (300 for age ≥ 70, or previous pelvic XRT)/over 90 minutes	Every 3 weeks

All chemotherapy doses need to be carefully adjusted for patient factors and toxicity.

Table 10–3B. IRINOTECAN COMBINED WITH 5-FU AND LEUCOVORIN
Irinotecan 125 mg/m² over 90 min on days 1, 8, 15, and 22, followed immediately by leucovorin 20 mg/m² IVP on days 1, 8, 15, and 22, followed immediately by 5-FU 500 mg/m² over 1–2 min on days 1, 8, 15, and 22. Give four weekly treatments followed by a 2-week rest period.[79]

All chemotherapy doses need to be carefully adjusted for patient factors and toxicity.

every 3 weeks regimen is utilized. A trial comparing both the toxicity and efficacy of these two regimens for patients with 5-FU refractory colorectal cancer is currently ongoing. Until the results of the randomized comparative trial are known, the choice of schedule remains physician and patient dependent.

Phase II studies utilizing irinotecan suggest response rates of approximately 15 percent and an average response duration of 6 months in patients with 5-FU refractory metastatic colorectal cancer.[43] In addition, a significant percentage of patients who do not respond appear to have stable disease for varying time periods. Irinotecan has been shown to offer an overall survival advantage at 1 year as compared with either best supportive care or infusional 5-FU treatment for patients who have progressed on previous 5-FU treatment.[41,42] It is approved for this indication in the United States. In addition (see below under combined therapy section for further discussion), the combination of 5-FU, LV, and irinotecan is now approved as initial therapy for patients with metastatic colorectal cancer by the FDA in the United States (Table 10–3B).[70]

Toxicity.   The most common toxicities associated with irinotecan are diarrhea, cholinergic syndrome (which usually occurs during or soon after the infusion), neutropenia, nausea/vomiting, asthenia, and

alopecia[44,45] (Table 10–4). The cholinergic syndrome consists of some combination of diaphoresis, abdominal cramping, diarrhea, nausea and vomiting, hyperlacrimation, and rhinorrhea. It is more frequently seen at higher doses, and the symptoms can be controlled by the administration of the anticholinergic drug, atropine.

The diarrhea that occurs later appears to be primarily due to direct toxicity of SN-38 to the GI tract. Aggressive use of loperamide has been critical for managing the late diarrhea (occurring 12 hours or more after drug administration) associated with irinotecan. Febrile neutropenia occurs in up to 10 to 15 percent of patients but has been manageable with appropriate use of antibiotics. As mentioned above, the most significant difference in the incidence of toxicities between the every 3 weeks and weekly schedules, appears to be in the occurrence of febrile neutropenia and the cholinergic syndrome, which are both more common in the every 3 weeks schedule.

Resistance.   Although characterization of mechanisms of resistance in patients still is pending, a number of potential mechanisms for resistance to irinotecan have been demonstrated preclinically. These include alterations in carboxylesterase levels, altered levels of topoisomerase I within tumor cells, and, perhaps most importantly, active efflux of irinotecan out of cells.[46–48]

Oxaliplatin

Currently 5-FU + LV and irinotecan are the major approved treatments for colorectal cancer in the United States. A third drug, oxaliplatin, is approved in France and is undergoing active study in the United States as well as other countries throughout the world (Figure 10–5). Oxaliplatin, oxalato trans-L-1,2-diaminocyclohexane platinum, is a platinum compound that is clinically active against a number of solid tumors.[49,50] As opposed to cisplatin and car-

Table 10–4. IRINOTECAN TOXICITIES	
Frequent	Diarrhea, nausea, vomiting, cholinergic syndrome, neutropenia, asthenia, alopecia
Infrequent	Dyspnea, flushing

All chemotherapy doses need to be carefully adjusted for patient factors and toxicity.

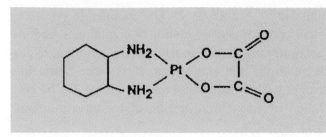

Figure 10–5. Oxaliplatin.

boplatin, it belongs to a second class of platinum compounds, those that have a diaminocyclohexane (DACH) carrier ligand. It has been shown to have both in vitro and in vivo antitumor activity against colon carcinoma cell lines, animal colon cancer tumor models, and in human colon cancer tumor cloning assays.[51–53]

Although it functions by forming intrastrand DNA adducts and interstrand DNA crosslinks, similar to cisplatin, there are several differences that may account for its increased antitumor activity against colorectal cancer as compared with cisplatin. The mismatched repair system in cells is much more efficient in recognizing the cisplatin-DNA complex structure as compared with the oxaliplatin-DNA complex.[54,55] Therefore, cells without a functional mismatched repair system are more resistant to cisplatin than to oxaliplatin. The relatively high frequency of altered mismatch repair enzyme function in colorectal cancer cells may explain the greater activity of oxaliplatin as opposed to cisplatin or carboplatin against these tumors. Oxaliplatin is more efficient than cisplatin at inducing DNA strand breaks and apoptosis at the same level of induction of primary DNA lesions[56] and has been shown to have activity in vitro against cisplatin-resistant cell lines.[57] Preliminary evidence suggests that oxaliplatin may inhibit dihydropyrimidine dehydrogenase (the primary enzyme involved in 5-FU metabolism), which may also contribute to its activity against colorectal carcinoma.[58] There is a significantly greater volume of distribution of oxaliplatin than cisplatin, suggesting that the lipophilic DACH moiety may increase tissue and potentially tumor penetration of oxaliplatin as compared with cisplatin.[59] Pharmacokinetic studies indicate that renal excretion is the primary route of elimination of oxaliplatin.[59]

Used alone on an every 3 weeks schedule, oxaliplatin produces objective tumor responses in approximately 20 to 25 percent of patients with chemotherapy naive metastatic colorectal cancer and 10 percent of patients with 5-FU refractory colorectal cancer.[10–12,60–62] Preclinical studies suggest synergistic antitumor activity when oxaliplatin and 5-FU are combined.[9,14,15,58,63,64] Clinical studies combining a variety of schedules of infusional 5-FU with oxaliplatin have produced responses in approximately 30 to 50 percent of chemotherapy naive and 10 to 46 percent of previously treated colorectal cancer patients[16–23,65–74] (Table 10–5). In these trials, 5-FU has been given as a 24-, 48-, 96-, or 120-hour infusion. Oxaliplatin has been given as either a continuous infusion or as a 2-hour infusion. Thus, there is evidence to suggest enhanced activity for oxaliplatin combined with 5-FU/LV as compared with oxaliplatin alone in both previously untreated patients as well as patients who have progressed on 5-FU/LV therapy.

A significant number of early trials evaluating oxaliplatin for colorectal cancer utilized chronomodulated drug delivery for both the 5-FU and oxaliplatin. In trials that have randomized between chronomodulated drug delivery and constant rate delivery, there has been a higher response rate in the chronomodulated delivery patients.[60,66,68,72] The initial study indicated an increased median survival with chronomodulation whereas the second did not. Crossover therapy was allowed in the latter trial, which makes the results more difficult to interpret. However, the exact role of the chronomodulated delivery in the efficacy of combined 5-FU, LV, and oxaliplatin remains unclear because of a number of issues, including the question of whether the oxaliplatin in the constant infusion arm might have been

Table 10–5. OXALIPLATIN REGIMENS		
Drug	**mg/m²**	**Frequency**
Oxaliplatin	130	Q 3 weeks
Oxaliplatin +	85–100 day 1 (B)	Q 2 weeks
LV +	200 days 1, 2 (B)	Q 2 weeks
5-FU+	400 days 1, 2 (B)	Q 2 weeks
5-FU	600 days 1, 2 (CI over 22 hrs)	Q 2 weeks

B = bolus; CI = continuous infusion.
All chemotherapy doses need to be carefully adjusted for patient factors and toxicity.

partially inactivated by the basic pH of the 5-FU. The questions raised about the exact role chronomodulation was playing in all of these studies made it difficult to be certain what role oxaliplatin itself was playing.

There have been, however, a number of randomized trials evaluating oxaliplatin that have not utilized chronomodulated delivery. These have shown higher response rates in both chemotherapy naive as well as 5-FU refractory colorectal cancer patients receiving combined 5-FU, LV, and oxaliplatin as opposed to 5-FU and LV.[49,50,71] This is consistent with the chronomodulated studies and argues that there is enhanced antitumor activity when oxaliplatin is added to 5-FU and LV. Most of these trials have had nonsignificant differences in median survival between the arms, but as many patients on the non-oxaliplatin arm eventually received oxaliplatin, it is still not certain what the additional benefit is in terms of survival when oxaliplatin is added to 5-FU/LV.

The optimal schedule and doses for combining 5-FU with oxaliplatin to produce an antitumor effect are not known. In addition to the still unresolved issue of whether chronomodulated delivery might be better than the constant schedules, one in vitro study suggests that shorter durations of 5-FU exposure may have the greatest synergistic effect with oxaliplatin.[58] There has been limited experience to date with combining oxaliplatin with the bolus 5-FU-based treatment schedules that are commonly employed in the United States. Based on the preclinical in vitro data mentioned above, this may be an effective schedule for combining these agents. Combinations with the weekly bolus regimen are just being evaluated in phase II studies to confirm tolerability and antitumor activity. Preliminary data from studies suggest that this approach has tolerable toxicity for once-weekly 5-FU bolus schedules. For the daily × 5 once monthly 5-FU + LV schedules, significant reductions in 5-FU and LV dose are necessary to prevent excessive toxicity.

Toxicity.   In general, oxaliplatin has very manageable toxicities when given alone.[49,73] The most frequently occurring toxicities of oxaliplatin include peripheral neuropathy (which is cumulative) and esophageal dysesthesia (Table 10–6). These are both significantly enhanced in the presence of cold. In addition, it is also associated with diarrhea, and this is enhanced when given with 5-FU and LV. In combination with 5-FU/LV oxaliplatin is also associated with a higher rate of neutropenia than when either treatment is delivered alone. The neutropenia may be ameliorated by chronomodulated delivery of the 5-FU/LV, but this needs to be confirmed in further studies. Nausea and vomiting are the other acute side effects. As opposed to cisplatin, oxaliplatin does not have significant renal or auditory toxicities.

Resistance.   As mentioned above, oxaliplatin's activity is not affected to the same degree as cisplatin's by deficiencies in mismatched repair enzymes, a relatively frequent occurrence in colorectal cancers.[49] This may at least in part explain the fact that cisplatin and oxaliplatin are not completely cross-resistant. In contrast, similar to cisplatin, elevations of glutathione levels in cells appear to correlate with oxaliplatin resistance.[74] Other potential mechanisms of resistance include decreased accumulation of oxaliplatin in cells and alteration of enzymes involved in controlling the cell cycle.[49]

Other Agents

Other agents with low-level activity against colorectal cancer include mitomycin C and the nitrosoureas. These are uncommonly used for the treatment of colorectal cancer patients. When they are used, it is usually in the setting of patients who have progressed on prior 5-FU- and irinotecan-based therapies. They are usually given in combination with a 5-FU-based regimen. With the availability of a number of new agents (such as irinotecan or oxaliplatin) their use has declined.

Table 10–6. OXALIPLATIN TOXICITIES	
Frequent	Laryngopharyngeal dysesthesia, peripheral neuropathy, which is cumulative (both enhanced by cold exposure), mild thrombocytopenia; in conjunction with 5-FU: increase in the frequency of diarrhea, nausea and vomiting, and neutropenia, which can be seen with 5-FU
Less frequent	Allergic reactions, venous irritation, fever, mild elevations in LFTs

All chemotherapy doses need to be carefully adjusted for patient factors and toxicity.

Combination Therapy

The availability of irinotecan and oxaliplatin in addition to 5-FU has led to the ability to test whether combinations of these agents have greater activity than single agents. In addition, combinations have been tested for whether they might provide a survival advantage in both patients with metastatic disease as well as in the adjuvant setting. Combinations of 5-FU with irinotecan are relatively recent.[75–80] Preclinical studies suggest synergy when 5-FU/LV is combined with irinotecan, with a suggestion that synergy is greatest when irinotecan precedes 5-FU/LV.[81] A number of phase I to III studies have utilized various schedules of these drugs in combination.[75–80] The toxicity profiles of the different schedules has been acceptable. Interestingly, diarrhea, which is a major side effect of both drugs, has not been significantly more prevalent than seen with either treatment alone, even when the drugs have been administered on concomitant schedules. Two recent studies have indicated that there is a survival advantage for the combination of 5-FU- and LV-based therapy combined with irinotecan as opposed to 5-FU and LV treatment alone.[79,80] One is a randomized phase III study that indicated a higher response rate, time to progression, and trend toward improved overall survival for the combination including irinotecan over 5-FU/LV alone for initial treatment of patients with metastatic disease.[79] Follow-up of this trial confirms that there is a survival advantage for the combined treatment group (FDA, public information). The second trial was a phase III trial that indicated longer time to tumor progression and improved overall survival in patients who received irinotecan in combination with 5-FU and LV as opposed to those who received the 5-FU and LV alone.[79,80] Based on the results of these two trials, the US FDA approved the combination of 5-FU, LV, and irinotecan as first-line therapy for patients with metastatic colorectal cancer. Additional phase III trials to evaluate this question further are ongoing. In addition, a phase III intergroup trial is evaluating whether adjuvant therapy with the combination of irinotecan, 5-FU, and LV will produce a survival advantage as compared with 5-FU and LV alone for patients with Dukes C colorectal cancer that has been resected.

Similar to the case with irinotecan, oxaliplatin has been shown to be synergistic with 5-FU/LV in preclinical studies.[49] As discussed above, the combination of these agents has been extensively studied in a number of trials.[50] Phase II trials have indicated response rates of approximately 30 to 50 percent in previously untreated patients and 20 to 46 percent in patients who have progressed on previous 5-FU-based therapy. Small phase III trials have suggested a significantly higher response rate and progression-free survival over that seen with 5-FU/LV therapy.[71] As is true for irinotecan, phase III trials are further evaluating the role of 5-FU, LV, and oxaliplatin combinations in the initial treatment of metastatic colorectal cancer.

The least tested of these combinations have been oxaliplatin and irinotecan. Preclinical studies suggest synergy when platinum compounds and irinotecan are given together, and there is a reasonable amount of experience combining irinotecan with cisplatin in other disease settings; this has been most extensively studied in lung cancer where there is a suggestion of enhanced activity. A number of phase I studies have recently been reported evaluating the combination of oxaliplatin with irinotecan.[82–84] The major toxicities seen were diarrhea, neutropenia, vomiting, and dose-cumulative neuropathy. Phase II studies are currently evaluating the efficacy of combined therapy. In addition, one of the three arms of the ongoing intergroup trial in the United States evaluating various combinations of 5-FU, LV, irinotecan, and oxaliplatin for the initial therapy of patients with metastatic colorectal

Table 10–7. NEW APPROACHES FOR COLORECTAL CANCER
Modulation of 5-FU/LV
Oral delivery of 5-FU or 5-FU precursors
Inhibition of DPD (metabolism)
Novel thymidylate synthase inhibitors
Irinotecan combinations with 5-FU and/or oxaliplatin
Oxaliplatin combinations with 5-FU and/or irinotecan
Other topoisomerase I inhibitors
Monoclonal antibodies (eg, 17-1A)
Targeting specific proteins or metabolic pathways (eg, farnesyl transferase inhibitors)
Biologic response modifiers
Antiangiogenic or antimetastatic agents
Gene therapy
Mechanical (hyperthermia, radiofrequency ablation, cryoablation)

All chemotherapy doses need to be carefully adjusted for patient factors and toxicity.

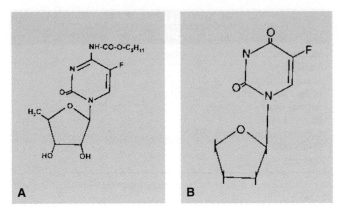

Figure 10–6. Oral 5-FU analogs. *A*, Capecitabine (Xeloda). *B*, Ftorafur.

cancer is a combination of irinotecan with oxaliplatin. The other two arms are the combination of (1) 5-FU, LV, and irinotecan and (2) 5-FU, LV, and oxaliplatin.

Finally, there is the potential for combining all three agents, which is in the early stages of development. Whether initial combinations of agents will prove to have an overall response and survival advantage over sequential use of the agents still needs to be tested. A number of large trials evaluating various combinations of these agents in both the metastatic and adjuvant settings are either ongoing or planned, and the answers should be available over the next 5 to 10 years.

Chemotherapeutic Agents as Radiation Sensitizers

Irinotecan and 5-FU are radiation sensitizers.[85–87] Oxaliplatin has not yet been adequately enough studied as a radiation sensitizer to know how effective it is at radiosensitization. 5-FU is by far the most extensively studied of these to date and the only one that has been shown in randomized trials to improve the survival of patients with rectal adenocarcinomas in the adjuvant setting.[88] Studies evaluating irinotecan as a radiation sensitizer are ongoing and oxaliplatin is being evaluated in combination with 5-FU for the treatment of locally advanced rectal cancer. Only future phase III studies will determine what role these agents may have alone, combined with radiation, or in combination with each other and radiation for the treatment of rectal cancer.

NEW AGENTS AND APPROACHES

A number of new compounds are actively being evaluated for their role in the treatment of patients with colorectal cancer (Table 10–7) and (Figure 10–6). The furthest along of these are the oral 5-FU analogues and precursors, a number of which are already approved for use in both Japan and Europe. Phase III trials of two of these agents (capecitabine and orzel) have indicated equivalence of the oral agents to the daily × 5 once-monthly 5-FU/LV schedule in the metastatic disease setting.[89,90] They are both being evaluated by the FDA for approval for this indication.

Capecitabine (N4-pentoxycarbonyl-5'-deoxy-5-fluorocytidine), an oral fluoropyrimidine carbamate, is converted by a three step enzymatic process to 5-FU.[91,92] The initial step in the liver converts it to 5'-deoxy-fluorocytidine, the next step to 5'-deoxy-5-fluorouridine, and the final step (by the enzyme thymidine phosphorylase that may be expressed at higher levels in tumor cells than normal tissues) to 5-FU. The fact that the enzyme involved in the final conversion may be present at higher levels in tumors has the potential advantage of increased drug levels at the sites of tumors, although this has not been established in patients.

UFT (4:1 ratio of uracil to ftorafur) combines the 5-FU prodrug Tegafur (ftorafur) with uracil (a competitive inhibitor of DPD), therefore enhancing the bioavailability of the 5-FU.[93] UFT has been combined with LV to make an agent called Orzel. Although the oral agents do not offer a response or survival advantage over currently available IV administration, they do offer a more convenient delivery method for chronic drug administration. This should also allow for easier combinations with other agents or treatment modalities (eg, radiation therapy) in the future, especially when the utilization of prolonged 5-FU therapy is being explored.

Another approach has utilized the combination of oral 5-FU with eniluracil that inactivates DPD, therefore significantly enhancing the bioavailability of the oral 5-FU.[94] In addition, by inhibiting DPD, one may eliminate issues related to variability in toxicity between patients due to the varying DPD levels in different individuals. However, this theoretical benefit still needs to be established in clinical trials. This combination clearly has antitumor activity and its potential role in the treatment of patients is currently undergoing phase III testing. A number of other oral 5-FU compounds are also currently being evaluated.

A number of new TS inhibitors are also undergoing evaluation for their potential roles in the treatment of patients with colorectal cancer. Raltitrexed has been most extensively studied.[95] Although some studies have shown equivalency to 5-FU/LV, others have not, and it is still not approved in the United States, though it has been approved for use in Europe and Canada. The multitargeted antifolate, LY 231514, has been shown to have activity against metastatic colorectal cancer in small phase II trials and is currently undergoing further evaluation.[96,97] It remains uncertain whether any of the new TS inhibitors will offer a therapeutic advantage over 5-FU/LV. These types of agents may also have additive or synergistic activity when used in combination with 5-FU.[22] This is being pursued in a number of early trials.

A number of new topoisomerase inhibitors are being evaluated in clinical trials. These include 9-NC, DX8951f, and GG-211.[98–100] The role any of these agents might have in treating colorectal cancer is yet to be determined.

Knowledge about the biology of colorectal tumors has provided a number of potential protein targets for the treatment of this disease. Since ras mutations occur in approximately 30 to 50 percent of patients with colorectal cancer, ras inhibitors are one of the logical candidates for development to potentially treat these patients.[101–103] A number of farnesyl transferase inhibitors (which block the farnesylation of ras that is required for its localization in the cell membrane and therefore activity) are currently undergoing various stages of clinical testing.[104–106] In addition, antisense oligonucleotides are being evaluated for their ability to inhibit the immediate downstream effector for ras, raf.[107] Various other signal transduction pathways are important for the survival, proliferation, or metastasis of malignant colorectal cells. Inhibition of some of these (eg, protein kinase C, growth factor receptors, or cyclin-dependent kinases) is currently undergoing early clinical testing.[108–110] It is too early to know whether they will have any role in the treatment of colorectal cancer patients (Table 10–8).

Table 10–8. POTENTIAL SPECIFIC TARGETS IN COLORECTAL CANCER
Mutant ras and downstream effectors
Mutant p53
Mutant APC gene
Mutant mismatched repair enzymes
Growth factor receptors
Protein kinase C
Cyclin-dependent kinases
Metastasis
Angiogenesis

All chemotherapy doses need to be carefully adjusted for patient factors and toxicity.

Biologic Response Modifiers

The most extensively studied of the biologic response modifiers for the treatment of colorectal cancer has been alpha interferon that has most commonly been given in combination with 5-FU/LV. A large number of randomized studies have shown no benefit for the combination of alpha interferon with 5-FU/LV.[20,111] Other biologic agents, such as IL-2, have also been evaluated, again without clear-cut benefit.[112,113] Vaccines against a number of proteins, including mutant p53, mutant ras, and CEA, are being evaluated both in the metastatic disease and minimal residual disease settings.[114–116] There is not yet convincing evidence that these have sufficient activity to be useful in patients with either the adjuvant or metastatic disease. However, continued evaluation of various vaccination approaches is ongoing both preclinically and in clinical trials.

Various inhibitors of the metastatic process or angiogenesis, such as metalloproteinase inhibitors (eg, marimistat, Bay-12-9566), continue to be evaluated for their potential role in the treatment of patients.[117–119] However, none has as of yet been shown to have clear clinical activity. Other inhibitors of angiogenesis (antibodies to vascular endothelial growth factor receptor [EGFR]) are either undergoing early clinical testing or will be evaluated in clinical trials in the near future.

Monoclonal antibodies have been evaluated in a number of settings for their potential therapeutic activity in treating patients with colorectal cancer. These have been targeted against a variety of antigens, including CEA, A33, fibroblast-activating protein, and the 17-1A monoclonal.[120–125] The latter of these has been most extensively studied, especially for the adjuvant treatment of patients with Dukes B and C disease. A small phase III study suggested survival benefit comparable to that seen with chemotherapy when 17-1A was given in the adjuvant setting, and a larger multinational confirmatory trial is ongoing.[120] In addition, it is being evaluated for its potential role in the treatment of patients with Dukes B disease in the adjuvant setting in an intergroup trial in the United States. A number of other monoclonal antibodies, either by themselves or coupled with radioactive or toxic compounds, are being evaluated in phase I and II trials, but it is too early to know if any of these will have clinical benefit.[120–125]

CURRENT UTILIZATION OF CHEMOTHERAPY IN SPECIFIC SETTINGS

Radiation plus Chemotherapy in the Adjuvant Setting for Rectal Cancer

A number of randomized trials have established a role for adjuvant radiation therapy and chemotherapy for patients with resected T3 and T4 rectal cancer and those with positive nodes (stages 2 and 3).[126–128] The standard approach in the United States has combined systemic 5-FU, followed by combined 5-FU and radiation therapy, followed by systemic 5-FU in a sandwich schedule. A number of trials attempting to define the optimum method for delivering the 5-FU are ongoing, and a better definition of the most effective approach awaits the results of these trials. Certainly, one acceptable approach is the regimen that incorporates infusional 5-FU with radiation as reported in 1994.[128]

Whether preoperative treatment might offer any advantage over postoperative treatment was evaluated in a randomized trial, but unfortunately this trial had to be closed before reaching adequate patient numbers for full evaluation because of poor accrual. Follow-up of this study is still ongoing, and this may give hints about the relative value of preoperative versus postoperative therapy. Certainly, there is no strong evidence at the present time to favor a pre- or postoperative approach from a survival or disease recurrence standpoint. Preoperative therapy may offer an advantage in terms of easier delivery of the radiation therapy and potential for ability to perform

a low anterior resection rather than abdominal perineal resection in patients who have a good response to the chemotherapy plus radiation therapy. A number of trials are under way evaluating the potential integration of irinotecan and/or oxaliplatin as well as other new chemotherapeutic agents into treatment of patients with rectal adenocarcinomas.

Radiation plus Chemotherapy in the Adjuvant Setting for Colonic Cancer

As opposed to the situation for rectal cancer, the potential role for the addition of radiation to chemotherapy in certain disease settings of colonic cancer patients remains unclear. Retrospective evaluations have suggested that certain disease settings may be associated with increased risk of local failure, and these might benefit from adjuvant radiation therapy in addition to chemotherapy.[129] A randomized study to evaluate this more definitively was closed early because of poor accrual and therefore was underpowered to evaluate the benefit from adjuvant radiation therapy.[130] At the level of accrual achieved, it did not suggest benefit for the addition of radiation therapy to chemotherapy in this setting. However, overall evidence remains inconclusive as to whether adjuvant radiation therapy in addition to chemotherapy produces a long-term survival advantage for those colon cancer patients at increased risk for local recurrence. Additional studies are needed to fully define the potential role of adding radiation therapy to chemotherapy in this setting.

Chemotherapy ± Radiation Therapy for Unresectable Patients

Definitive radiation therapy is not curative for the majority of patients with colorectal cancer whose tumors cannot be resected or who have a local recurrence after a low anterior resection. However, it can palliate symptoms and produce survival prolongation with a small percentage of patients surviving 5 years.[131–134] There is no consistent experience for the addition of 5-FU-based chemotherapy to radiation therapy alone in this setting. Thus, the question of whether addition of chemotherapy to radiation therapy would provide any survival benefit for patients who cannot be surgically resected remains open.

Adjuvant Chemotherapy for Colon Cancer

Chemotherapy has clearly been shown to improve the overall survival of patients with Dukes C colon cancer in the adjuvant setting.[26,135–138] A number of schedules of 5-FU either with LV or levamisole have been utilized. At the present time, 6 months of 5-FU/LV given by either the 5 days per week each month or once weekly for 6 weeks on/2 weeks off schedules and 5-FU plus levamisole given initially for 5 days in a row followed 1 month later by once-weekly therapy for 1 year are acceptable regimens (see Table 10–1). The question of whether immediate perioperative systemic 5-FU at the time of resection of the colon cancer enhances the survival benefit of adjuvant 5-FU and LV is being evaluated in a prospective randomized trial. In addition, currently the role of integrating irinotecan and/or oxaliplatin into the adjuvant treatment of these patients is being explored. The potential role of the monoclonal antibody 17-1A in this setting is also under investigation.[139]

Although there is a trend toward improved survival, none of the major individual randomized studies has shown a statistically significant overall survival benefit for chemotherapy in the adjuvant treatment of patients with Dukes B disease. However, most of these were underpowered to evaluate a small difference. There are subsets of patients with Dukes B disease (those who present with obstructive symptoms or perforation) who are at sufficiently high risk for development of recurrent or metastatic disease that consideration of adjuvant chemotherapy on a case-by-case basis is warranted. As is the case for patients with Dukes C disease mentioned above, studies evaluating the monoclonal antibody 17-1A in the adjuvant treatment of patients with Dukes B disease are ongoing. Future studies will evaluate combinations of chemotherapeutic agents, new agents, or other approaches.

Chemotherapy for Resectable Metastatic Disease

Preliminary data from two recent studies suggest that the combination of hepatic arterial infusion (HAI) delivery of FUDR (see Figure 10–1B) and systemic 5-FU/LV enhances the survival of patients with metastatic disease confined to the liver that can be surgically resected.[140,141] If confirmed with further follow-up, this would become the standard approach for patients in this setting.

Chemotherapy for Unresectable Metastatic Disease

Treatment of patients with metastatic disease remains disappointing. The most active single agents produce response rates in the 20 to 25 percent range, and there is no impact of treatment on 5-year survival.[2,5,8,35,40,49,50] 5-FU/LV remains the standard initial treatment approach. Other agents with activity against colorectal cancer include irinotecan and oxaliplatin as discussed above. As discussed above, the combination of 5-FU/LV and irinotecan has been shown to produce a survival advantage over 5-FU/LV alone with tolerable toxicity and is now approved for front-line therapy of patients with metastatic colorectal cancer in the United States.[79,80] A number of trials are evaluating combinations of agents, especially irinotecan and oxaliplatin, with 5-FU or each other.[76] The results of these studies should help better define the clinical benefit of these combinations seen in initial trials and which of these combinations ultimately will have the greatest efficacy with tolerable toxicity.[49,66,71,78–80]

Based on suggestions of higher response rates when chemotherapy is given directly into the liver for patients with unresectable hepatic metastases, an intergroup trial is evaluating response rates, response durations, and survival for patients treated with intrahepatic FUDR versus 5-FU/LV in a prospectively randomized study.[142]

Other means of local delivery of 5-FU or FUDR (eg, via the portal vein or intraperitoneally) have not yet been convincingly shown to provide benefit over systemic delivery in either the adjuvant or metastatic disease settings. These alternative means of delivery are continuing to be explored in clinical trials.

FUTURE THERAPEUTIC DIRECTIONS

For surgically resectable patients who are at high risk for recurrence or development of metastatic disease as well as patients with locally advanced disease, the major focus remains evaluation of combined modality approaches. Phase II and III trials of combined modality therapy (chemotherapy, radiation therapy, and surgery) are ongoing.

For patients with unresectable metastatic disease, phase II and III trials of combinations of current agents remain a major area of clinical investigation. In addition, trials of new agents are attempting to identify active compounds. In addition to continued evaluation of alternative schedules of delivering 5-FU/LV, irinotecan, and oxaliplatin these include topoisomerase I inhibitors (such as 9-NC or DX8951f), thymydilate synthase (TS) inhibitors (such as D1694 and LY231514), and oral 5-FU-related compounds.

Although proof is still lacking that targeted therapies will be clinically useful for patients with colorectal cancer, the success of targeted therapies against several other malignancies (eg, trastuzumab for breast cancer and rituximab for non-Hodgkin's lymphomas) as well as increased understanding of the biologic processes important for survival and proliferation of neoplastic colorectal cells clearly indicates the potential therapeutic utility of this approach. Compounds developed using biochemic and molecular biologic approaches to modulate specific targets are providing new agents for testing in the treatment of colorectal cancer. Biologic processes that might be important in the survival and proliferation of neoplastic colorectal cells include (1) ras mutations that occur in approximately 30 to 50 percent of colorectal neoplasms, making this highly suitable for approaches targeting ras function (see above); (2) p53 (critical in controlling a number of cellular processes, including DNA integrity, progression through the cell cycle, and apoptosis), which is mutated in approximately 50 percent of colorectal cancers[143,144]; (3) various growth factor receptors (such as epidermal growth factor receptor [EGFR], HER2/Neu receptors, fibroblast growth factor [FGF] receptors, or insulin-like growth factor receptors) or growth factors (such as transforming growth factor α [TGF-α] or FGFs) that may be involved in autocrine or paracrine proliferation of neoplastic colorectal cells or development of angiogenesis or metastases[145–148]; (4) intracellular signalling pathways, such as the COX-2 pathway,

which is important in the proliferation of colonic polyps and may play a role in malignant cells as well[29]; and (5) the expression of specific splice variants of CD44 that may be involved in the metastatic process (although there still remain questions about its exact role in colorectal cancer).[149,150] In addition, preclinical studies indicate that a significant immune response may be generated against tumor cells, including colonic adenocarcinoma cells, that express altered mucin 1.[151]

Approaches being explored to take advantage of the biology of colorectal cancer include (1) Vaccines: (a) against tumor-specific mutant p53 and ras; (b) targeting CD44 splice variants; and (c) altered mucin constructs (such as Muc1) that, if expressed on the surface of a high percentage of colorectal cancer cells, might make them more immunogenic; (2) Gene therapy (such as with viral vector constructs) attempting to inhibit mutant ras function or restore normal p53 function; (3) Small molecule inhibitors of ras function, such as farnesyl transferase inhibitors; (4) Inhibitors of tyrosine kinases to block function of growth factor receptors (as well as other tyrosine kinases such as src family kinases) that might be involved in proliferation of colorectal cancer cells; (5) Antibodies or fusion toxins targeted against growth factor receptors or other cell surface antigens; (6) Monoclonal antibodies that can inhibit the function of mutated oncogenes; (7) Antisense oligonucleotides targeting growth factors or their receptors, or mutant ras, p53, DCC, or other mutant genes that might be important in the proliferation of colorectal cancer cells; (8) Peptides or peptidomimetics that can interfere with or modulate the function of growth factor receptors or mutated oncogenes; and (9) COX-2 inhibitors alone and in combination with other agents, such as chemotherapy.

Other new approaches being studied include (1) liposome delivery systems to enhance delivery of cytotoxic agents to colorectal tumor cells; (2) differentiating agents (retinoic acid, vitamin D analogs, butyric acid); (3) antiangiogenesis agents; (4) photodynamic therapy; (5) hyperthermia; (6) radiofrequency ablation (which has recently been approved for use in treating hepatic metastases); and (7) cryosurgery.[151–153]

CONCLUSION

Trials have established that optimal integration of surgery and chemotherapy (+ radiation therapy for rectal cancer patients) can impact on the survival of certain patients who can be surgically resected but are at high risk for recurrent or metastatic disease. These would include patients with Dukes C (stage 3) colon cancer and those with stage 2 or 3 rectal cancers. Recent evidence suggests that chemotherapy delivered directly into the liver after resection of metastatic disease to the liver may also offer a survival benefit. Although there are effective therapies for palliation and short-term prolongation of survival, the long-term prognosis remains poor for patients with colorectal cancer who cannot be surgically resected. Increased understanding of the biology of colorectal cancer has provided a number of leads that are being pursued in an attempt to improve treatment for this malignancy.

REFERENCES

1. Landis SH, Murray T, et al. Cancer statistics, 1999. CA Cancer J Clin 1999;49:8–31.
2. Grem JL. Systemic treatment options in advanced colorectal cancer: perspectives on combination 5-fluorouracil plus leucovorin. Semin Oncol 1997;24(5 Suppl 18):8–18.
3. Bertino JR. Chemotherapy of colorectal cancer: history and new themes. Semin Oncol 1997;24(5 Suppl 18): 3–7.
4. Grem J, Chabner B, et al. Fluoropyrimidine. Cancer Chemotherapy and Biotherapy 1996;(ed 2):149–211.
5. Kamm YJ, Wagener DJ, et al. 5-Fluorouracil in colorectal cancer: rationale and clinical results of frequently used schedules. Anticancer Drugs 1998;9:371–80.
6. de Gramont A, Louvet C, et al. A review of GERCOD trials of bimonthly leucovorin plus 5-fluorouracil 48-h continuous infusion in advanced colorectal cancer: evolution of a regimen. Groupe d'Etude et de Recherche sur les Cancers de l'Ovaire et Digestifs (GERCOD). Eur J Cancer 1998;34:619–26.
7. Wils JA. High-dose infusional 5-FU in the treatment of advanced colorectal cancer: a summary of the European experience. J Infus Chemother 1996;6:145–8.
8. Machover D. A comprehensive review of 5-fluorouracil and leucovorin in patients with metastatic colorectal carcinoma. Cancer 1997;80:1179–87.
9. Labianca R, Pessi A, et al. (1996). Modulated 5-fluorouracil (5-FU) regimens in advanced colorectal cancer: a critical review of comparative studies. Eur J Cancer 1996;32A(Suppl 5):S7–12.
10. Benson AB 3rd. Regional and systemic therapies for advanced colorectal carcinoma: randomized clinical trial results. Oncology 1998;12(10 Suppl 7):28–34.
11. Ardalan B, Luis R, et al. Biomodulation of fluorouracil in colorectal cancer. Cancer Invest 1998;16:237–51.
12. Rustum YM, Cao S, et al. Rationale for treatment design: biochemical modulation of 5-fluorouracil by leucovorin. Cancer J Sci Am 1998;4(1):12–8.
13. Anonymous. Modulation of fluorouracil by leucovorin in patients with advanced colorectal cancer, evidence in terms of response rate. Advanced Colorectal Cancer Meta-Analysis Project. J Clin Oncol 1992;10: 896–903.
14. Thomas DM, Zalcberg JR. 5-Fluorouracil: a pharmacological paradigm in the use of cytotoxics. Clin Exper Pharmacol Physiol 1998;25:887–95.
15. Van Cutsem E, Peeters M. Developments in fluoropyrimidine therapy for gastrointestinal cancer. Curr Opin Oncol 1999;11:312.
16. Mini E, Coronnello M, Carotti S. Biochemical modulation of fluoropyrimidines by antifolates and folates in an in vitro model of human leukemia. J Chemother 1990;2(Suppl 1):17–27.
17. Anonymous. Meta-analysis of randomized trials testing the biochemical modulation of fluorouracil by methotrexate in metastatic colorectal cancer. Advanced Colorectal Cancer Meta-Analysis Project. J Clin Oncol 1994;12:960–9.
18. Blanke CD, Messenger M, et al. Trimetrexate: review and current clinical experience in advanced colorectal cancer. Semin Oncol 1997;24(5 Suppl 18):57–63.
19. Punt C, Keizer H, et al. Multicenter ranadomized trial of 5-fluorouracil (5-FU) and leucovorin (LV) with or without trimetrexate (TMTX) as first line treatment in patients (pts) with advanced colorectal cancer. ASCO 18.
20. Raderer M, Scheithauer W. Treatment of advanced colorectal cancer with 5-fluorouracil and interferon-alpha: an overview of clinical trials. Eur J Cancer 1995;31A:1002–8.
21. Ardalan B, Luis R, et al. Biomodulation of fluorouracil in colorectal cancer. Cancer Invest 1998;16:237–51.
22. Longo GS, Izzo J, et al. Pretreatment of colon carcinoma cells with Tomudex enhances 5-fluorouracil cytotoxicity. Clin Cancer Res 1998;4:469–73.
23. Izzo J, Zielinski Z, et al. Molecular mechanisms of the synergistic sequential administration of D1964 (Tomudex) followed by FUra in colon carcinoma cells [meeting abstract]. Proceedings of the Annual Meeting American Association of Cancer Research (201995) 1995. 36.
24. Falcone A, Danesi R, et al. Intravenous azidothymidine with fluorouracil and leucovorin: a phase I-II study

in previously untreated metastatic colorectal cancer patients. J Clin Oncol 1996;14:729–36.

25. Clark J, Sikov W, et al. Phase II study of 5-fluorouracil leucovorin and azidothymidine in patients with metastatic colorectal cancer. J Cancer Res Clin Oncol 1996;122:554–8.

26. Casillas S, Pelley RJ, et al. Adjuvant therapy for colorectal cancer: present and future perspectives. Dis Colon Rectum 1997;40:977–92.

27. Bleiberg H. Colorectal cancer: the challenge. Eur J Cancer 32A(Suppl 5):S2–6.

28. Sinicrope FA, Pazdur R, et al. Phase I trial of sulindac plus 5-fluorouracil and levamisole: potential adjuvant therapy for colon carcinoma. Clin Cancer Res 1996;2(1):37–41.

29. Aschele C, Debernardis D, et al. Immunohistochemical quantitation of thymidylate synthase expression in colorectal cancer metastases predicts for clinical outcome to fluorouracil-based chemotherapy. J Clin Oncol 1999;17:1760–70.

30. Peters GI, van der Wilt GL, et al. Predictive value of thymidylate synthase and dihydropyrimidine dehydrogenase. Eur J Cancer 1994;30A:1408–11.

31. Leichman CG, Lenz HJ, et al. Quantitation of intratumoral thymidylate synthase expression predicts for disseminated colorectal cancer response and resistance to protracted-infusion fluorouracil and weekly leucovorin. J Clin Oncol 1997;15:3223–9.

32. Minderman H, Cao S, et al. Rational design of irinotecan administration based on preclinical models. Oncology 1998;12(8 Suppl 6):22–30.

33. Pommier Y, Pourquier P, et al. Mechanism of action of eukaryotic DNA topoisomerase I and drugs targeted to the enzyme. Biochim Biophys Acta 1998;1400: 83–105.

34. Iyer L, Ratain MJ. Clinical pharmacology of camptothecins. Cancer Chemother Pharmacol 1998;42 (Suppl):S31–43.

35. Muggia FM, Dimery I, et al. Camptothecin and its analogs. An overview of their potential in cancer therapeutics. Ann N Y Acad Sci 1996;803:213–23.

36. Takimoto CH, Wright J, et al. Clinical applications of the camptothecins. Biochim Biophys Acta 1998; 1400:107–19.

37. Iyer L, King CD, et al. Genetic predisposition to the metabolism of irinotecan (CPT-11). Role of uridine diphosphate glucuronosyltransferase isoform 1A1 in the glucuronidation of its active metabolite (SN-38) in human liver microsomes. J Clin Invest 1998;101: 847–54.

38. Wadler S, Benson AB 3rd, et al. Recommended guidelines for the treatment of chemotherapy-induced diarrhea. J Clin Oncol 1998;16:3169–78.

39. Kuhn JG. Pharmacology of irinotecan. Oncology 1998;12(8 Suppl 6):39–42.

40. Pitot HC. US pivotal studies of irinotecan in colorectal carcinoma. Oncology 1998;12(8 Suppl 6):48–53.

41. Rougier P, Van Cutsem E, et al. Randomised trial of irinotecan versus fluorouracil by continuous infusion after fluorouracil failure in patients with metastatic colorectal cancer. Lancet 1998;352:1407–12.

42. Cunningham D, Pyrhonen S, et al. Randomised trial of irinotecan plus supportive care versus supportive care alone after fluorouracil failure for patients with metastatic colorectal cancer. Lancet 1998;352: 1413–8.

43. Van Cutsem E, Cunningham D, et al. Clinical activity and benefit of irinotecan (CPT-11) in patients with colorectal cancer truly resistant to 5-fluorouracil (5-FU). Eur J Cancer 1999;35:54–9.

44. Rothenberg M, Cox J, et al. A multicenter, phase II trial of weekly irinotecan (CPT-11) in patients with previously treated colorectal carcinoma. Cancer 1999;85: 786–95.

45. Bleiberg H, Cvitkovic E. Characterisation and clinical management of CPT-11 (irinotecan)-induced adverse events: the European perspective. Eur J Cancer 1996;32A(Suppl 3):S18–23.

46. Rothenberg ML. Topoisomerase I inhibitors: review and update. Ann Oncol 1997;8:837–55.

47. Kojima A, Hackett NR, et al. Reversal of CPT-11 resistance of lung cancer cells by adenovirus-mediated gene transfer of the human carboxylesterase cDNA. Cancer Res 1998;58:4368–74.

48. Chu X, Suzuki H, et al. Active efflux of CPT-11 and its metabolites in human KB-derived cell lines. J Pharmacol Exp Ther 1999;288:735–41.

49. Raymond E, Chaney SG, et al. Oxaliplatin: a review of preclinical and clinical studies. Ann Oncol 1998;9:1053–1071.

50. Bleiberg H. Oxaliplatin (L-OHP): a new reality in colorectal cancer. Br J Cancer 1998;77(Suppl 4):1–3.

51. Rixe O, Ortuzar W, Alvarez M, et al. Oxaliplatin, tetraplatin, cisplatin and carboplatin: spectrum of activity in drug-resistant cell lines and in the cell lines of the national cancer institute's anticancer drug screen panel. Biochem Pharmacol 1996;52:1855–65.

52. Tashiro T, Kawada Y, Sakurai Y, Kidani Y. Antitumour activity of a new platinum complex, oxalato (trans-1-1,2-diaminocyclohexane) platinum (II), new experimental data. Biomed Parmacother 1989;43:251–60.

53. Raymond E, Lawrence R, Izbicki E, et al. Effects of oxaliplatin (OxPt) in human tumor cloning assay. Proc AACR 1998;39:158 (Abs 1083).

54. Scheeff ED, Howell SB. Computer modeling of the primary cisplatin and oxaliplatin DNA adducts and relevance to mismatch repair recognition. Proc AACR 1998;39:158 (Abs 1082).

55. Vaisman A, Varchenko M, Umar A, et al. Defects in hMSH6, but not in hMSH3, correlate with increased

resistance and enhanced replicative bypass of cis-platin, but not oxaliplatin, adducts. Proc AACR 1998;39:159 (Abs 1085).

56. Faivre S, Woynoarowski JM. Oxaliplatin effects on DNA integrity and apoptosis induction in human tumor cells. Proc AACR 1998;39:158 (Abs 1081).

57. Rixe O, Ortuzar W, et al. Oxaliplatin, tetraplatin, cis-platin, and carboplatin: spectrum of activity in drug-resistant cell lines and in the cell lines of the National Cancer Institute's Anticancer Drug Screen panel. Biochem Pharmacol 1996;52:1855–65.

58. Fischel JL, Etienne MC, Formento P, et al. Search for an optimal schedule combining fluorouracil (FU) and oxaliplatin (LOHP)-experimental data. Proc AACR 1998;39:159 (Abs 1087).

59. Graham MA, Gamelin E, Missett JL, et al. Clinical pharmacokinetics of oxaliplatin. Proc AACR 1998;39:159 (Abs 1088).

60. Levi F, Perpoint B, Carufi C, et al. Oxaliplatin activity against metastatic colorectal cancer: a phase against metastatic colorectal cancer: a phase II study of 5-day continuous venous infusion at circadian rhythm modulated rate. Eur J Cancer 1993;29:1280–4.

61. Machover D, Diaz-Rubio E, De Gramont A, et al. Two consecutive phase II studies of oxaliplatin (L-OHP) for treatment of patients with advanced colorectal carcinoma who were resistant to previous treatment with fluoropyrimidines. Ann Oncol 1996;7:95–8.

62. Moreau S, Machover D, de Gramont A, et al. Phase II trial of oxaliplatin (L-OHP) in patients with colorectal carcinoma previously resistant to 5-fluorouracil and folinic acid. Proc Am Soc Clin Oncol 1993;12:214.

63. Raymond E, Buguet-Fagot C, Djelloul S, et al. Anti-tumor activity of oxaliplatin in combination with 5-fluorouracil and the thymidylate synthase inhibitor AG337 in human colon, breast, and ovarian cancers. Anticancer Drugs 1987;8:876–5.

64. Mathe G, Kidani Y, Segiguchi M, et al. Oxalato-platinum or L-OHP, a third-generation platinum complex: an experimental and clinical appraisal and preliminary comparison with cis-platinum and carboplatinum. Biomed Pharmacother 1989;43:237–50.

65. de Gramont A, Vignoud J, Tournigand C, et al. Oxali-platin with high-dose leucovorin and 5-fluorouracil 48-hour continuous infusion in pretreated metastatic colorectal cancer. Eur J Cancer 1997;33:214–9.

66. Levi F, Zidani R, Misset J-L. Randomized multicentre trial of chemotherapy with oxaliplatin, fluorouracil, and folinic acid in metastatic colorectal cancer. Lancet 1997;350:681–6.

67. Bertheault-Cvitkovic F, Jami A, Ithzaki M, et al. Biweekly intensified ambulatory chronomodulated chemotherapy with oxaliplatin, 5-fluorouracil and folinic acid in patients with metastatic colorectal cancer. J Clin Oncol 1996;14:2950–8.

68. Levi F, Zidani R, Vannetzel JM, et al. Chronomodulated versus fixed infusion rate delivery of ambulatory chemotherapy with oxaliplatin, 5-fluorouracil and folinic acid in patients with colorectal cancer metas-tases: a randomized multiinstitutional trial. J Natl Cancer Inst 1994;86:1608–17.

69. Bleiberg H. Oxaliplatin (L-OHP): a new reality in col-orectal cancer. Br J Cancer 1998;77(Suppl 4):1–3.

70. Andre T, Bensmaine MA, Louvet C, et al. Addition of oxaliplatin (EloxatineR) to the same leucovorin (LV) and 5-fluorouracil (5FU) bimonthly regimens after progression in patients (pts) with metastatic colorec-tal cancer (MRCC): preliminary report. Proc Am Soc Clin Oncol 1997;16:270a (Abs 958).

71. Giacchetti S, Zidani R, Perpoint B, et al. Phase III trial of 5-fluorouracil (5-FU), folinic acid (FA), with or without oxaliplatin (OXA) in previously untreated patients (pts) with metastatic colorectal cancer (MCC). Proc Am Soc Clin Oncol 1997;16:228a (Abs 805).

72. Levi F, Dogliotti L, Perpoint B, et al. A multicenter phase II trial of intensified chronotherapy with oxali-platin (L-OHP), 5-fluorouracil (5-FU) and folinic acid (FA) in patients (pts) with previously untreated metastatic colorectal cancer (MCC). Proc Am Soc Clin Oncol 1997;16:266a (Abs 945).

73. Raymond E, Chaney SG, et al. Oxaliplatin: a review of pre-clinical and clinical studies. Ann Oncol 1998; 9:1053–71.

74. Gerard B, Bleiberg H, Michel J, et al. Oxaliplatin com-bined to 5-FU and folinic acid (5-FU/FA) as second- or third-line treatment in patients with advanced colorectal cancer. Proc Am Soc Clin Oncol 1997; 16:288a (Abs 1025).

75. Khayat D, Gil-Delgado M, et al. European experience with irinotecan plus fluorouracil/folinic acid or mit-omycin. Oncology 1998;12(8 Suppl 6):64–7.

76. Goldberg RM, Erlichman C. Irinotecan plus 5-FU and leucovorin in advanced colorectal cancer: North American trials. Oncology 1998;12(8 Suppl 6):59–63.

77. Vanhoefer U, Harstrick A, et al. Phase I study of a weekly schedule of irinotecan, high-dose leuco-vorin, and infusional fluorouracil as first-line chemotherapy in patients with advanced colorectal cancer. J Clin Oncol 1999;17:907–13.

78. Kalbakis K, Kandylis N, et al. First line chemotherapy with 5-fluorouracil (5-FU), leucovorin (LV) and irinotecan (CPT-11) in advanced colorectal cancer (CRC): a multicenter phase II study. ASCO 1999; 18:257a.

79. Saltz L, Locker P, et al. Weekly irinotecan (CPT-11), leucovorin (LV), and fluorouracil (FU) is superior to daily x5 LV/FU in patient's (pts) with previously untreated metastatic colorectal cancer. ASCO 2000;18:233a.

80. Douillard J, Cunningham D, et al. A randomized phase III trial comparing irinotecan (IRI)+5-FU/folic acid (FA) to the same schedule of 5-FU/FA in patients (pts) with metastatic colorectal cancer (MCRC) as front line chemotherapy (CT). ASCO 2000;18:233a.

81. Guichard S, Cussac D, et al. Sequence-dependent activity of the irinotecan-5FU combination in human colon-cancer model HT-29 in vitro and in vivo. Int J Cancer 1997;73:729–34.

82. Wasserman E, Cuvier C, et al. Combination of oxaliplatin plus irinotecan in patients with gastrointestinal tumors: results of two independent phase I studies with pharmacokinetics. J Clin Oncol 1999; 17:1751–1759.

83. Wasserman E, Kalla S, et al. Oxaliplatin (L-OHP) and irinotecan (CPT11) phase I/II studies: results in 5 FU refractory (FR) colorectal cancer (CRC) patients (pts). ASCO 1999;18:238.

84. Scheithauer W, Lathan B, et al. Irinotecan plus oxaliplatin ± G-CSF as second line therapy in patients with advanced 5-FU/leucovorin-refractory colorectal cancer.

85. Koutcher JA, Alfieri AA, et al. Radiation enhancement by biochemical modulation and 5-fluorouracil. Int J Radiat Oncol Biol Phys 1997;39:1145–52.

86. Rich TA, Kirichenko AV. Camptothecin radiation sensitization: mechanisms, schedules, and timing. Oncology 1998;12(8 Suppl 6):114–20.

87. Lawrence T, Tepper J, et al. Fluoropyrimidine-radiation interactions in cells and tumors. Semin Radiat Oncol 1998;4:260–6.

88. Minsky B. Adjuvant therapy for rectal cancer: results and controversies. Oncology 1999;August.

89. Twelves C, Harper P, et al. A phase III trial (SO14796) of Xeloda (Capecitabine) in previously untreated advanced/metastatic colorectal cancer. ASCO 1999;18:236a.

90. Douillard J, Cunningham D, et al. A randomized phase III trial comparing irinotecan (IRI)+5-FU/folic acid (FA to the same schedule of 5-FU/FA in patients (pts) with metastatic colorectal cancer (MCRC) as front line chemotherapy (CT). ASCO 1999;18:233a.

91. Pazdur R, Hoff PM, et al. The oral fluorouracil prodrugs. Oncology 1998;12(10 Suppl 7):48–51.

92. Meropol NJ. Oral fluoropyrimidines in the treatment of colorectal cancer. Eur J Cancer 1998;34:1509–13.

93. Hoff PM, Pazdur R, et al. UFT and leucovorin: a review of its clinical development and therapeutic potential in the oral treatment of cancer. Anticancer Drugs 1998;9:479–90.

94. Clark JW. Perspectives on new chemotherapeutic agents in the treatment of colorectal cancer. Semin Oncol 1997;24(5 Suppl 18):19–24.

95. Cunningham D. Mature results from three large controlled studies with raltitrexed ('Tomudex'). Br J Cancer 1998;77(Suppl 2):15–21.

96. Shih C, Habeck LL, et al. Multiple folate enzyme inhibition: mechanism of a novel pyrrolopyrimidine-based antifolate LY231514 (MTA). Adv Enzyme Regul 1998;38:135–52.

97. Calvert AH, Walling JM. Clinical studies with MTA. Br J Cancer 78(Suppl 3):35–40.

98. Herben VM, Ten Bokkel Huinink WW, et al. Clinical pharmacokinetics of camptothecin topoisomerase I inhibitors. Pharm World Sci 1998;20:161–72.

99. Rothenberg ML. Topoisomerase I inhibitors: review and update. Ann Oncol 1997;8:837–55.

100. Gerrits CJ, de Jonge MJ, et al. Topoisomerase I inhibitors: the relevance of prolonged exposure for present clinical development. Br Cancer 1999;76: 952–62.

101. Tortola S, Marcuello E, et al. p53 and K-ras gene mutations correlate with tumor aggressiveness but are not of routine prognostic value in colorectal cancer. J Clin Oncol 1999;17:1375–81.

102. Zhang H, Nordenskjold B, et al. K-ras mutations in colorectal adenocarcinomas and neighbouring transitional mucosa. Eur J Cancer 1998;34:2053–7.

103. Kressner U, Bjorheim J, et al. Ki-ras mutations and prognosis in colorectal cancer. Eur J Cancer 1998; 34:518–21.

104. Britten C, Rowinsky E, et al. The farnesyl protein transference (FPTase) inhibitor L-

105. Awada A, Punt CJ, et al. Phase I study of Carzelesin (U-80,244) given (4-weekly) by intravenous bolus schedule. Br J Cancer 1999;79:1454–61.

106. Hudes G, Schol J, et al. (1999). Phase I clinical and pharmacokinetic trial of the farnesyltransferance inhibitor R115777 on a 21-day dosing schedule. ASCO 1999;18:156a.

107. Holmlund JT, Rudin CM, et al. Phase I trial of ISIS 5132/ODN, a 20-Mer phosphorothioate antisense Oligonucleotide inhibitor of C-RAF kinase, administered by a 24-hour weekly intravenous (IV) infusion to patients with advanced cancer. ASCO 1999;18: 157a.

108. Senderowicz AM, Headlee D, et al. Phase I trail of infusional UNC-01, a novel protein kinase inhibitor, in patients with refractory neoplasms. ASCO 1999;18:159a.

109. Sausville E. Cyclin-dependant kinase: novel targets for cancer tretaments. ASCO (ASCO Oncology Educational Book): 1999. p. 8–21.

110. Siu LL, Hidalgo M, et al. Dose and schedule-duration escalation of the epidermal growth factor receptor (EGFR) tyrosine kinase (TK) inhibitor CP-358, 774: a phase I and pharmacokinetic (PK) study. ASCO 1999;18:388a.

111. Kjaer M. Combining 5-fluorouracil with interferon-alpha in the treatment of advanced colorectal cancer: optimism followed by disappointment. Anticancer Drugs 1996;7:35–42.

112. Brivio F, Lissoni P, et al. Preoperative interleukin-2 subcutaneous immunotherapy may prolong the survival time in advanced colorectal cancer patients. Oncology 1996;53:263–8.

113. Goey SH, Gratama JW, et al. Interleukin 2 and interferon alpha-2a do not improve anti-tumor activity of 5-fluorouracil in advanced colorectal cancer. Br J Cancer 1996;74:2018–23.

114. Khleif S, Abrams S, et al. The generation of CD8+Tcell responses from patients vaccinated with mutant ras peptides corresponding to the patient's own ras mutation. Proc Am Soc Clin Oncol 1997; 16:437a.

115. Zitvogel L, Mayordomo JI, et al. Therapy of murine tumors with tumor peptide-pulsed dendritic cells: dependence on T cells, B7 costimulation, and T helper cell 1-associated cytokines. J Exp Med 1996;183(1):87–97.

116. Hodge JW. Carcinoembryonic antigen as a target for cancer vaccines. Cancer Immunol Immunother 1996;43:127–34.

117. Zaknoen S, Wolff R, et al. Marimastat in advanced progressive colorectal cancer— a dose finding study. Proc Am Soc Clin Oncol 1997;16:237a.

118. Konno H, Tanaka T, et al. Efficacy of an angiogenesis inhibitor, TNP-470, in xenotransplanted human colorectal cancer with high metastatic potential. Cancer 1996;77(8 Suppl):1736–40.

119. Rowinsky E, Hammond L, et al. Prolonged administration of bay 12-9566, an oral peptidic biphenyl matrix metalloproteinase (MMP) inhibitor: a phase I and pharmacokinetic (PK) study. ASCO 1998;17: 216a.

120. Diaz-Canton EA, Pazdur R. Adjuvant medical therapy for colorectal cancer. Surg Clin North Am 1997;77(1):211–28.

121. Welt S, Divgi CR, et al. Antibody targeting in metastatic colon cancer: a phase I study of monoclonal antibody F19 against a cell-surface protein of reactive tumor stromal fibroblasts. J Clin Oncol 1994;12: 1193–203.

122. Roselli M, Buonomo O, et al. Novel clinical approaches in monoclonal antibody-based management in colorectal cancer patients: radioimmunoguided surgery and antigen augmentation. Semin Surg Oncol 1998;15:254–62.

123. Lane D, Eagle K, et al. Radioimmuno-therapy of metastic colorectal tumors with iodine-131-labled antibody to carcinoembryonic antigen: phase I/II study with comparative biodistribution for intact and F (ab') 2 antibodies. Br J Cancer 197;70:521–5.

124. Bodey B, Siegel SE, et al. Human cancer detection and immunotherapy with conjugated and non-conjugated monoclonal antibodies. Anticancer Res 1996;16:661–74.

125. Dillman R. Unconjugated monoclonal antibodies for the treatment of hematologic and solid malignancies. Am Soc Clin Oncol Educational Book: 1999. p. 460–82.

126. NIH Consensus Conference. Adjuvant therapy for patients with colon and rectal cancer. JAMA 1990; 264:1444–50.

127. O'Connell MJ, Martenson JA, et al. Improving adjuvant therapy for rectal cancer by combining protracted-infusion fluorouracil with radiation therapy after curative surgery. N Engl J Med 1994;331: 502–7.

128. Rockette H, Deutsch M, et al. Effective of postoperative radiation therapy (RTX) when used with adjuvant chemothrapy in Dukes' B and C rectal cancer: results from NSABP-RO2 [abstract]. Proc Am Soc Clin Oncol 1994;13:193.

129. Willett CG, Fung CY, et al. Postoperative radiation therapy for high-risk colon carcinom. J Clin Oncol 1993;11:1112–7.

130. Martenson J, Willet C, et al. A phase III study of adjuvant radiation therapy (RT), 5-fluorouracil with resected high risk colon cancer; initial results of Int 0130. ASCO 18:235.

131. Accarpio G, Scopinaro G, et al. Experience with local rectal cancer excision in light of two recent preoperative diagnostic methods. Dis Colon Rectum 1987;30:296–8.

132. Brierley JD, Cummings BJ, et al. Adenocarcinoma of the rectum treated by radical external radiation therapy. Int J Radiat Oncol Biol Phys 1995;31:255–9.

133. Overgaard M, Overgaard J, et al. Dose-response relationship for radiation therapy of recurrent, residual, and primarily inoperable colorectal cancer. Radiother Oncol 1984;1:217–25.

134. Minsky BD, Cohen AM, et al. Radiation therapy for unresectable rectal cancer. Int J Radiat Oncol Biol Phys 1991;21:1283–9.

135. Stewart JM, Zalcberg JR. Update on adjuvant treatment of colorectal cancer. Curr Opin Oncol 1998; 10:367–74.

136. Kemeny N, Saltz L, et al. Adjuvant therapy of colorectal cancer. Surg Oncol Clin N Am 1997;6:699–722.

137. Vaughn DJ, Haller DG. The role of adjuvant chemotherapy in the treatment of colorectal cancer. Hematol Oncol Clin North Am 1997;11:699–719.

138. Casillas S, Pelley RJ, et al. Adjuvant therapy for colorectal cancer: present and future perspectives. Dis Colon Rectum 1997;40:977–92.

139. Stocchi L, Nelson H. Diagnostic and therapeutic applications of monoclonal antibodies in colorectal cancer. Dis Colon Rectum 1998;41:232–50.

140. Kemeny N, Cohen A, et al. Randomized study of hepatic arterial infusion (HAI) and systemic chemotherapy (SYS) versus SYS alone as adjuvant

therapy after resection of hepatic metastases from colorectal cancer. ASCO 1999;18:236a.

141. Kemeny MM, Adak S, et al. Results of the intergroup [Eastern Cooperative Oncology Group (ECOG) and Southwest Oncology Group (SWOG)] perspective randomized study of surgery alone versus continous hepatic artery infusion of FUDR and continous systematic infusion of 5-FU after hepatic resection for colorectal liver metastases. ASCO 1999;18:264a

142. Cohen AM, Kemeny NE, et al. Is intra-arterial chemotherapy worthwhile in the treatment of patients with unresectable hepatic colorectal cancer metastases? Eur J Cancer 1996;32A:2195–205.

143. Kressner U, Inganas M, et al. Prognostic value of p53 genetic changes in colorectal cancer. J Clin Oncol 1999;17:593–9.

144. Tortola S, Marcuello H, et al. p53 and K-ras gene mutations correlate with tumor aggressiveness but are not of routine prognostic value in colorectal cancer. J Clin Oncol 1999;17:1375–81.

145. Kawamoto K, Onodera H, et al. Possible paracrine mechanism of insulin-like growth factor-2 in the development of liver metastases from colorectal carcinoma. Cancer 1999;85(1):18–25.

146. Messa C, Russo F, et al. EGF, TGF-alpha, and EGF-R in human colorectal adenocarcinoma. Acta Oncol 1998;37:285–9.

147. el-Hariry I, Pignatelli M, et al. Fibroblast growth factor 1 and fibroblast growth factor 2 immunoreactivity in gastrointestinal tumours. J Pathol 1997;181 (1):39–45.

148. Saclarides TJ. Angiogenesis in colorectal cancer. Surg Clin North Am 1997;77(1):253–60.

149. Neumayer R, Rosen HR, et al. CD44 expression in benign and malignant colorectal polyps. Dis Colon Rectum 1999;42(1):50–5.

150. Weg-Remers S, Schuder G, et al. CD44 expression in colorectal cancer. Ann N Y Acad Sci 1998;859: 304–6.

151. Tanimoto T, Tanaka S, et al. MUC1 expression in intramucosal colorectal neoplasms. Possible involvement in histogenesis and progression. Oncology 1999;56:223–31.

152. Choti MA, Bulkley GB. Management of hepatic metastases. Liver Transpl Surg 1999;5(1):65–80.

153. Dale PS, Souza JW, et al. Cryosurgical ablation of unresectable hepatic metastases. J Surg Oncol 1998; 68:242–5.

11

Surgical Management of Metastatic Colon and Rectal Cancer

SAM S. YOON, MD

KENNETH K. TANABE, MD

Colon and rectal cancer can disseminate to several sites or spread to one or two isolated organs.[1] The most common sites of metastases are the liver and lung. In an autopsy series of over 1,500 patients who died of colon carcinoma, liver metastases were identified in 44 percent of cases and lung metastases were identified in 21 percent of cases.[2] Other organs with metastases included the adrenal glands (7%), bone marrow (6%), spleen (3.4%), pleura (2.8%), and brain (2.5%).

At the time of initial diagnosis of primary colon or rectal carcinoma, 70 percent of patients have disease that is potentially curable and the remaining 30 percent of patients have advanced disease in the form of unresectable local disease or distant metastases.[1] Following potentially curative surgical resection, about 35 percent of these patients develop recurrent disease.[1] The management of primary colon carcinoma, primary rectal carcinoma, and local recurrences is addressed in other sections. The treatment of isolated metastases with surgical resection, hepatic cryosurgery, radio frequency ablation, and hepatic arterial infusion chemotherapy is reviewed in this section.

SURVEILLANCE FOLLOWING RESECTION OF PRIMARY COLON AND RECTAL CARCINOMA

Hematogenous metastases in many patients will be detected synchronously with the diagnosis of their primary colon carcinoma; however, in many other patients, metastases will subsequently be detected following treatment of their primary carcinoma. Several strategies have been proposed to screen these patients for detection of metastases. Surveillance following curative resection for colorectal cancer is intended to discover recurrences early in their course in hopes of optimizing the results of subsequent therapy. Because many patients do not harbor hematogenous metastases and because early detection of recurrences in the remaining patients is unlikely to alter survival, it is difficult to demonstrate cost-efficacy for most surveillance strategies in this patient population. Nonetheless, many organizations, such as the National Comprehensive Cancer Network (NCCN) and the American Society of Clinical Oncology (ASCO), have published guidelines for surveillance.[3,4] Interestingly, the recommendations of these two organizations differ significantly, and this disparity results from the absence of good data on which to base the recommendations. Another factor that must be taken into consideration is patient expectations concerning the diligence with which their physician searches for recurrences. The simplest strategy involves only a periodic physical examination and colonoscopy, whereas more intensive strategies include carcinoembryonic antigen (CEA), liver function tests, complete blood counts, fecal occult blood testing, abdominal and pelvic computed tomography (CT) scans, and chest radiographs.

NATURAL HISTORY

Knowledge of the natural history of metastatic colon and rectal carcinoma allows one to form a baseline from which the value of various treatments can be determined. The natural history of metastases isolated to the liver has been well studied retrospectively.[5-9] Median survival of patients in these studies ranged from 5 to 9 months. As a result of the lack of modern-day imaging modalities, the majority of patients in these older studies had advanced disease, and thus patients diagnosed today with isolated liver metastases probably experience longer survival merely due to earlier diagnosis. To assess the value of surgical resection for liver metastases, several studies have attempted to determine the natural history of patients with potentially resectable liver metastases that were left untreated. In one study of patients who underwent only a biopsy of their liver metastases, no patient was observed to survive 5 years while 28 percent of similar patients who underwent liver resection survived 5 years.[10] Wood and colleagues reviewed 13 patients with untreated but potentially resectable liver metastases and found that only 1 patient survived 5 years.[11] The survival time for these patients ranged from 17 to 25 months. In a study of patients with solitary liver metastasis, unresected patients had a median survival of 19 months and no patients survived 5 years, while resected patients had a median survival of 36 months and 25 percent of patients survived 5 years.[12] Finally, one large retrospective study of 393 patients found that 5-year survival with and without surgical resection of colon carcinoma liver metastases was 25 percent and 2 percent, respectively.[13] Despite the inherent biases in these retrospective studies, most oncologists now generally accept that surgical resection of isolated liver metastases improves survival of patients with colon or rectal carcinoma.

The natural history of isolated lung metastases from colon and rectal carcinoma is less well studied, presumably because this occurs much less frequently than isolated liver metastases. In one autopsy study, only 2 percent of patients had isolated lung metastases, 20 percent had isolated liver metastases, and another 7 percent had both liver and lung metastases without other sites of metastasis.[2] The median survival of patients with unresectable pulmonary metastases is less than 10 months.[14] The median survival of patients with resectable pulmonary metastases is more favorable than this,

which is a reflection of the smaller tumor burden compared to patients with unresectable pulmonary metastases. Unfortunately, there are no good data on the natural history of patients with resectable pulmonary metastases who do not undergo resection.

Patients with brain metastases from colon or rectal carcinoma usually have widely disseminated disease and their prognosis is very poor. A recent series reported a median survival of 2 months in patients who received only supportive care.[15] Even with aggressive therapy, including surgical resection of brain metastases, median survival is still less than 1 year.[16]

PREOPERATIVE ASSESSMENT

Liver or lung metastases may be detected synchronously or metachronously relative to the diagnosis of a primary colon or rectal carcinoma. In patients who are considered candidates for surgical resection of their metastases, the goals of preoperative assessment are to (1) detect any extrahepatic metastases, (2) define the relationship of the liver metastases to the segmental liver anatomy and adjacent vital structures, and (3) evaluate the ability of the patient to tolerate partial hepatectomy. Initial evaluation should include a history and physical examination, hematology and chemistry panels, coagulation profiles, liver function tests, CEA level, electrocardiogram, chest x-ray, and abdominal and pelvic CT scans. Chest CT scans may be obtained to rule out lung metastases. In a recent study of patients with colon or rectal carcinoma liver metastases and normal chest x-rays, 11 of 100 patients had a positive chest CT.[17] Four of these 11 patients had malignant lesions of the lung (3 with colorectal carcinoma metastases and 1 with a primary lung cancer), thus providing a positive yield of 4 percent. Colonoscopy should be performed if not done within the past 12 months to rule out an anastomotic recurrence or the development of a metachronous primary colon or rectal carcinoma, which occurs at some point in 5 percent of patients.[18]

There is currently no consensus among surgeons as to which test best images the liver and abdomen prior to resection of metastases. Abdominal CT scan is the most commonly used test to initially identify liver metastases. With noncontrast-enhanced CT scan, liver tumors usually appear hypoattenuated relative to normal liver, but the difference in attenuation is low. Intravenous contrast increases the sensitivity of CT scans for liver metastases to about 80 percent.[19,20] The liver has a dual blood supply from the portal vein and the hepatic artery and receives 75 percent of its blood flow from the portal vein,[21] whereas liver metastases receive the majority of their blood flow from the hepatic artery.[22] For this reason, metastases are hypoattenuated relative to the enhanced normal liver on contrast-enhanced CT scan images that are acquired during the portal venous phase of enhancement.[23]

CT arterioportography (CTAP) combines contrast injection into the superior mesenteric or splenic artery and dynamic CT imaging. This produces greater contrast dye enhancement of normal liver during the portal venous phase than is observed following intravenous contrast administration, and the sensitivity for detection of tumors with CTAP exceeds 90 percent.[24] Disadvantages of CTAP include complications from catheter placement into the mesenteric arteries as well as the relatively low *specificity* of this test for diagnosis of liver metastases[20] (Figure 11–1).

Magnetic resonance imaging (MRI) of the liver is being used with increasing frequency for the assessment of liver tumors primarily due to the development of liver-specific contrast agents and dynamic scanning techniques. For example, superparamagnetic iron oxide particles (SPIO) are used with MRI because they are taken up by reticuloendothelial cells and reduce the enhancement of normal liver on T_2-weighted images, allowing easier identification of metastases[25] (Figure 11–2). One study found that MRI with the use of SPIO was as sensitive as CTAP in the identification of liver metastases.[26] Another contrast agent, manganese-pyridoxal diphosphate (Mn-DPDP), is a paramagnetic agent that enhances normal liver but not metastases on T_1-weighted images.[27] MRI with Mn-DPDP is currently the study of choice at the Massachusetts General Hospital for preoperative evaluation of liver metastases (Figure 11–3).

Laparoscopy and laparoscopic ultrasound allows detection of peritoneal implants[28] and small liver metastases.[29] One study found that laparoscopy with laparoscopic ultrasound detected unresectable disease in 6 of 24 patients with liver tumors that were preoperatively judged to be resectable.[30] However, the development of more sensitive and specific preoperative imaging studies such as MRI with Mn-DPDP has decreased the rate of unresectability in patients who undergo laparotomy for possible resection of liver metastases.

RADIOIMMUNODETECTION AND RADIOIMMUNOGUIDED SURGERY

Radioimmunodetection (RAID), otherwise known as immunoscintigraphy, uses radiolabeled antibodies against tumor-associated antigens such as CEA or

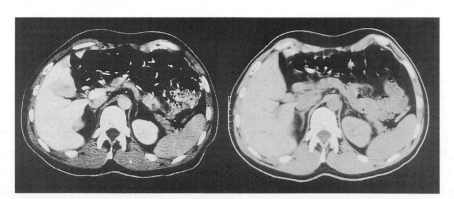

Figure 11–1.   CTAP study in a patient with colon carcinoma liver metastases. Excellent opacification of portal venous structures by contrast material is noted in the portal venous phase image (*left*). The hypodense lesion observed on images obtained in the portal venous phase is a false-positive finding that results from perfusion abnormalities that are observed commonly on CTAP. This lesion is not observed on images obtained in the equilibrium phase (*right*).

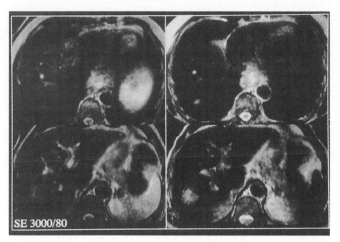

Figure 11–2. T$_2$-weighted MRI images obtained before (*left*) and following (*right*) administration of ferrumoxide intravenous contrast.

TAG-72 as a diagnostic study for cancer. After intravenous injection of radiolabeled antibody, the locations of tumor deposits are observed by either planar scintigraphy or single-photon emission computed tomography (SPECT). The use of RAID in the diagnosis and treatment of colon and rectal carcinoma has recently been reviewed,[31] and this modality has been extensively studied in the evaluation of primary, recurrent, and metastatic cancer. In general, RAID is more accurate in the identification of extrahepatic and pelvic disease, while CT scan is more accurate in the identification of liver metastases.[31] The sensitivity of RAID for detection of liver metastases has ranged between 18 and 87 percent, with a specificity of 57 to 100 percent, accuracy of 28 to 91 percent, and positive predictive value of 88 to 100 percent.[32–42] The wide variability in these parameters results from differences in the specific radiolabeled antibody used, study design, and imaging techniques.[31]

In a recent study by Serafini and colleagues using a technetium-labeled antibody 88BV59 (HumaSPECT-Tc), sensitivities for liver metastases detected by HumaSPECT-Tc and CT scan in patients with positive CT scans were 97 and 74 percent, respectively, while specificities were 14 and 63 percent, respectively.[41] For extrahepatic and pelvic disease, HumaSPECT-Tc was slightly more sensitive (77% vs 73%) but much less specific (36% vs 73%). For patients with negative CT scans, HumaSPECT-Tc had an overall sensitivity of 59 percent and a specificity of 88 percent. The authors further reported that the diagnostic accuracy of

HumaSPECT-Tc in predicting resectability at all sites was 98 percent and in predicting nonresectability at all sites was 60 percent, compared to 91 and 29 percent, respectively, for CT scan.

As noted previously, RAID is not as accurate as CT scans in detection of liver metastases but is more accurate in detection of extrahepatic abdominal and pelvic disease. Most patients with liver metastases considered for surgical resection receive further liver imaging with CT arterioportography or MRI, which are even more accurate than CT scan in detecting liver metastases. Thus, the benefit of RAID for patients with liver metastases would be to discover extrahepatic or pelvic disease to spare patients noncurative liver resection. As determined by Stocchi and Nelson, if RAID was used in this manner, 17 percent of patients would incorrectly be considered to have extrahepatic disease and be denied a potentially curative hepatic resection. An additional 35 percent of patients would be deemed free of extrahepatic disease by

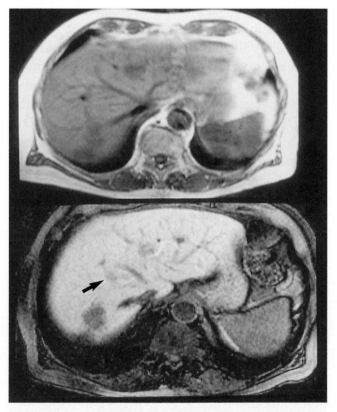

Figure 11–3. T$_1$-weighted MRI image without contrast (*above*) and following administration of Mn-DPDP intravenous contrast administration (*below*). Two colon carcinoma metastases are observed equally well using either technique; however, a third metastasis (*arrow*) is seen much more clearly following administration of Mn-DPDP.

RAID but subsequently found to have extrahepatic disease during surgical exploration.[31] Thus, the routine use of RAID in the preoperative assessment of patients with isolated, resectable liver metastases is controversial. The use of RAID for patients with isolated lung metastases has not been extensively studied.

Radioimmunoguided surgery (RIGS) is another modality that has primarily been utilized in patients with primary or recurrent colon or rectal carcinoma to identify foci of cancer that have in the past been invisible to modern-day imaging techniques and standard surgical exploration. RIGS utilizes one of a variety of radiolabeled monoclonal antibodies that target tumor-specific antigens.[43] Most monoclonal antibodies used presently target TAG-72, which is expressed by a variety of tumors including colorectal carcinomas and is not present in appreciable amounts in normal tissues except for transitional colonic epithelium and secretory phase endothelium.[44]

A typical RIGS procedure with I^{125}-radiolabeled TAG-72 involves oral administration of a saturated solution of potassium iodide (SSKI) daily starting 2 days prior to intravenous administration of I^{125}-radiolabeled TAG-72. The SSKI is continued for 3 to 4 weeks preoperatively. Patients are periodically monitored until background radioactivity falls below a specified level that will allow selective intraoperative identification of tumor (usually 2 or 3 weeks). During the operation, patients undergo routine surgical exploration with visual inspection and manual palpation. A hand-held gamma detection probe is used to locate foci of radiolabeled antibody, which are then biopsied or resected as clinically indicated.[45]

As noted previously, RIGS studies have examined patients with either primary or recurrent colorectal carcinoma. Localization rates have been 60 to 90 percent for primary tumors and 63 to 100 percent for recurrences.[45-58] The surgical procedure was modified based on RIGS findings in 15 to 50 percent of cases in these published reports. Several studies have demonstrated that patients with removal of all metastases identified by RIGS have improved survival compared to patients with RIGS-positive tissue left behind.[59-61]

Martin and colleagues reported that RIGS correctly localized tumor in 17 of 22 (77%) patients with colon or rectal carcinoma liver metastases,[48] and DiCarlo and colleagues reported correct localization in 36 of 45 (80%) similar patients.[56] Bakalakos and colleagues recently analyzed their results of surgical resection of colorectal carcinoma liver metastases with and without RIGS.[62] Only 28 percent of patients operated on without RIGS were found to have no extrahepatic metastases compared to 65 percent of patients operated on with RIGS. However, there are no data from prospective trials that demonstrate improved survival in patients staged with RIGS. There are currently two Phase III trials under way to compare RIGS with traditional diagnostic modalities in the treatment of primary, recurrent, and metastatic colon or rectal carcinoma.[31]

There are few studies on the use of RIGS in patients with lung metastases. One study with only four patients reported that RIGS identified additional lung metastases compared to preoperative CT scan, chest x-ray, and intraoperative inspection and palpation.[63]

Given that the majority of patients who undergo resection of liver or lung metastases from colon or rectal carcinoma experience recurrent disease, better diagnostic techniques are needed to identify potentially resectable but undetected disease and to exclude patients with disseminated disease not amenable to resection. Further studies are needed to determine if RIGS may aid the surgeon in these matters.

SURGICAL RESECTION OF LIVER METASTASES

The liver is divided into sectors by the hepatic veins, and these are further divided into segments by the branches of the portal triad (Figure 11–4). In addition to the main hepatic veins, small hepatic veins drain directly from the posterior surface of the liver (including the caudate) directly into the vena cava. The left and right triangular ligaments and the falciform ligament secure the liver to the diaphragm. Precise knowledge of the surgical anatomy of the liver, its blood vessels, and its biliary drainage system are mandatory for liver surgery.

Laparoscopy is often initially performed in an attempt to avoid an unnecessary laparotomy in patients who are candidates for resection of their liver metastases. Peritoneal implants that are too small to be detected radiographically may be detected laparoscopically,[30] and liver resection is contraindicated in patients with peritoneal metastases. In addition, unsuspected liver metastases may be detected laparoscopically either by direct inspection or by laparoscopic ultrasound examination. Patients who undergo only laparoscopy can generally be discharged on the same day, whereas patients who undergo a laparotomy generally spend several days in the hospital postoperatively. Accordingly, even if laparoscopy detects unsuspected metastases infrequently, it is generally cost effective.

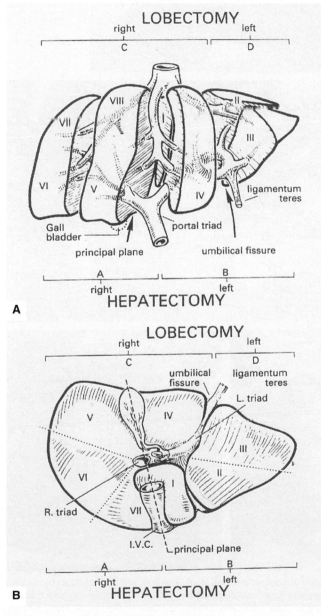

Figure 11–4. Functional anatomy of the liver. A schematic view of the liver demonstrates sectors or segments I through VIII, as described by Couinand. Adapted from Blumgart LH.[141]

The patient should be positioned supine with a small roll underneath the right chest to elevate the right upper quadrant. Both arms may be positioned out on arm boards to allow adequate access by the anesthesiologists. A large-bore, rapid-infusion intravenous catheter is placed in an antecubital vein. Placement of a central venous catheter and arterial catheter is often indicated. The abdomen should be prepped and draped from the nipples down to the pubis. A bilateral subcostal incision (also referred to as a chevron incision) generally provides adequate exposure. Only rarely is it necessary to extend the incision superiorly to the xyphoid, thereby creating a T at the apex. This is most often necessary for patients whose costal angle is quite sharp, or whose tumors are located such that they limit access and view of the suprahepatic vena cava. Similarly, it is rare that extension of the incision into the right chest is required. This is most often indicated for large and bulky tumors of the right lobe that limit access and view of the retrohepatic vena cava through a standard chevron incision.

The abdomen is carefully explored for any extrahepatic metastases. The ligamentum teres is divided and the falciform ligament is divided close to the liver (Figure 11–5). As the dissection proceeds superiorly toward the suprahepatic vena cava, the inferior phrenic veins should be identified to avoid injury and bleeding. Division of the right and left triangular ligaments will further mobilize the right and left lobes. If tumor on the dome of liver has invaded the diaphragm, a section of diaphragm should be resected en bloc with the specimen. This will require entry into the chest during division of the triangular ligaments. The diaphragmatic defect is closed in two layers. To evacuate air from the pleural space, a red rubber catheter positioned under a water seal is gradually withdrawn with the lungs at 30 cm H_2O positive pressure, and a purse-string suture around the catheter is tightened as the catheter is removed.

Intraoperative ultrasonography is performed to identify unsuspected metastases and to determine the anatomic relationship between metastases and major vascular structures (Figure 11–6). The liver should be carefully scanned from both anterior and posterior surfaces. Complete mobilization of the liver by division of the falciform ligament and trian-

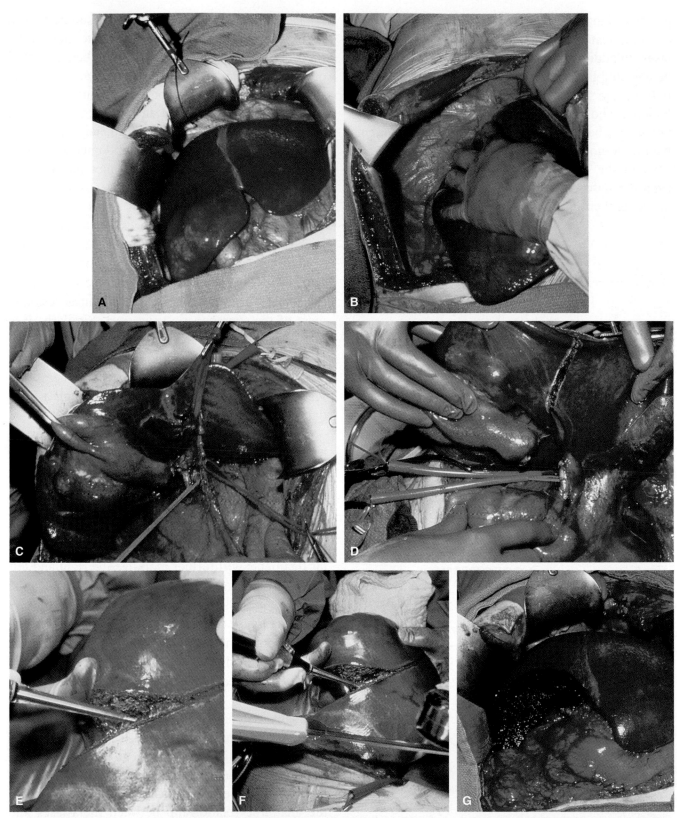

Figure 11–5. Resection of hepatic segments V and VI. *A,* A tumor is located in segments V and VI. *B,* The liver is fully mobilized by division of the falciform and right triangular ligaments. Complete mobilization is necessary for adequate palpation and intraoperative ultrasound examination. *C,* A vessel loop is placed around the portal vein and hepatic artery to allow intermittent vascular inflow occlusion. *D,* The liver capsule is incised with electrocautery along the intended resection lines. *E,* In this operation, an ultrasonic surgical aspirator was used to dissect through the hepatic parenchyma. *F,* Hemoclips and suture ligatures are used to ligate vessels and ducts. *G,* After removal of the specimen, the raw surface of the liver is cauterized with an argon beam coagulator. Photos courtesy of Fred Ames.

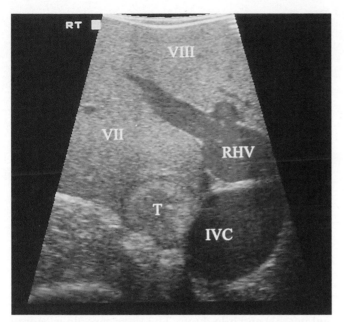

Figure 11–6. Intraoperative ultrasound image demonstrating the relationship between the tumor (T) located in segment VII and the inferior vena cava (IVC) and right hepatic vein (RHV).

gular ligaments greatly improves the ease of liver ultrasound examination.

Once a decision is made to embark upon a liver resection, a cholecystectomy is performed. Following cholecystectomy, a catheter is placed in the cystic duct to aid in the detection of small bile duct leaks following liver resection. A tourniquet is placed around the portahepatis, for intermittent occlusion to restrict blood flow in the portal vein and hepatic artery. If the planned procedure includes a right or left hepatectomy, careful dissection of the portahepatis is performed to identify the left and right hepatic arteries, hepatic ducts, and portal veins. The right or left portal structures are divided as indicated. It is important to avoid injury to the confluence of the left and right hepatic ducts during this maneuver. It is also important to know the location of replaced or accessory hepatic arteries. A replaced right hepatic artery arising from the superior mesenteric artery is most commonly located posterolaterally in the portahepatis. A replaced or accessory left hepatic artery arising from the left gastric artery is generally located in the gastrohepatic ligament a few centimeters medial to portahepatis.

In situations where tumor is located well away from the portahepatis, the entire right or left portal pedical may be ligated en mass.[64] The liver must

first be completely mobilized by division of its avascular attachments to the retroperitoneum and diaphragm. The hilar plate is then lowered with sharp dissection. To isolate the main right portal pedical, incisions into the liver are made in the gallbladder fossa and in the caudate lobe immediately parallel to and 5 mm to the right of the inferior vena cava (Figure 11–7). An umbilical tape is passed around to completely encircle the right portal pedicle, which may be either clamped or stapled with a TI-30 stapler with a vascular cartridge. It is important to keep the umbilical tape between the stapler and the confluence of the hepatic ducts to avoid injury to the left hepatic duct (Figure 11–8). It is important to have the right liver fully mobilized prior to performing this maneuver, as it is possible to inadvertently injure a hepatic vein. The left main portal pedicle may be similarly ligated en mass by incising the liver at the base of segment IV anterior to the left portal pedical and incising the liver in the caudate lobe posterior to the left portal pedical.

Prior to division of the right hepatic vein, short hepatic veins that drain directly from the caudate lobe into the vena cava are first divided. It is important to identify and avoid injury to the right adrenal vein. A ligamentous structure from the right lobe of

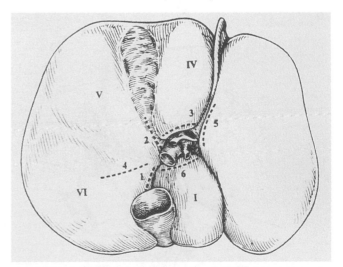

Figure 11–7. Sites for hepatotomy in portal pedicle isolation. The undersurface of the liver is illustrated. The dotted lines indicate sites for hepatotomy if control of the intrahepatic portal pedicles is desired. Incision at 3 allows lowering of the hilar plate. Incisions at 1 and 2 allow control of the main right pedicle. Incisions at 1 and 4 allow control of the right posterior pedicle. Incisions at 2 and 4 allow control of the right anterior pedicle. Incisions at 3 and 5 allow control of the left pedicle. Reproduced from Fong Y and Blumgart LH.[64]

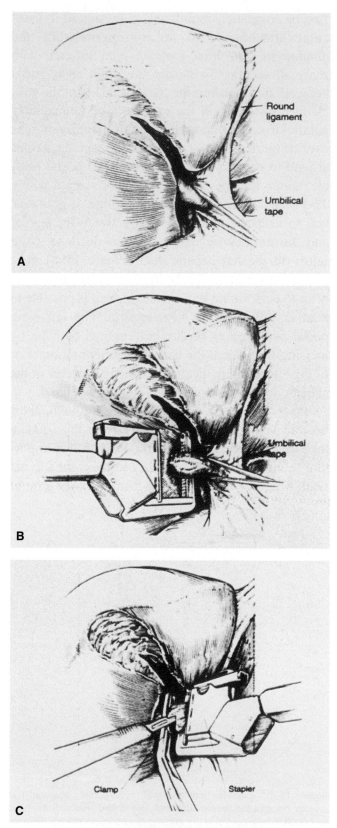

Figure 11–8. Control of the right portal pedicle. After an umbilical tape is passed around the main pedicle, it is retracted medially and the stapler is placed away from the bifurcation to avoid injury to the hilus. A clamp is subsequently placed to control bleeding from the specimen side. Reproduced from Fong Y and Blumgart LH.[64]

the liver arches across the lateral aspect of the vena cava just inferior to the right hepatic vein and must be identified and sharply divided to gain full access to the right hepatic vein. It is safe and usually simple to divide the right hepatic vein itself using a laparoscopic endo GIA 30 stapler with a vascular cartridge (Figure 11–9). This type of stapler may also be used for the left hepatic vein (Figure 11–10). Vascular control of the suprahepatic and intrahepatic vena cava should be obtained prior to isolation of the hepatic veins if the size and location of metastases reduce visualization and exposure of the hepatic veins.

Several methods exist for dividing liver parenchyma, and all are designed to divide liver tissue but allow identification and ligation of individual vessels and bile ducts. The liver capsule is scored with electrocautery. Many surgeons use a device that ultrasonically disrupts and aspirates tissue. These devices can be adjusted to minimize disruption of blood vessels and bile ducts. The technique of finger fracture is quicker, and achieves similar results; however, precise finger fracture is either not possible or awkward in some regions of the liver. Clamp fracture is another quick and hemostatic method of parenchymal transection. Most liver surgeons employ a combination of these techniques in any single operation. Bleeding vessels are oversewn as they are encountered, and an argon beam coagulator is useful for obtaining hemostasis along the transected edge of the liver. Blood loss can be reduced by using a tourniquet to impede hepatic vascular inflow for 15-minute periods with intervening 5-minute periods of normal perfusion. Bleeding from hepatic veins may be reduced by maintaining low central venous pressure during hepatic transection.[65] While many anesthesiologists feel more secure keeping the central venous pressure high, this maneuver will only increase blood loss. Placement of the patient in a 15-degree Trendelenberg position during hepatic transection will lower the hepatic vein pressure and simultaneously reduce the chances of air embolism. Finally, circumferential compression of the unresected portion of liver along the transection line using a penrose drain will reduce hepatic venous bleeding. By employing these maneuvers, it is only very rarely necessary to position clamps or tourniquets to achieve complete vascular isolation (Figure 11–11).

Liver resections for colon and rectal carcinoma metastases should be performed such that the minimum surgical margin is 1 cm. This goal does not apply to nonsurgical margins such as the liver capsule. With the realization that portal structures are enveloped by the liver capsule, it is reasonable to resect metastases immediately adjacent to major portal structures that will not be resected. However, if tumor invasion into a major portal branch is detected, it must be resected in order to achieve a satisfactory surgical margin. There is no advantage to performing a major resection when removal of one or more segments can remove all metastases with an adequate margin. In fact, segmental resections often spare more normal liver tissue than a major resection. Multiple segmental resections may also allow resection of multiple metastases that would not otherwise be encompassed by a traditional major resection. Recognition of hepatic veins is critical in determining which segments may be surgically excised. A large inferior right hepatic vein is present in approximately 20 percent of individuals and is usually identified on preoperative MRI or CT images (Figure 11–12). The presence of this vein permits resection of segments VII and VIII without sacrifice of segments V and VI. With the use of intraoperative ultrasound, the anatomic segments are quickly and accurately delineated.

To identify small bile duct leaks following completion of a liver resection, the cystic duct is cannulated and saline or methylene blue dye is injected with the distal common bile duct occluded. All bile duct leaks along the transected edge of the liver are oversewn. When feasible, the greater omentum is mobilized off of the transverse colon and draped over the transected edge of the liver. It is generally not necessary to reapproximate the liver capsule,

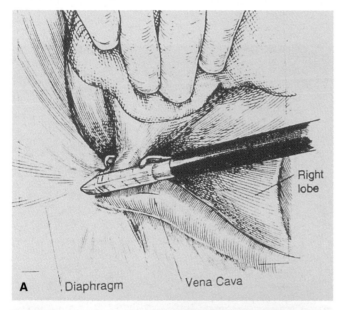

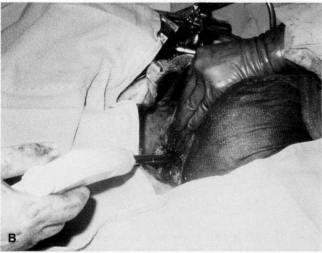

Figure 11–9. Stapling the right hepatic vein. *A,* The liver is rotated clockwise to provide exposure to place an endo GIA 30 vascular stapler to the junction of the right hepatic vein and vena cava. Reproduced from Fong Y and Blumgart LH.[64] *B,* Intraoperative photo of this technique being applied.

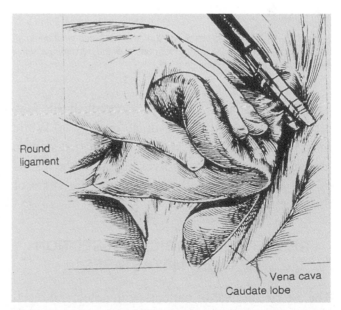

Figure 11–10. In stapling the left hepatic vein, the liver is rotated to the right and an Endo GIA 30 vascular stapler is applied at the junction of the left hepatic vein and the vena cava. Reproduced from Fong Y and Blumgart LH.[64]

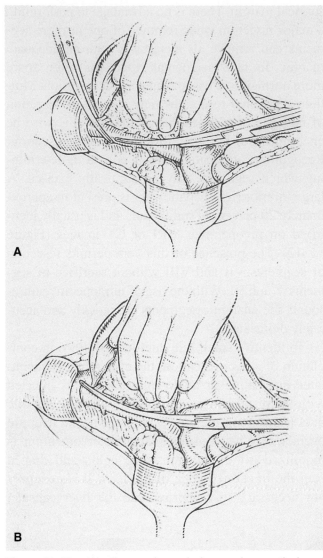

Figure 11–11.   Hepatic vascular exclusion requires postioning of either one or two vascular clamps for control of the retrohepatic vena cava. Reproduced from Blumgart LH.[141]

and the use of large sutures to accomplish this may inadvertently constrict bile ducts or vessels. While most liver surgeons routinely leave a closed suction in place following a major liver resection, the results of one clinical trial call into question the value of this practice.[66]

RESULTS OF SURGICAL RESECTION OF LIVER METASTASES

The 5-year survival of patients with colon and rectal carcinoma liver metastases is very low except in patients who undergo surgical resection of their metastases. Numerous studies have consistently

demonstrated that complete surgical resection of isolated liver metastases results in 5-year survival rates of 24 to 38 percent and median survivals of 28 to 46 months (Table 11–1).[67–73] The operative mortality has consistently improved as a result of advances in operative technique and postoperative care. Operative mortality rates in recent studies range from 0 to 7 percent. Morbidity following major hepatic resections continues to be frequent (22% to 39%), and the most common causes of morbidity are bleeding, bile leak or fistula, liver failure, abdominal abscess, wound infection, pneumonia, and myocardial infarction.

Despite these impressive surgical results in patients with distant metastatic disease, the majority

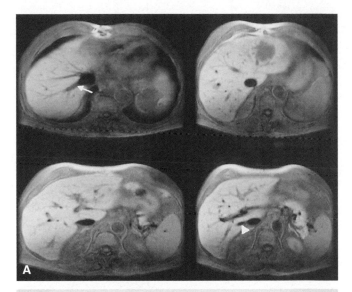

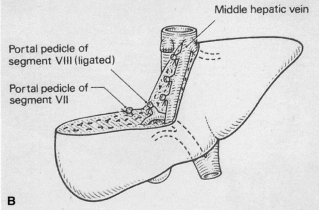

Figure 11–12.   *A,* MRI examination demonstrates the location of the right hepatic vein (*arrow*) as well as the presence of an inferior right hepatic vein (*arrowhead*), which is present in approximately 20% of patients. *B,* The presence of an inferior right hepatic vein permits resection of segments VII and VIII without resection of segments V and VI. Line drawing reproduced from Franco D and Borgonovo G.[412]

Table 11–1. RESULTS OF RESECTION OF COLON AND RECTAL CARCINOMA LIVER METASTASES

Study (Year)	Number of Patients	Operative Mortality (%)	Operative Morbidity (%)	Median Survival (months)	5-Year Survival (%)
Schlag[67] (1990)	122	4	34	28	—
Doci[68] (1991)	100	5	39	—	30
Rosen[69] (1992)	280	4	—	33.6	25
Gajowski[70] (1994)	204	0	—	33	32
Scheele[71] (1995)	434	4.4	22	—	33
Wanebo[74] (1996)	74	7	38	35	24
Fong[73] (1997)	456	2.8	24	46	38

of patients who undergo surgical resection of their liver metastases subsequently die of recurrent disease. There are two strategies to address this problem: (1) improve diagnostic modalities so that small foci of malignancy can be detected and (2) improve patient selection so that those who are unlikely to benefit from surgical resection are spared a major operation. Recent improvements in diagnostic tests have been described above. In terms of improving patient selection, numerous retrospective studies have tried to identify prognostic factors to aid in patient selection. Table 11–2 lists negative prognostic factors that have been found to be statistically significant by univariate or multivariate analysis in surgical series from the past decade.[68–71,73–75,140] Only factors that were found to be statistically significant in at least two studies have been included. Some general conclusions can be made regarding the negative prognostic factors for patients with liver metastases who undergo liver resection. Patient characteristics such as age or sex do not consistently influence survival. The majority of

negative prognostic factors listed are associated with unfavorable tumor biology. For example, metastases from poorly differentiated cancers and those with lymph node metastases are biologically more aggressive than metastases from well-differentiated tumors without lymph node metastases. More extensive tumor burden, as suggested by the presence of metastases that are larger in size or greater in number, suggests both unfavorable tumor biology and the requirement of a more difficult liver resection. The presence of extrahepatic metastases is also associated with more aggressive tumors. While the majority of prognostic factors listed in Table 11–2 cannot be altered with surgical therapy, one factor that can be controlled is the surgical resection margin. Cady and colleagues have emphasized that surgical resection margins should be at least 1 cm, and that margins less than 1 cm adversely affect survival.[75]

A report from the Memorial Sloan-Kettering Cancer Center reviewed the outcome of 456 patients who underwent surgical resection for liver metastases from colon or rectal carcinoma.[73] They reported a 5-year survival of 38 percent and a median survival of 46 months. The operative mortality and morbidity rates were 2.8 and 24 percent, respectively. In an analysis of prognostic variables, the presence of extrahepatic metastases and metastases larger than 10 cm were the strongest negative prognostic factors; the authors suggested that these may be strong contraindications to resection.

In several series, the presence of four or more metastases is a negative prognostic factor,[70,73–76] and some surgeons have suggested that this may be an absolute contraindication to resection.[75,76] This is a point of some controversy. In the largest single-institution series reported to date, the group of patients who had four or more metastases resected had a 5-

Table 11–2. NEGATIVE PROGNOSTIC FACTORS AFTER SURGICAL RESECTION OF COLON AND RECTAL CARCINOMA LIVER METASTASES[68,71,73,74,140]

Primary Colorectal Tumor Characteristics	Metastases Characteristics	Surgical Resection Characteristics
Advanced stage	Lymph node involvement	Less than 1-cm tumor-free margin
High grade	Extrahepatic metastases	Extensive resection
	Large size	
	Increased number	
	Satellitosis	
	Bilobar distribution	
	Short disease-free interval	
	Synchronous metastases	
	Elevated CEA level	

Data from Doci R et al.,[68] Rosen CG et al.,[69] Gajowski TJ et al.,[70] Schecle J et al.,[71] Fong Y et al.,[73] Wanebo HJ et al.,[74] and Younes RN et al.[140]

year survival of 24 percent.[73] In contrast, Cady and colleagues reported that no patients with four or more metastases resected survived for even 4 years.[75] While patients with four or more metastases appear to have a less favorable prognosis, surgical resection when safe may lead to long-term survival.

SURGICAL RESECTION OF RECURRENT LIVER METASTASES

Of patients who undergo resection for colon or rectal liver metastases, 65 to 80 percent will experience a recurrence of their cancer. About 20 to 30 percent of these patients will experience a recurrence only in the liver and 40 to 50 percent in the liver and another site.[72] Of the 20 to 30 percent of patients with a recurrence only in the liver following hepatectomy, some will be candidates for repeat hepatic resection. Several studies have addressed the issue of whether further liver resection of such patients would be beneficial.

The majority of published reports regarding this topic have fewer than 30 patients, and thus it is difficult to draw meaningful conclusions from these studies. Three groups have reported series of between 64 and 170 patients.[77–79] The 5-year survival rates in these studies were 16 percent, 32 percent, and 41 percent, which are similar to 5-year survival rates following first hepatectomy (see Table 11–1). The 41 percent 5-year survival reported in the study by Adam and colleagues may be related to the high proportion of patients who received adjuvant chemotherapy in addition to hepatic resection.[79] The mortality and morbidity rates for repeat liver resections for metastases are similar to those observed following the first liver resection.[72] The morbidity rates in the three largest series ranged from 19 to 27 percent (compared to 11% to 20% following the first hepatectomy), and the causes of morbidity were similar to those after first hepatic resection.[77–79] The only negative prognostic factor found to be statistically significant in the Fernandez-Trigo and colleagues study was an incomplete resection that left disease behind. Adam and colleagues found that, based on univariate analysis, negative prognostic factors were noncurative surgery, an interval between hepatectomies of less than 1 year, three or more metastases, CEA level greater than 30 IU/L, and the presence of extrahepatic metastases. In a multivariate analysis, only noncurative surgery and short interval between hepatectomies were statistically significant factors.

The number of patients who have undergone repeat hepatectomies for metastases is far fewer than the number who have had only one hepatectomy and so the available literature is limited. In general, the indications for repeat hepatectomy are the same as the indications for initial hepatectomy. Repeat hepatectomy offers a reasonable chance at long-term survival, and, in experienced centers, this procedure can be performed with low morbidity and mortality.

HEPATIC CRYOSURGERY

Hepatic cryosurgery refers to destruction of liver tumors in situ by freezing. The procedure is usually performed under general anesthesia through an abdominal incision, although recent technological advances have enabled surgeons to perform the procedure laparoscopically in some instances. The abdomen is explored to identify any extrahepatic disease, and the liver is mobilized by dissection of its supporting ligaments. After inspection and palpation, intraoperative ultrasound is performed to identify liver metastases and their relationship to vital structures. A cryoprobe is then inserted into the lesion. For superficial lesions, this can be done under direct vision. For deeper lesions, ultrasound guidance is used to place a needle into the lesion followed by placement of a guidewire (Figure 11–13). The tract is dilated and a cryoprobe is passed. Following placement of the cryoprobe, liquid nitrogen is circulated through the cryoprobe, which generates an expanding iceball observed by ultrasound. The liquid nitrogen is circulated until the iceball grows at least 1 cm beyond the limits of the tumor.[80,81]

The world literature on hepatic cryosurgery has been reviewed recently.[82] Two freeze-thaw cycles result in more effective killing of tumor cells than a single cycle[83] but may increase morbidity[84] and are associated with an increased risk of cryoshock phenomenon (coagulopathy and multisystem organ failure).[85–87] One of the problems with hepatic cryotherapy is that large vessels in the liver may prevent adequate freezing of adjacent tumor due to a heat

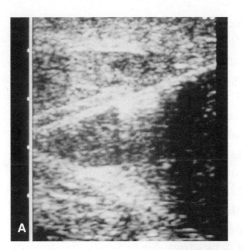

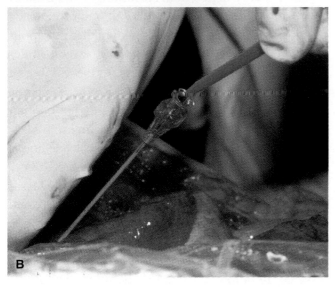

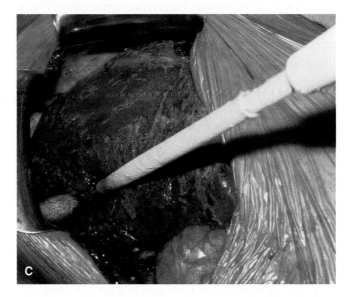

Figure 11–13. Cyrosurgery. A needle is positioned in the tumor under ultrasound guidance (*A*) and a guidewire is threaded into the needle (*B*) to allow subsequent enlargement of the tract with a dilator. Freezing of the liver tumor and surrounding tissues is accomplished by placement of a cryoprobe (*C*). Photos courtesy of Charles Staley.

sink effect of warm blood circulating through the vessel.[88] Hepatic inflow occlusion decreases blood flow, and this maneuver allows more rapid and larger iceball formation.[89,90] Despite more effective ablation of tumors adjacent to large vessels using hepatic inflow occlusion,[91] recurrence of tumors adjacent to these vessels continues to be a problem.[80] In addition, hepatic inflow occlusion may increase the risk of injury to vessel walls and bile ducts leading to hemorrhage and bile leaks.

Because hepatic cryosurgery has not yet been demonstrated to be as effective as surgical removal of metastases, most patients treated with this technique have been considered unresectable by conventional criteria. Published reports on cryotherapy for colon and rectal carcinoma liver metastases have reported widely different results primarily due to varied patient selection, small numbers, or, most commonly,

lack of long-term follow-up.[82,92] Two groups recently reported on their large experience with cryosurgery for colorectal carcinoma liver metastases with reasonably long follow-up.[80,93] These two studies have reported on 116 and 158 patients and began accrual of patients between 1987 and 1990. The median survival in these studies was 26 to 30 months. The overall 5-year survival was reported in only one study and was 13.4 percent. Operative mortality in these series was 0.9 to 3.7 percent. The most commonly reported complications included bleeding, acute renal failure, pleural effusions requiring drainage, biloma or bile fistula, and abdominal abscess. In the study by Seifert and colleagues, the following factors were found to have negative prognostic value in both univariate and multivariate analyses: serum CEA level greater than 5 ng/dL, lymph node metastases in the primary tumor resection specimen, unresectable extrahepatic metastases, incomplete cyrosurgical ablation, and an iceball size greater than 3 cm.[80] Weaver and colleagues found a CEA level greater than 100 ng/dL to be a significant negative prognostic factor.[93]

In general, patients who have been treated with hepatic cryosurgery have had more advanced disease than patients treated by surgical resection, but they have had less advanced disease than patients treated with regional or systemic chemotherapy. Therefore, it is not surprising that the median survival of patients treated with hepatic cryosurgery lies between the median survivals of patients treated with surgical resection or chemotherapy. Selection bias may explain in part the reported improvement in survival with cryosurgery compared to chemotherapy. However, survival for 5 years is uncommon in patients with liver metastases left untreated or treated with chemotherapy. Cryosurgery may provide some benefit given that some patients treated with cryosurgery survive 5 years.

It is unknown whether cryosurgical liver tumor ablation will provide equivalent results to surgical resection in patients who are currently treated with resection. When surgical resection can be performed safely, it is the preferred modality over cryosurgery given the good results observed in mature studies. Hepatic cryosurgery of liver metastases is most commonly performed in patients whose liver metastases are not surgically resectable but limited in extent such that all metastases can be treated completely cryosurgically. In certain cases, surgical resection of larger tumors combined with cryosurgical ablation of smaller tumors is feasible.[84,85] Cryosurgery may also be useful following surgical resection when there is an involved or inadequate surgical margin.[81,94] Lastly, hepatic cryosurgery may be useful for patients who have metastases that are surgically resectable but have poor liver function or comorbid conditions that preclude a major liver resection.[82]

RADIOFREQUENCY ABLATION

One of the more promising technologies for in situ ablation of hepatic malignancies involves delivery of radiofrequency (RF) energy to produce hyperthermia and coagulation necrosis of tumors. Radiofrequency ablation involves percutaneous or intraoperative insertion of an RF electrode into the center of a liver tumor under ultrasound or CT guidance. The electrode is connected to a radiofrequency generator, and the patient and the generator are both electrically grounded (Figure 11–14). As electrical current flows from the electrode toward the grounding pad, the tissue surrounding the electrode absorbs the energy, which creates ion agitation, which in turn produces heat. Excessive heating results in coagulation necrosis, but tissue desiccation also results in increased electrical impedance, which thereby reduces the current and energy deposition. Accordingly, the zone of coagulation necrosis induced with radiofrequency ablation was limited to 1.5 cm in diameter per application in initial experiments. However, several strategies have been developed to increase the volume of coagulation necrosis per application. These include saline infusion during RF ablation, internal cooling of the electrode to avoid desiccation, multiple electrode arrays, and needles that deploy electrode hooks out into the tumor (Figure 11–15).

In a recent clinical trial conducted at the Massachusetts General Hospital, liver tumors were treated with RF ablation using either percutaneous electrode insertion or intraoperative electrode insertion (Figure 11–16). Most of the tumors were subsequently resected to allow correlation between pathologic

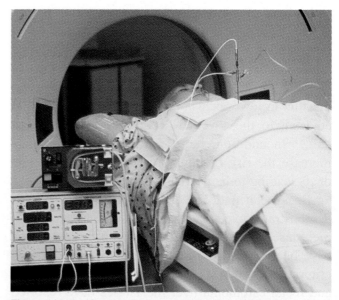

Figure 11–14. Percutaneous placement of an RF electrode into a liver tumor under CT guidance. The RF generator that delivers energy and perfusion pump that cools the electrode are seen to the left.

observations and radiographic images (Figure 11–17). CT scans obtained following RF ablation accurately estimated the area of coagulation necrosis observed in the subsequently resected lesions.[95]

To date, only small series of patients with limited follow-up after RF ablation have been reported in the literature[96,97] Further studies and longer follow-up are clearly necessary before RF ablation should be offered outside the context of a clinical trial. Nonetheless, RF ablation offers several theoretical advantages over cryosurgery. First, unlike cryosurgery, RF ablation can be performed percutaneously under image guidance with relative ease. This results in significantly less expensive treatments that can be administered in an outpatient setting. Second, the complication rate of hepatic tumor RF ablation appears to be much lower than that observed with cryosurgery.[96–101] Third, the time that is required for RF ablation is significantly less than that required for cryosurgical ablation. Finally, equipment costs are significantly less for RF ablation than for cryosurgery.

HEPATIC ARTERIAL INFUSION CHEMOTHERAPY

The majority of patients with colon and rectal carcinoma metastases confined to the liver have diffuse metastases that cannot be treated by surgical resection or ablative therapies such as cryosurgery or RF ablation. Hepatic arterial infusion (HAI) chemotherapy is an effective therapy for these patients. Several rationales exist that support this therapeutic approach. Liver metastases larger than a few millimeters derive most of their blood supply from the hepatic arterial system,[22] while normal liver receives most of its blood from the portal venous system.[21] Accordingly, chemotherapy infused into the hepatic artery is delivered preferentially to the metastases. In addition, some chemotherapeutic agents, such as floxuridine (FUDR), undergo first-pass clearance by the liver, and this limits systemic drug exposure following infusion directly into the hepatic artery. Intratumoral levels of FUDR are 100 to 400 times greater following administration into the hepatic artery compared to intravenous administration.[102] Systemic FUDR levels following administration into the

hepatic artery are one-fourth that observed following intravenous FUDR administration.[103]

HAI chemotherapy is generally reserved for patients with isolated liver metastases who have no clinical evidence of extrahepatic metastases. Rare exceptions are made for patients with a large tumor burden in the liver and minimal extrahepatic metastases and would likely die soon from their liver tumor burden without effective therapy.[104] HAI chemotherapy is delivered through a surgically placed pump connected to a catheter that is inserted into the hepatic arterial blood supply. Prior to the operation, an arteriogram of the branches supplied

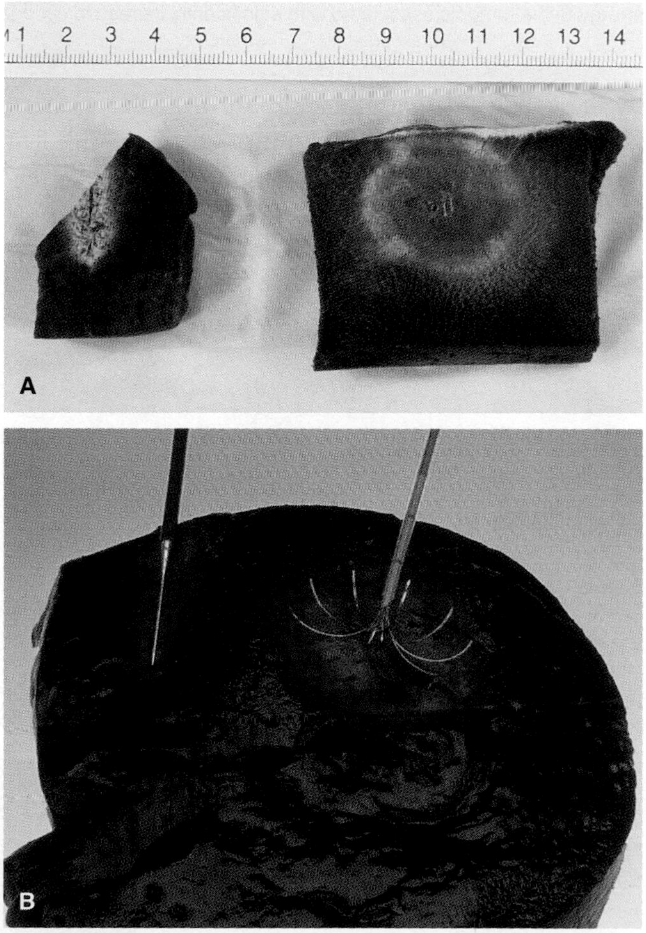

Figure 11–15. *A,* Coagulation necrosis induced by RF energy delivery via a conventional (non-cooled) electrode (*left*) compared to that observed using a cooled electrode (*right*). Tissue vaporization and carbonization adjacent to the conventional electrode creates electrical impedance that limits energy delivery. Active cooling of the electrode during RF ablation energy deposition prevents tissue vaporization and carbonization, which permits maintenance of low electrical impedance and allows delivery of more energy. *B,* Coagulation necrosis induced by RF energy delivery via a conventional electrode (*left*) compared to that observed using an electrode with hooks deployed out into the tissue.

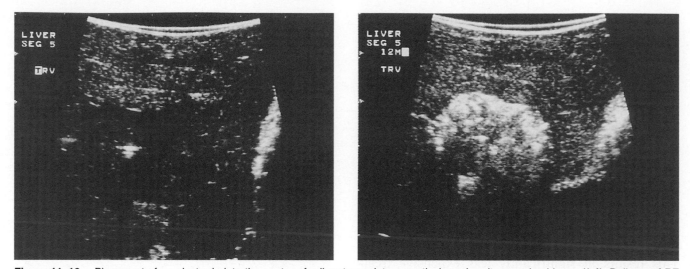

Figure 11–16.   Placement of an electrode into the center of a liver tumor intraoperatively under ultrasound guidance (*left*). Delivery of RF energy to the tumor is associated with significantly increased echogenicity in the treated area (*right*). This typically resolves within 15 minutes.

by the celiac axis and the superior mesenteric artery is obtained for surgical planning. Over one-third of patients will have atypical anatomy of hepatic arter-

ies.[105] Patients are explored through either a right subcostal or midline incision, and the abdomen is explored to exclude the presence of extrahepatic

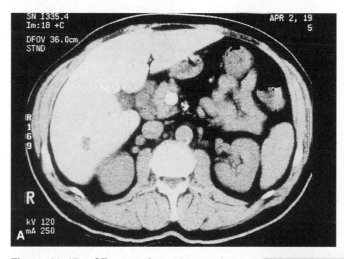

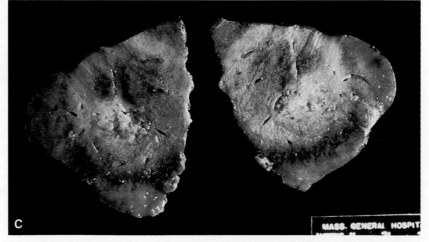

Figure 11–17.   CT scan of a colon carcinoma liver metastases in the right lobe prior to (*A*) and following RF ablation (*B*). The tumor was resected several days later (*C*), and coagulation necrosis was observed throughout the tumor.

metastases. The gallbladder is removed to prevent chemical cholecystitis. Careful dissection is performed to isolate the hepatic arterial blood supply in order to prevent misperfusion of the stomach, duodenum, or pancreas with chemotherapy. The catheter is placed into the hepatic arterial circulation (usually into the gastroduodenal artery) and attached to an infusion pump, which is implanted into a subcutaneous pocket in the abdominal wall. Fluorescein is injected into the pump sideport and the abdominal organs are observed with a Wood's lamp to confirm complete liver perfusion and exclude extrahepatic perfusion. Postoperatively, technetium-labeled macroaggregated albumin is injected into the sideport and a scintillation scan is obtained to again verify full liver perfusion and exclude extrahepatic perfusion. Several HAI chemotherapy regimens have been developed. A typical regimen consists of a 14-day continuous infusion of FUDR 0.15 mg/kg/day, leucovorin 4 mg/m²/day, and dexamethasone 20 mg/14 days followed by a continuous infusion of heparinized saline for 14 days. The cycle is then repeated.

Patients require close monitoring when receiving HAI chemotherapy. Because hepatobiliary toxicity is common, liver function tests are obtained every 2 weeks. Infusions are withheld when liver function tests are abnormal and can be resumed at a lower dose when these tests normalize. An abdominal CT scan is generally obtained after three cycles to assess tumor response. Treatment can be continued for patients with stable disease or disease regression but should be discontinued for patients with disease progression during therapy.

Complications of HAI chemotherapy can be divided into technical complications and chemotherapy-related complications. Technical complications include misperfusion leading to gastritis, duodenitis, or pancreatitis; catheter and arterial thrombosis; catheter migration or dislodgment; and pump pocket seromas or infections.[104] Chemotherapy-related complications include biliary sclerosis, chemical hepatitis, bile duct strictures, and chemotherapy-induced gastritis, duodenitis, or pancreatitis.[104] In a surgical series by Curley and colleagues, there was a 5.5 percent early technical complication rate and a 28.8 percent late technical complication rate.[105]

The results of five randomized trials comparing HAI of FUDR to intravenous administration of FUDR or 5-fluorouracil (5-FU) are shown in Table 11–3.[106–110] Response rates for HAI chemotherapy were consistently higher than for systemic chemotherapy (42 to 62% vs 10 to 21%), but none of the studies showed a statistically significant increase in median survival. Two trials compared HAI of FUDR to best supportive care and both demonstrated a survival advantage, but most of the control patients did not receive chemotherapy.[111,112] These studies have all suffered from high rates of hepatobiliary toxicity and frequent surgical complications. In addition, some of these studies allowed crossover between treatment groups. Harmantas and colleagues performed a meta-analysis of six studies and found a statistically significant survival advantage for HAI chemotherapy, but this analysis included one study in which some patients in the control group received no therapy.[113] In a separate meta-analysis performed by the Meta-analysis Group in Cancer, no statistically significant survival advantage was observed in patients treated with HAI chemotherapy.[114] The Cancer and Leukemia Group B (CALGB) is currently conducting a prospective, randomized trial without crossover that may determine whether there is a survival advantage for HAI chemotherapy compared to intravenous chemotherapy.

One area of current investigation is the combination of HAI chemotherapy using an FUDR-based regimen together with intravenous chemotherapy with agents such as CPT-11. Another area of active investigation is the administration of HAI chemotherapy following curative liver resection for metastases. In one trial conducted by the Eastern Cooperative Oncology Group (ECOG), patients were randomized following curative liver resection of colon and rectal metastases to sequential administration of HAI chemotherapy and intravenous chemotherapy or observation. In a separate prospective randomized trial conducted at Memorial Sloane-Kettering Cancer Center, patients were randomized following curative liver resection of colon and rectal carcinoma metastases to either HAI chemotherapy combined with intravenous chemotherapy or intravenous chemotherapy alone. Data from these trials are not yet mature.

Table 11–3. PROSPECTIVE RANDOMIZED CLINICAL TRIALS OF HAI CHEMOTHERAPY VERSUS SYSTEMIC CHEMOTHERAPY*

Study (Year)	Study Size	HAI Treatment (sample size)	Systemic Treatment (sample size)	Median Survival HAI vs. Systemic (months)	p Value
Kemeny[106] (1987)	99	FUDR (48)	FUDR (51)	17 vs 12	NS
Chang[107] (1987)	64	FUDR (32)	FUDR (32)	17 vs 12	NS
Hohn[108] (1989)	143	FUDR (67)	FUDR (76)	15.5 vs 15.8	NS
Martin[110] (1990)	69	FUDR (33)	5-FU (36)	12.6 vs 10.5	NS
Wagman[109] (1990)	41	FUDR (31)	5-FU (10)	13.8 vs 11.6	NS

*Adapted from Harmantas A et al.

SURGICAL RESECTION OF LUNG METASTASES

Patients with colon and rectal carcinoma lung metastases require a preoperative assessment similar to patients with liver metastases. Patients should initially undergo a history and physical examination, laboratory tests including a CEA level, electrocardiogram, chest x-ray, and abdominal and pelvic CT scans, as well as colonoscopy if not done within the past 12 months. A chest CT scan is required to identify the number and location of metastases. Chest CT is more sensitive than chest x-ray in identification of metastases; however, since chest CT scans identify nodules as small as 3 mm, the specificity of this test for diagnosis of metastases is low.[115] It is important to bear in mind that a solitary lung nodule is most likely a metastasis in any patient with a history of malignancy.[116] Chest MRI is as sensitive as chest CT for identification of pulmonary metastases, but provides little additional information and is more expensive.[117] Pulmonary function tests may be required in some patients to assess lung function.

The minimum criteria that must be met by patients considered candidates for resection of their pulmonary metastases are as follows: (1) no evidence of other metastases, (2) no evidence of a local recurrence, (3) all pulmonary metastases can be safely resected, and (4) the patient has adequate pulmonary reserve and is healthy enough to recover from a thoracotomy.[116] Additional factors that may be useful in patient selection have been examined in several studies (Table 11–4). As is the case with factors influencing outcome following resection of liver metastases, negative prognostic factors for survival following resection of pulmonary metastases are generally associated with aggressive tumor biology. These include larger size of metastases (> 3 cm), more than

a single metastasis, and synchronous clinical presentation. In addition, two studies have reported reduced survival in patients with elevated CEA levels who undergo resection of lung metastases.[118,119] Lastly, at least two studies have emphasized the importance of obtaining clear surgical margins.[119,120]

Percutaneous needle biopsy of lung lesions in patients with colon and rectal carcinoma is rarely indicated. In most patients with a history of colon or rectal carcinoma, the interval development of new pulmonary lesions is sufficient to render a diagnosis of pulmonary metastases. In patients who are good candidates for resection, a wedge excision with clear margins should be performed with intraoperative frozen section analysis. Lung metastases can generally be easily differentiated from primary lung cancers based on the histologic appearance.[118]

Historically, patients with metastases in only one lung frequently underwent a posterolateral thoracotomy, and patients with bilateral metastases underwent either median sternotomy, clamshell bilateral thoracotomy, or staged bilateral posterolateral thoracotomies. In patients with bilateral lesions, the patient's pulmonary reserve and location of lesions determine the surgical approach. Median sternotomy generally results in less postoperative pain and morbidity than bilateral thoracotomies.[121] Staged posterolateral thoracotomies allow better exposure to each lung for posterior lesions or lesions in the left lower lobe.[122] For these procedures, patients are initially intubated with a single-lumen endotracheal tube and bronchoscopy is performed to evaluate the tracheobronchial tree. Subsequently, a double-lumen endotracheal tube is inserted. Following exposure of the desired lung, the lung is inspected and palpated thoroughly for lesions. The lung can be deflated to aid with exposure and palpation. All nodules should be resected with a margin of normal tissue.

Table 11–4. RESULTS OF RESECTION OF COLON AND RECTAL CARCINOMA LUNG METASTASES

Study (Year)	Number of Patients	Operative Mortality (%)	Operative Morbidity (%)	5-Year Survival (%)	10-Year Survival (%)	Negative Prognostic Factors
Goya[123] (1989)	62	—	4.8	42	22	Tumor > 3 cm
Mori[124] (1991)	35	—	—	38	—	Tumor > 3 cm > 1 metastasis
McAfee*[118] (1992)	139	1.4	12.2	30.5	19.1	> 1 metastasis CEA > 5 ng/mL
McCormack[122] (1992)	144	0	2.1	44	26	None
Regnard[120] (1995)	101	—	—	21*	—	Synchronous disease Incomplete resection
van Halteren†[125] (1995)	38	—	—	43	—	Disease-free interval < 24 months
Girard[119] (1996)	86	1.2	—	24	20	Incomplete resection CEA > 5 ng/mL

*Survival rate only for those with curative resections.
†Series included only curative resections.

The largest surgical series published in the past decade generally used the surgical approaches described above.[118–120,122–125] The survival of patients with resected isolated lung metastases is comparable to that of patients with resected liver metastases, with 5- and 10-year survivals ranging from 24 to 44 percent and 19 to 26 percent, respectively (see Table 11–4). The morbidity and mortality in most reports are quite low. In seven series of 35 or more patients reported in the past 10 years, the operative morbidity has ranged from 2.1 to 12.2 percent and the operative mortality has ranged from 0 to 1.4 percent.

The introduction of video-assisted thoracoscopic surgery (VATS) provides a new tool for removal of lung metastases. Recovery from this procedure is much quicker than from a full thoracotomy and is associated with significantly less postoperative pain. It is more difficult to identify and palpate lesions using VATS than thoracotomy. This is important in that some patients may have additional metastases that can only be detected intraoperatively, and, accordingly, some thoracic surgeons have argued against its routine use for resection of metastases.[126] However, with the advent of high-resolution spiral CT scans of the chest, the accuracy of lung imaging in patients with one or two lesions is now greater than 90 percent.[127] Several groups have reported encouraging results with VATS for pulmonary metastases.[127–131] Watanabe and colleagues reported on a series of 27 patients who underwent VATS resection of one or two lung metastases (mostly from colorectal carcinoma), and the 3-year survival was 56 per-

cent.[127] In another recent study of 24 patients who underwent VATS resection of a single colorectal carcinoma lung metastasis, a 49.5 percent estimated 5-year survival was reported.[131] Larger studies are required to confirm these initial encouraging results of VATS resection.

SURGICAL RESECTION OF LIVER AND LUNG METASTASES

A few groups have reported broader criteria and more aggressive approaches to liver and lung resections for colorectal carcinoma metastases than those outlined above. Some patients will present with resectable pulmonary and hepatic metastases. Alternatively, patients who have undergone metastectomy in one of these sites may subsequently present with resectable metastases in the other site. The results of metastectomy in both organs have been reported in several small series.[119,123,132–136] These studies included a total of 77 patients, and so the degree to which one can make general conclusions is limited. The reported median survival in these studies ranged between 16 and 27 months.[133,135,136]

The largest of these published series retrospectively analyzed 25 patients who underwent resection of both liver and lung metastases and compared them to 23 patients with metastases at both sites who did not undergo resection.[136] The median survival of patients who were resected versus control patients was 16 months versus 6 months. The 5-year survival was 9 and 0 percent. As might be expected, improved survival was observed in those patients with younger age, single metastases, metachronous presentation, and longer disease-free intervals. However, these retrospective comparisons are undoubtedly influenced by selection bias. Given the small number of patients in published reports and the retrospective nature of all of the studies, the question of whether it is beneficial to resect synchronous or metachronous metastases to both the liver and lung remains unanswered. The decision to perform resections in both sites should be made on an individualized basis.

SURGICAL TREATMENT OF BRAIN METASTASES

Colon and rectal carcinoma metastasizes to the brain infrequently. In three large autopsy series, only 1.8 to 2.9 percent of patients had brain metastases.[2,137–139] In the majority of patients with brain metastases, metastases are also present in other organs, and treatment is therefore directed toward slowing the progression of disease and palliation of symptoms. The prognosis in these patients is poor. Treatments include steroids, whole-brain radiation therapy, and surgical resection. The median survival in patients managed with supportive care is 1 to 2 months and median survival is 3 to 4 months in patients treated with radiation therapy.[15,139]

Hammoud and colleagues reported that the median survival of patients with colorectal carcinoma brain metastases treated with surgery (with or without other forms of therapy) was 9 months compared to 3 months following treatment with radiation and 1 month following treatment with steroids alone.[139] In another study comprised of 24 patients with brain metastases who survived for more than 1 year, the investigators observed that 19 patients had undergone resection (16 in conjunction with radiation therapy) and the remaining 5 patients had been treated with radiation therapy alone.[15] Of note, 2 patients who underwent surgery were still alive after 10 years.

In addition to numerous small series, there are three studies of more than 30 patients who underwent resection of their brain metastases.[15,16,139] The median interval between diagnosis of the primary colorectal carcinoma and the diagnosis of brain metastases ranged between 26 and 28 months.[16,139] The 30-day operative mortality rate was reported in only one study and was 4.1 percent.[16] None of the three studies reported morbidity rates. The median survival after resection ranged from 8.7 to 10 months. A significant proportion of surgical patients in all studies received additional therapy including steroids and whole-brain radiation therapy. Significant negative prognostic factors included systemic disease, memory loss,[15] early onset of brain metastases,[139] and infratentorial location.[16] It must be emphasized that these are retrospective analyses, and the results are undoubtedly heavily influenced by selection bias. However, the small possibility for cure in patients treated with surgical resection combined with radiation therapy makes this treatment an option that should be considered in appropriately selected patients.

CONCLUSION

This chapter has presented a discussion of management of patients with colon and rectal carcinoma who have limited metastases. About one-third of these patients experience long-term survival following resection of their hepatic or pulmonary metastases. Several prognostic factors have been identified that aid in selection of patients who are appropriate for surgical resection. Most of these prognostic factors reflect the underlying tumor biology. When disease in the liver has advanced such that surgical resection cannot be accomplished but is limited enough for ablative techniques, cryosurgery and RF ablation are promising alternatives to chemotherapy. Patients with metastases isolated to the liver may benefit from HAI chemotherapy, either as primary therapy or as adjuvant therapy following curative liver resection. Highly selected patients with limited pulmonary metastases may benefit from surgical resection.

REFERENCES

1. August D, Ottow R, Sugarbaker P. Clinical perspectives of human colorectal cancer metastasis. Cancer Metastasis Rev 1984;3:303–24.
2. Weiss L, Grundmann E, Torhorst J, et al. Haematogenous metastatic patterns in colonic carcinoma: an analysis of 1541 necropsies. J Pathol 1986;150: 195–203.

3. Desch CE, Benson AB, Smith TJ, et al. Recommended colorectal cancer surveillance guidelines by the American Society of Clinical Oncology. J Clin Oncol 1999;17:1312–21.

4. Engstrom PF, Benson AB 3rd, Cohen A, et al. NCCN Colorectal Cancer Practice Guidelines. The National Comprehensive Cancer Network. Oncology 1996; 10:140–75.

5. Jaffe BM, Donegan WL, Watson F, Spratt JS. Factors influencing survival in patients with untreated hepatic metastases. Surg Gynecol Obstet 1968;127:1–11.

6. Oxley EM, Ellis H. Prognosis of carcinoma of the large bowel in the presence of liver metastases. Br J Surg 1969;56:149–52.

7. Bengmark S, Hafstrom L. The natural history of primary and secondary malignant tumors of the liver. Cancer 1969;23:198–202.

8. Abrams MS, Lerner HJ. Survival of patients at Pennsylvania Hospital with hepatic metastases from carcinoma of the colon and rectum. Dis Colon Rectum 1971;14:431–4.

9. Bengtsson G, Carlsson G, Hafstrom L, Jonsson P-E. Natural history of patients with untreated liver metastases from colorectal cancer. Am J Surg 1981; 141:586–9.

10. Wilson SM, Adson MA. Surgical treatment of hepatic metastases from colorectal cancer. Arch Surg 1976;111:330–3.

11. Wood CB, Gillis CR, Blumgart LH. A retrospective study of the natural history of patients with liver metastases from colorectal cancer. Clin Oncol 1976; 2:285–8.

12. Wanebo HJ, Semoglou C, Attiyeh F, Stearns MJ. Surgical management of patients with primary operable colorectal cancer and synchronous liver metastases. Am J Surg 1978;135:81–5.

13. Wagner JS, Adson MA, Van Heerden JA, et al. The naural history of hepatic metastases from colorectal cancer. Ann Surg 1984;199:502–8.

14. Pestana C, Reitemeier RJ, Moertel CG, et al. The natural history of carcinoma of the colon and rectum. Am J Surg 1964;108:826–9.

15. Farnell G, Buckner J, Cascino T, et al. Brain metastases from colorectal carcinoma. The long term survivors. Cancer 1996;78:711–6.

16. Wronski M, Arbit E. Resection of brain metastases from colorectal carcinoma in 73 patients. Cancer 1999;85:1677–85.

17. Povoski SP, Fong Y, Sgouros SC, et al. Role of chest CT in patients with negative x-rays referred for hepatic colorectal metastases. Ann Surg Oncol 1998;5:9–15.

18. Evans JT, Dayton MT. Colon, rectum, and anus. In: Lawrence PF, editor. Essentials of general surgery. 2nd ed. Baltimore, MD: Williams & Wilkins; 1992. p. 219–43.

19. Heiken JP, Weyman PJ, Lee JKT, et al. Detection of focal hepatic masses: prospective evaluation with CT, delayed CT, CT during arterial portography, and MR imaging. Radiology 1989;171:47–51.

20. Nelson RC, Thompson GH, Chezmar JL, et al. CT during arterial portography: diagnostic pitfalls. Radiographics 1992;12:705–18.

21. Greenway C, Stark R. Hepatic vascular bed. Physiol Rev 1971;51:23–45.

22. Breedis C, Young G. The blood supply of neoplasms in the liver. Am J Pathol 1954;30:969–85.

23. Kemmerer SR, Mortele KJ, Ros PR. CT scan of the liver. Radiol Clin North Am 1998;36:247–60.

24. Soyer P, Bluemke DA, Hruban RH, et al. Hepatic metastases from colorectal cancer: detection and false-positive findings with helical CT during arterial portography. Radiology 1994;193:71–4.

25. Paley MR, Ros PR. Hepatic metastases. Radiol Clin North Am 1998;36:349–63.

26. Seneterre E, Taourel P, Bouvier Y, et al. Detection of hepatic metastases: ferumoxide-enhanced MR imaging versus unenhanced MR imaging and CT during arterial portography. Radiology 1996;200:785–92.

27. Taylor HM, Ros PR. Hepatic imaging: an overview. Radiol Clin North Am 1998;36:237–45.

28. Bezzi M, Silecchia G, De Leo A, et al. Laparoscopic and intraoperative ultrasound. Eur J Radiol 1988;27 (Suppl 2):S207–14.

29. Kolecki R, Schirmer B. Intraoperative and laparoscopic ultrasound. Surg Clin North Am 1998;78:251–71.

30. Barbot DJ, Marks JH, Feld RI, et al. Improved staging of liver tumors using laparoscopic intraoperative ultrasound. J Surg Oncol 1997;64:63–7.

31. Stocchi L, Nelson H. Diagnostic and therapeutic applications of monoclonal antibodies in colorectal cancer. Dis Colon Rectum 1998;41:232–50.

32. Beatty JD, Williams LE, Yamauchi D, et al. Presurgical imaging with indium-labeled anti-carcinoembryonic antigen for colon cancer staging. Cancer Res 1990;50:922s–6s.

33. Corbisiero RM, Yamauchi DM, Williams LE, et al. Comparison of immunoscintigraphy and computerized tomography in identifying colorectal cancer: individual lesion analysis. Cancer Res 1991;51:5704–11.

34. Leinsinger G, Kirsch C, Denecke H, Pletzer G. Immunoscintigraphy using SPECT and I-131 labeled monoclonal antibodies to CEA/CA19-9 in the follow-up of colorectal cancer. Antib Immunoconj Radiopharm 1991;4:577–85.

35. Doerr R, Abdel-Nabi H, Krag D, Mitchell E. Radiolabeled antibody imaging in the management of colorectal cancer: results of a multicenter clinical study. Ann Surg 1991;214:118–214.

36. Haseman M, Brown D, Keeling C, Reed N. Radioimmunodetection of occult carcinoembryonic antigen-producing cancer. J Nucl Med 1992;33:1750–6.

37. Granowska M, Britton KE, Mather SJ, et al. Radioimmunoscintigraphy with technetium-99m labelled monoclonal antibody, 1A3, in colorectal cancer. Eur J Nucl Med 1993;20:690–8.

38. Divgi CR, McDermott K, Griffin TW, et al. Lesion-by-lesion comparison of computerized tomography and indium-111-labeled monoclonal antibody C110 radioimmunoscintigraphy in colorectal carcinoma: a multicenter trial. J Nucl Med 1993;34:1656–61.

39. Steinstrasser A, Oberhausen E. Anti-CEA labelling kit BW 431/26: results of the European multicenter trial. Nuklearmedizin 1995;34:232–42.

40. Moffat FL, Jr., Pinsky CM, Hammershaimb L, et al. Clinical utility of external immunoscintigraphy with the IMMU-4 technetium-99m Fab' antibody fragment in patients undergoing surgery for carcinoma of the colon and rectum: results of a pivotal, phase III trial. The Immunomedics Study Group. J Clin Oncol 1996;14:2295–305.

41. Serafini AN, Klein JL, Wolff BG, et al. Radioimmunoscintigraphy of recurrent, metastatic, or occult colorectal cancer with technetium 99m-labeled totally human monoclonal antibody 88BV59: results of pivotal, phase III multicenter studies [published erratum appears in J Clin Oncol 1998 16:2575]. J Clin Oncol 1998;16:1777–87.

42. Wolff BG, Bolton J, Baum R, et al. Radioimmunoscintigraphy of recurrent, metastatic, or occult colorectal cancer with technetium Tc 99m 88BV59H21-2V67-66 (HumaSPECT-Tc), a totally human monoclonal antibody. Patient management benefit from a phase III multicenter study. Dis Colon Rectum 1998;41:953–62.

43. Aftab F, Stoldt HS, Testori A, et al. Radioimmunoguided surgery and colorectal cancer. Eur J Surg Oncol 1996;22:381–8.

44. Thor A, Ohuchi N, Szpak CA, et al. Distribution of oncofetal antigen tumor-associated glycoprotein-72 defined by monoclonal antibody B72.3. Cancer Res 1986;46:3118–24.

45. Manayan RC, Hart MJ, Friend WG. Radioimmunoguided surgery for colorectal cancer. Am J Surg 1997;173:386–9.

46. O'Dwyer PJ, Mojzisik CM, Hinkle GH, et al. Intraoperative probe-directed immunodetection using a monoclonal antibody. Arch Surg 1986;121:1391–4.

47. Sickle-Santanello BJ, O'Dwyer PJ, Mojzisik C, et al. Radioimmunoguided surgery using the monoclonal antibody B72.3 in colorectal tumors. Dis Colon Rectum 1987;30:761–4.

48. Martin EW Jr, Mojzisik CM, Hinkle GH Jr, et al. Radioimmunoguided surgery using monoclonal antibody. Am J Surg 1988;156:386–92.

49. Sardi A, Workman M, Mojzisik C, et al. Intra-abdominal recurrence of colorectal cancer detected by radioimmunoguided surgery (RIGS system). Arch Surg 1989;124.

50. Nieroda CA, Mojzisik C, Sardi A, et al. The impact of radioimmunoguided surgery (RIGS) on surgical decision-making in colorectal cancer. Dis Colon Rectum 1989;32:927–32.

51. Cohen AM, Martin EW Jr, Lavery I, et al. Radioimmunoguided surgery using Iodine 125 B72.3 in patients with colorectal cancer. Arch Surg 1991;126:349–52.

52. Nieroda CA, Mojzisik C, Hinkle G, et al. Radioimmunoguided surgery (RIGS) in recurrent colorectal cancer. Cancer Detect Prev 1991;15:225–9.

53. Dawson PM, Blair SD, Begent RH, et al. The value of radioimmunoguided surgery in first and second look laparotomy for colorectal cancer. Dis Colon Rectum 1991;34:217–22.

54. Arnold MW, Schneebaum S, Berens A, et al. Radioimmunoguided surgery challenges traditional decision making in patients with primary colorectal cancer. Surgery 1992;112:624–30.

55. Arnold MW, Schneebaum S, Berens A, et al. Intraoperative detection of colorectal cancer with radioimmunoguided surgery and CC49, a second-generation monoclonal antibody. Ann Surg 1992;216:627–32.

56. Di Carlo V, Badellino F, Stella M, et al. Role of B72.3 iodine 125-labeled monoclonal antibody in colorectal cancer detection by radioimmunoguided surgery. Surgery 1994;115:190–8.

57. Paganelli G, Stella M, Zito F, et al. Radioimmunoguided surgery using iodine-125-labeled biotinylated monoclonal antibodies and cold avidin. J Nucl Med 1994;35:1970–5.

58. Stella M, De Nardi P, Paganelli G, et al. Avidin-biotin system in radioimmunoguided surgery for colorectal cancer. Advantages and limits. Dis Colon Rectum 1994;37:335–43.

59. Martin E, Carey L. Second look surgery for colorectal cancer. Ann Surg 1991;214:321–7.

60. Arnold MW, Young DC, Hitchcock CL, et al. Radioimmunoguided surgery in primary colorectal carcinoma: an intraoperative prognostic tool and adjuvant to traditional staging. Am J Surg 1995;170:315–8.

61. Bertsch DJ, Burak WE Jr, Young DC, et al. Radioimmunoguided surgery system improves survival for patients with recurrent colorectal cancer. Surgery 1995;118:634–9.

62. Bakalakos EA, Young DC, Martin EW Jr. Radioimmunoguided surgery for patients with liver metastases secondary to colorectal cancer. Ann Surg Oncol 1998;5:590–4.

63. Prati U, Roveda L, Scoppetta N, et al. Radioimmunoassisted surgery for lung metastases from colorectal cancer: results and perspectives. Semin Surg Oncol 1998;15:223–5.

64. Fong Y, Blumgart LH. Useful stapling techniques in liver surgery. J Am Coll Surg 1997;185:93–100.

65. Melendez JA, Arslan V, Fischer ME, et al. Perioperative outcomes of major hepatic resections under low central venous pressure anesthesia: blood loss, blood transfusion, and the risk of postoperative renal dysfunction. J Am Coll Surg 1998;187:620–5.

66. Fong Y, Brennan MF, Brown K, et al. Drainage is unnecessary after elective liver resection. Am J Surg 1996;171:158–62.

67. Schlag P, Hohenberger P, Herfarth C. Resection of liver metastases in colorectal cancer—competitive analysis of treatment results in synchronous versus metachronous metastases. Eur J Surg Oncol 1990; 16:360–5.

68. Doci R, Gennari L, Bignami P, et al. One hundred with hepatic metastases from colorectal cancer treated by resection: analysis of prognostic determinants. Br J Surg 1991;78:797–801.

69. Rosen CB, Nagorney DM, Taswell HF, et al. Perioperative blood transfusion and determinants of survival after liver resection for metastatic colorectal carcinoma. Ann Surg 1992;216:493–505.

70. Gajowski TJ, Iwatsuki S, Madariaga JR, et al. Experience in hepatic resection for metastatic colorectal cancer: analysis of clinical and pathologic risk factors. Surgery 1994;116:703–11.

71. Scheele J, Stang R, Altendorf-Hofmann A, Paul M. Resection of colorectal liver metastases. World J Surg 1995;19:59–71.

72. Wanebo HJ, Chu QD, Avradopoulos KA, Vezeridis MP. Current perspectives on repeat hepatic resection for colorectal carcinoma: a review. Surgery 1996;119: 361–9.

73. Fong Y, Cohen AM, Fortner JG, et al. Liver resection for colorectal metastases. J Clin Oncol 1997;15:938–46.

74. Wanebo HJ, Chu QD, Vezeridis MP, Soderberg C. Patient selection for hepatic resection of colorectal metastases. Arch Surg 1996;131:322–9.

75. Cady B, Jenkins RL, Steele GD Jr, et al. Surgical margin in hepatic resection for colorectal metastasis: a critical and improvable determinant of outcome. Ann Surg 1998;227:566–71.

76. Hughes KS, Simon R, Songhorabodi S, et al. Resection of the liver for colorectal carcinoma metastases: a multi-institutional study of patterns of recurrence. Surgery 1986;100:278–84.

77. Nordlinger B, Jaeck D, Guiguet M, et al. Surgical resection of hepatic metastases: multicentric retrospective study by the French Association of Surgery. In: Nordlinger B, Jaeck D, editors. Treatment of hepatic metastases of colorectal cancer. New York: Springer-Verlag; 1992. p. 129–46.

78. Fernandez-Trigo V, Shamsa F, Sugarbaker PH. Repeat liver resection from colorectal metastasis. Surgery 1995;117:296–304.

79. Adam R, Bismuth H, Castaing D, et al. Repeat hepatectomy for colorectal liver metastases. Ann Surg 1997;225:51–62.

80. Seifert JK, Morris DL. Prognostic factors after cryotherapy for hepatic metastases from colorectal cancer. Ann Surg 1998;228:201–8.

81. Seifert JK, Morris DL. Cryotherapy of the resection edge after liver resection for colorectal cancer metastases. Aust N Z J Surg 1998;68:725–8.

82. Seifert JK, Junginger T, Morris DL. A collective review of the world literature on hepatic cryotherapy. J R Coll Surg Edinb 1998;43:141–54.

83. Whittaker DK. Mechanisms of tissue destruction following cryosurgery. Ann R Coll Surg Engl 1984; 66:313–8.

84. Morris DL, Ross WB, Iqbal J, et al. Cryoablation of hepatic malignancy: an evaluation of tumour marker data and survival in 110 patients. GI Cancer 1996;1:247–51.

85. Weaver ML, Atkinson D, Zemel R. Hepatic cryosurgery in treating colorectal metastases. Cancer 1995;76: 210–4.

86. Cozzi P, Stewart G, Morris D. Thrombocytopenia after hepatic cryotherapy for colorectal metastases: correlates with hepatocellular injury. World J Surg 1994; 18:774–7.

87. Stewart GJ, Preketes A, Horton M, et al. Hepatic cryotherapy: double-freeze cycles achieve greater hepatocellular injury in man. Cryobiology 1995;32: 215–9.

88. Ravikumar TS, Steele G, Kane R, King V. Experimental and clinical observations on hepatic cryosurgery for colorectal metastases. Cancer Res 1991;51:6323–7.

89. Kane RA. Ultrasound-guided hepatic cryosurgery for tumour ablation. Semin Interven Radiol 1993;10: 132–42.

90. Dilley AV, Warlters A, Dy D, et al. Hepatic cryotherapy: is portal clamping worth it? Aust N Z J Surg 1991; 61:A522.

91. Onik GM, Atkinson D, Zemel R, Weaver ML. Cryosurgery of liver cancer. Semin Surg Oncol 1993;9: 309–17.

92. Tandan VR, Harmantas A, Gallinger S. Long-term survival after hepatic cryosurgery versus surgical resection for metastatic colorectal carcinoma: a critical review of the literature. Can J Surg 1997;40:175–81.

93. Weaver M, Ashton J, Zemel R. Treatment of colorectal liver metastases by cryotherapy. Semin Surg Oncol 1998;14:163–70.

94. Dwerryhouse SJ, Seifert JK, McCall JL, et al. Hepatic resection with cryotherapy to involved or inadequate resection margin (edge freeze) for metastases from colorectal cancer. Br J Surg 1998;85:185–7.

95. Goldberg SN, Gazelle GS, Compton CC, et al. Treatment of intrahepatic malignancy with radiofre-

quency ablation: radiologic-pathologic correlation. Cancer (in press).

96. Solbiati L, Goldberg SN, Ierace T, et al. Hepatic metastases: percutaneous radio-frequency ablation with cooled-tip electrodes. Radiology 1997;205:367–73.

97. Solbiati L, Ierace T, Goldgerb SN, et al. Percutaneous US-guided radio-frequency tissue ablation of liver metastases: treatment and follow-up in 16 patients. Radiology 1997;202:195–203.

98. Livraghi T, Goldgerb SN, Monti F, et al. Saline-enhanced radio-frequency tissue ablation in the treatment of liver metastases. Radiology 1997;202:205–10.

99. Rossi S, Di Stasi M, Buscarini E, et al. Percutaneous RF interstitial thermal ablation in the treatment of hepatic cancer. AJR Am J Roentgenol 1996;167:759–68.

100. Siperstein AE, Rogers SJ, Hansen PD, Gitomirsky A. Laparoscopic thermal ablation of hepatic neuroendocrine tumor metastases. Surgery 1997;122:1147–55.

101. Curley SA, Izzo F, Delrio P, et al. Radiofrequency ablation of unresectable primary and metastatic hepatic malignancies: results in 123 patients. Ann Surg 1999;230:1–8.

102. Ensminger WD, Gyves JW. Clinical pharmacology of hepatic arterial chemotherapy. Semin Oncol 1983;10:176–82.

103. Collins JM. Pharmacologic rationale for regional drug delivery. J Clin Oncol 1984;2:498–504.

104. Knol JA. Colorectal cancer metastatic to the liver: hepatic arterial infusion chemotherapy. In: Cameron JL, editor. Current surgical therapy. 6th ed. St. Louis, MO: Mosby; 1998. p. 355–61.

105. Curley SA, Chase JL, Roh MS, Hohn DC. Technical considerations and complications associated with the placement of 180 implantable hepatic arterial infusion devices. Surgery 1993;114:928–35.

106. Kemeny N, Daly J, Reichman B, et al. Intrahepatic or systemic infusion of fluorodeoxyuridine in with liver metastases from colorectal carcinoma. Ann Intern Med 1987;107:459–65.

107. Chang AE, Schneider PD, Sugarbaker PH, et al. A prospective randomized trial of regional versus systemic continuous 5-fluorodeoxyuridine chemotherapy in the treatment of colorectal liver metastases. Ann Surg 1987;206:685–93.

108. Hohn DD, Stagg RJ, Friedman MS, et al. A randomized trial of continuous intravenous versus hepatic intraarterial floxuridine in patients with colorectal cancer metastatic to the liver: the Northern California Oncology Group Trial. J Clin Oncol 1989;7:1646–54.

109. Wagman LD, Kemeny MM, Leong G, et al. A prospective randomized evaluation of the treatment of col-

orectal cancer metastatic to the liver. J Clin Oncol 1990;8:1885–93.

110. Martin KJ, O'Connell MJ, Wieand HS, et al. Intra-arterial floxuridine vs systemic fluorouracil for hepatic metastases from colorectal cancer. Arch Surg 1990;125:1022–7.

111. Rougier P, Laplanche A, Huguier M, et al. Hepatic arterial infusion of floxuridine in patients with liver metastases from colorectal carcinoma: long-term results of a prospective randomized trial. J Clin Oncol 1992;10:1112–8.

112. Allen-Mersh T, Earlam S, Fordy C, et al. Quality of life and survival with continuous hepatic-artery floxuridine infusion for colorectal liver metastases. Lancet 1994;344:1255–60.

113. Harmantas A, Rotstein LE, Langer B. Regional versus systemic chemotherapy in the treatment of colorectal carcinoma liver metastatic to the liver. Cancer 1996;78:1639–45.

114. Reappraisal of hepatic arterial infusion in the treatment of unresectable liver metastases from colorectal cancer. Meta-Analysis Group in Cancer. J Natl Cancer Inst 1996;88:252–8.

115. Chang AE, Schaner EG, Conkle DM, et al. Evaluation of computed tomography in the detection of pulmonary metastases: a prospective study. Cancer 1979;43:913–6.

116. Putnam J, Roth J. Secondary tumors in the lung. In: Shields T, editor. General thoracic surgery. 4th ed. Baltimore: Williams & Wilkins; 1994. p. 1334–52.

117. Feuerstein I, Jicha D, Pass H, et al. Pulmonary metastases: MR imaging with surgical correlation—a prospective study. Radiology 1992;182:123–9.

118. McAfee MK, Allen MS, Trastek VF, et al. Colorectal lung metastases: results of surgical excision. Ann Thorac Surg 1992;53:780–6.

119. Girard P, Ducreux M, Baldeyrou P, et al. Surgery for lung metastases from colorectal cancer: analysis of prognostic factors. J Clin Oncol 1996;14.

120. Regnard JF, Nicolosi M, Coggia M, et al. Colorectal lung metastases: results of surgical resection. Gastroenterol Clin Biol 1995;19:378–84.

121. van der Veen AH, van Geel AN, Hop WC, Wiggers T. Median sternotomy: the preferred incision for resection of lung metastases. Eur J Surg 1998;164:507–12.

122. McCormack PM, Burt ME, Bains MS. Lung resection for colorectal metastases. 10-year results. Arch Surg 1992;127:1403–6.

123. Goya T, Miyazawa N, Kondo H, et al. Surgical resection of pulmonary metastases from colorectal cancer: 10-year follow-up. Cancer 1989;64:1418–21.

124. Mori M, Tomoda H, Ishida T, et al. Surgical resection of pulmonary metastases from colorectal adenocarcinoma. Arch Surg 1991;126:1297–302.

125. van Halteren H, van Geel A, Hart A, Zoetmulder F.

Pulmonary resection for metastases of colorectal origin. Chest 1995;107:1526–31.

126. McCormack PM, Ginsberg KB, Bains MS, et al. Accuracy of lung imaging in metastases with implications for the role of thoracoscopy. Ann Thorac Surg 1993;56:863–6.

127. Watanabe M, Deguchi H, Sato M, et al. Midterm results of thoracoscopic surgery for pulmonary metastases especially from colorectal cancer. J Laparoendosc Adv Surg Tech A 1998;8:195–200.

128. Togo S, Fujii S, Yamaguchi S, et al. Thoracoscopic lung resection for lung metastasis of colorectal cancer. Surg Laparosc Endosc 1996;6:480–84.

129. Dowling RD, Landreneau RJ, Miller DL. Video-assisted thoracoscopic surgery for resection of lung metastases. Chest 1998;113(1 Suppl):2S–5S.

130. Maniwa Y, Okada M, Yamamoto H, et al. An availability of video-assisted thoracic surgery for the resection of pulmonary metastases. Ann Thorac Cardiovasc Surg 1999;5:69–73.

131. De Giacomo T, Rendina EA, Venuta F, et al. Thoracoscopic resection of solitary lung metastases from colorectal cancer is a viable therapeutic option. Chest 1999;115:1441–3.

132. Griffith KD, Sugarbaker PH, Chang AE. Repeat hepatic resections for colorectal metastases. Surgery 1990;107:101–4.

133. Smith JW, Fortner JG, Burt M. Resection of hepatic and pulmonary metastases from colorectal cancer. Surg Oncol 1992;1:399–404.

134. Yano T, Hara N, Ichinose Y, et al. Results of pulmonary resection of metastatic colorectal cancer and its application. J Thorac Cardiovasc Surg 1993;106:875–9.

135. Gough DB, Donohue JH, Trastek VA, Nagorney DM. Resection of hepatic and pulmonary metastases in patients with colorectal cancer. Br J Surg 1994;81:94–6.

136. Robinson BJ, Rice TW, Strong SA, et al. Is resection of pulmonary and hepatic metastases warranted in patients with colorectal cancer? J Thorac Cardiovasc Surg 1999;117:66–76.

137. Floyd CE, Stirling CT, Cohn I. Cancer of the colon, rectum, and anus: review of 1687 cases. Ann Surg 1966;166:829–37.

138. Temple DF, Ledesma EJ, Mittelman A. Cerebral metastases. From adenocarcinoma of the colon and rectum. N Y State J Med 1982;82:1812–4.

139. Hammoud M, McCutcheon I, Elsouki R, et al. Colorectal carcinoma and brain metastases: distribution, treatment, and survival. Ann Surg Oncol 1996;3:453–63.

140. Younes RN, Rogatko A, Brennan MF. The influence of intraoperative hypotension and perioperative blood transfusion on disease-free survival in patients with complete resection of colorectal liver metastases. Ann Surg 1991;214:107–13.

141. Blumgart LH. Liver resection—liver and biliary tumors. In: Blumgart LH, editor. Surgery of the liver and biliary tract. 2nd ed. Edinburgh: Churchill Livingstone; 1994. p. 1495–535.

12

Anal Cancer

DAVID P. RYAN, MD
CHRISTOPHER G. WILLETT, MD

Anal cancer comprises only 1.5 percent of all digestive system malignancies in the United States; 3,300 new cases were anticipated in 1999.[1] Nevertheless, our pathophysiologic understanding and ability to successfully treat patients with anal cancer has undergone profound change. Thirty years ago, anal cancer was believed to be caused by chronic, local inflammation of the perianal area[2,3] and was treated by abdominoperineal resection.[4] As a result of carefully conducted epidemiologic and clinical studies, we now know that the development of anal cancer is associated with infection by human papillomavirus (HPV) and patients with anal cancer can be cured with preservation of the anal sphincter in a majority of patients.

ANATOMY AND HISTOLOGY

The anus can be divided into the mucosa-lined anal canal and the epidermis-lined anal margin. The proximal end of the anal canal begins anatomically at the junction of the puborectalis portion of the levator ani muscle with the external anal sphincter and extends to the anal verge over approximately 4 cm (Figure 12–1). The anal canal is divided by the dentate line, a macroscopic landmark overlying the transition from glandular to squamous mucosa that is often referred to as the transitional zone. The anal margin begins approximately at the anal verge and represents the transition from the squamous mucosa to the epidermis-lined perianal skin.

In part due to the lack of an easily identifiable landmark between the rectum and the anus and in part due to the widely variable histologic appearance of the transitional zone, there is much confusion regarding the pathologic classification of tumors arising in this area. In some people, abrupt transition from rectal glandular mucosa to anal squamous mucosa is present. In others, an intervening segment of junctional, basaloid, or so-called cloacogenic mucosa is present. Cloacogenic mucosa referred to areas consisting of pseudostratified epithelium with cuboidal or polygonal surface cells that closely resembles urothelium (Figure 12–2). Basaloid features are identified in approximately 25 percent of squamous cell cancers[5] and should be distinguished from basal cell carcinomas of the anal margin, which behave biologically as skin cancers. The terms junctional, basaloid, and cloacogenic have been abandoned and are referred to now as non-keratinizing squamous cell carcinomas. Tumors arising within the anal canal distal to the dentate line usually lack these features and are known as keratinizing squamous cell carcinomas (Figures 12–3 and 12–4; Table 12–1).

Since the transitional zone can vary widely among individual patients, the critical distinction between a rectal cancer and an anal cancer depends upon the pathologic classification and not the judgment of the surgeon. Adenocarcinomas arising in the transitional zone have the same natural history as other rectal adenocarcinomas and should be treated accordingly. Squamous cell carcinomas arising in the transitional zone (Figure 12–5) may vary morphologically but there are no discernible differences in biology, natural history, and treatment outcome among subtypes.[6,7]

The anal margin extends from the anal verge to the perianal skin. Distinguishing between tumors of the anal canal and anal margin can be very difficult

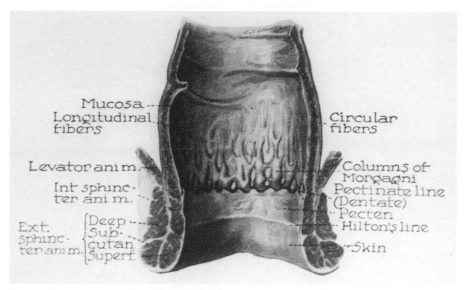

Figure 12–1. Anatomy of the anal canal.

clinically. Figure 12–6 shows a photograph of an anal canal cancer with involvement of the anal verge. Tumors of the anal margin are most often squamous cell neoplasms, but other types of cutaneous malignancies may occur in this region. Squamous cell cancers of the anal margin should be treated according to the same principles as squamous cell cancers of the anal canal. Tumors of the hair-bearing perianal skin should be considered skin cancers with a natural history and biology distinct from squamous cell carcinoma of the anus. Melanoma can arise in either the anal canal or anal margin and should be treated according to the same principles commonly applied to this tumor at other sites. Bowen's disease is an in situ squamous cell carcinoma that can occur on the anal margin, as well as

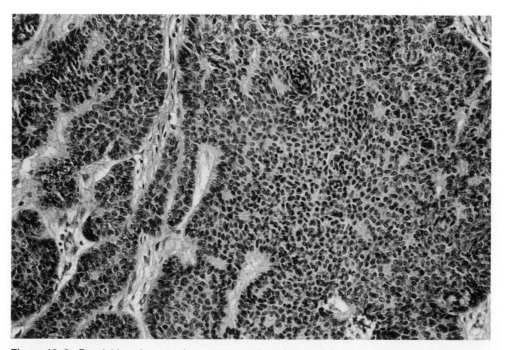

Figure 12–2. Basaloid or cloacogenic squamous cell carcinoma of the anus. Infiltrating squamous cell carcinoma consisting of basaloid cells composed entirely of small cells with scanty cytoplasm arranged in nests and trabeculae.

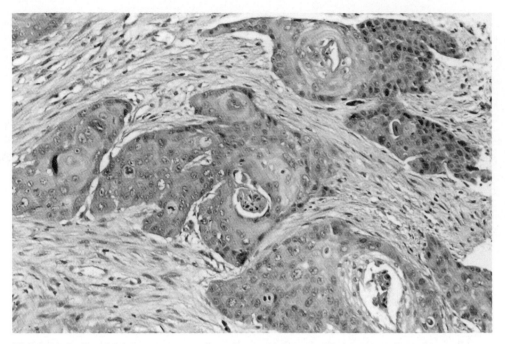

Figure 12–3. Keratinizing squamous cell carcinoma of the anus. Squamous cell carcinoma demonstrating keratin pearl formation that consists of large cells with abundant eosinophilic cytoplasm and central keratinization.

other areas of the skin that lack sun exposure. Paget's disease of the anus is an intraepithelial adenocarcinoma that is subclassified into two types: a primary cutaneous malignancy in which the malignant cells show sweat gland differentiation and an underlying adenocarcinoma of the rectum or perianal glands involving the adjacent squamous epithelium by lateral intramucosal/intraepithelial spread (Figure 12–7).

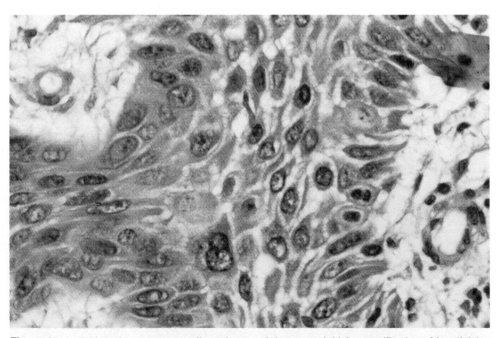

Figure 12–4. Bridges in squamous cell carcinoma of the anus. A high magnification of keratinizing squamous cell carcinoma of the anus that shows fine hairlike projections between cells called bridges. These represent the numerous desmosomal attachments between adjacent cells characteristic of this tumor type.

Table 12–1. WHO CLASSIFICATION OF CARCINOMA OF THE ANUS

Anal Canal
  Malignant epithelial tumors:
    Squamous cell (cloacogenic) carcinoma
      – large cell keratinizing
      – large cell nonkeratinizing (transitional)
      – basaloid
    Adenocarcinoma
      – rectal type
      – of anal glands
      – within anorectal fistula
    Small-cell carcinoma
    Undifferentiated

Anal Margin
  Malignant epithelial tumors:
    Squamous cell carcinoma
    Giant condyloma
    Basal cell carcinoma
    Others
    Bowen's disease
    Paget's disease

Lymphatic drainage of anal cancers is dependent upon the tumor's anatomic site of origin. Above the dentate line, drainage flows to perirectal and paravertebral nodes in a manner similar to rectal adenocarcinoma, while below the dentate line, lymphatics drain to the inguinal and femoral nodes. The inguinal, femoral, and iliac nodes are the most fre-

quent sites of nodal metastases.[8–11] Figure 12–8 shows the pelvic CT scan of a patient with metastases to the right inguinal nodes. These anatomic areas are rarely involved by rectal cancer.

The American Joint Committee on Cancer and the International Union Against Cancer have established a TNM staging system for anal cancer (Table 12–2). At presentation, approximately 50 percent of patients will have a superficial mass (ie, a T1 or T2 lesion), while approximately 25 percent of patients will have involvement of regional lymph nodes.[8,9,11–14] Tumor size has been shown in multivariate analysis to represent the most significant prognostic factor for patients with squamous cell cancers.[11,14] The probability of nodal spread is directly related to tumor size and location, occurring far more commonly in anal canal cancers than anal margin cancers.

EPIDEMIOLOGY

Initially, anal cancer was believed to develop in areas of chronic irritation associated with benign anal conditions such as hemorrhoids, fissures, and fistulae. Furthermore, case reports of anal cancer developing in patients with inflammatory bowel disease led to the assumption that anal cancer resulted

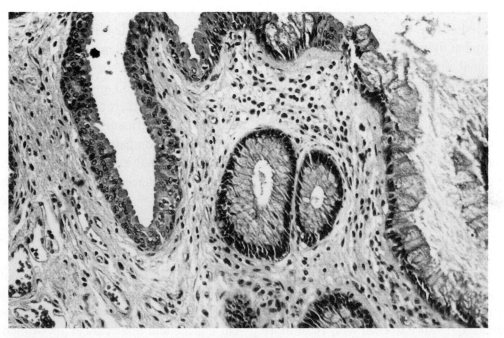

Figure 12–5. Squamous cell carcinoma of the anus arising in the transitional zone. This figure demonstrates normal rectal mucosa on the right transitioning into a pseudostratified epithelium on the left that resembles urothelium.

from chronic inflammation similar to the relationship between inflammatory bowel disease and colorectal neoplasia.[15-17]

Anal Cancer and Sexual Activity

Recent case-control studies have demonstrated that while the presence of anogenital condylomata places patients at higher risk for the development of anal cancer, a history of hemorrhoids, fistulae, and fissures has little, if any, impact on the subsequent development of anal cancer.[18,19] Moreover, Frisch and colleagues linked a Danish hospital registry with the Danish Cancer Registry and none of the 651 patients with Crohn's disease or 509 patients with ulcerative colitis in this assessment of 68,549 patients developed anal cancer.

Pursuing reports of an increased incidence of anal cancer in homosexual men,[20,21] Daling and colleagues reported the results of a population-based, case-control study of anal cancer conducted between 1978 and 1985 that utilized patients with colon cancer in the same geographic area as controls.[22] Women with anal cancer were more likely than controls to have a history of genital warts (relative risk or RR − 32.5), herpes simplex 2 (RR = 4.1), and chlamydia trachomatou (RR = 2.3). The men with anal cancer were more likely than controls to have never been married (RR = 8.6), to have engaged in homosexual sexual activity (RR = 50), to have practiced receptive anal intercourse (RR = 33), and to have a history of genital warts (RR = 27) or gonorrhea (RR = 17.2). These findings were mostly free of the impact of AIDS as the epidemic was still in its early stages. Subsequent studies confirmed the relationship between anal cancer and receptive anal intercourse in men.[18,23-26]

To better define which sexual activities are associated with anal cancer in heterosexual men and women, Frisch and colleagues conducted a case-control study of 417 patients with anal cancer compared with 534 patients with adenocarcinoma of the rectum and 554 normal controls.[27] For women, multivariate analysis demonstrated that the greatest relative risk of anal cancer occurred in those women with 10 or more lifetime sexual partners (RR = 4.5); a history of anal warts (RR = 11.7), genital warts (RR = 4.6), gonor-

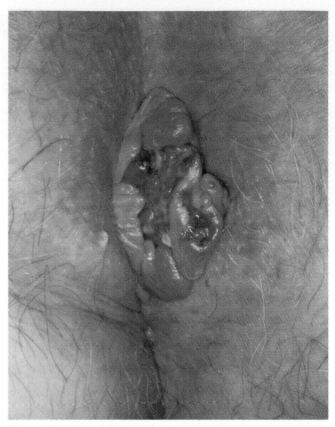

Figure 12–6. Squamous carcinoma of the anal canal arising at the anal margin.

rhea (RR = 3.3), or cervical dysplasia (RR = 2.3); and women who had undergone testing for HIV (RR = 1.7) or whose sexual partners had a history of a sexually transmitted disease (RR = 2.4). Of the 321 women with anal cancer, 10 percent of women reported engaging in receptive anal intercourse before the age of 30 and 4 percent of women had at least two anal intercourse partners. These women also had a significantly elevated risk of anal cancer on multivariate analysis. Among heterosexual men, multivariate analysis revealed significantly elevated risks of anal cancer with 10 or more lifetime sexual partners (RR = 2.5) or a history of anal warts (RR = 4.9) or syphilis/hepatitis (RR = 4.0). These findings strongly implicate anal cancer as being a sexually transmitted disease.

Lending more support to the role of sexual activity in the development of anal cancers are the reports demonstrating a strong relationship between cervical cancer and anal cancer in women.[28-31] A study from the Danish Cancer Registry demonstrated that the odds ratio for developing anal or vulvar cancer

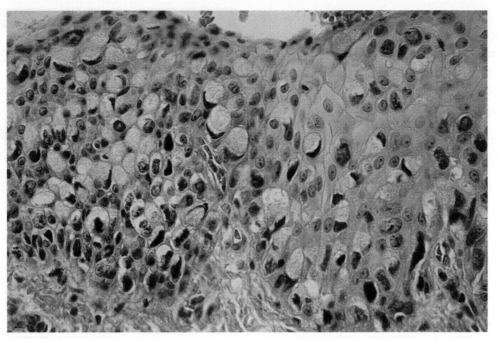

Figure 12–7. Paget's disease of the anus. This figure demonstrates large, mucin-containing, signet-like cells with hyperchromatic nuclei that are characteristic of Paget's disease of the anus. Note the location within the epithelium.

after a diagnosis of cervical cancer was much higher than that for stomach or colon cancer.[29] Furthermore, patients with anal cancer had a greater likelihood of having had previous vulvar, vaginal, and cervical cancers.[30]

Rabkin and colleagues reviewed the data from the Surveillance, Epidemiology, and End Results Program (SEER), which collects cancer incidence and survival data from population-based cancer registries representing approximately 14 percent of the

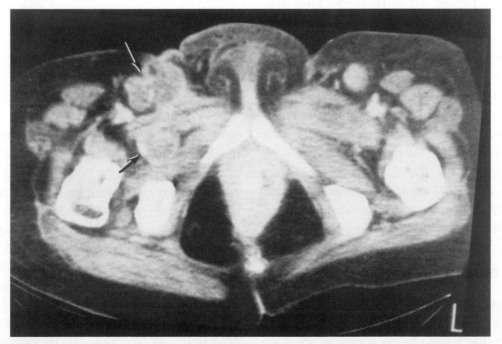

Figure 12–8. Clinical N2 disease. Pelvic CT scan from a patient with anal cancer demonstrating metastases to the right inguinal lymph nodes.

United States population. They found the relative risks of developing anal cancer and vaginal cancer after a diagnosis of invasive cervical cancer were 4.6 and 5.6, respectively.[31] Neither the Danish nor SEER observations could be explained by the use of prior radiation therapy to manage cervical cancer.

Anal Cancer and HPV

The known association between cervical cancer and HPV, the emerging relationship between cervical and anal cancer, and the linkage with sexual activity led to speculation that anal cancer might be caused by HPV. HPV DNA has been isolated by polymerase chain reaction (PCR) in 46 to 100 percent of in situ and invasive squamous cell carcinomas of the anus.[32] The premalignant condition of cervical intraepithelial neoplasia (CIN) associated with cervical HPV infection also occurs in anal HPV infection. As in CIN, anal intraepithelial neoplasia (AIN) can be morphologically low grade or high grade. These lesions are often polypoid condylomata acuminata. Evidence suggests that high-grade AIN is a precursor for anal carcinoma. AIN sometimes progresses from low grade to high grade, exists in areas adjacent to squamous cell carcinoma, and is associated with HPV infection.[33] Similar to the setting of cervical cancer, HPV 16 is the most frequently isolated type in anal malignancies and its presence predicts for high-grade AIN and invasive cancer, whereas low-grade AIN frequently shows other types of HPV.[26,34,35] In a recent case-control study by Frisch and colleagues, HPV DNA was isolated by PCR in 88 percent of 394 patients with anal cancer in contrast to 0 of 20 control patients with rectal adenocarcinoma.[27] Of these anal cancers, 73 percent contained HPV 16. No difference between HPV-positive and HPV-negative tumors has been found in regards to patient age, presence of adjacent dysplasia, ductal differentiation, or prognosis.[36]

Anal Cancer and HIV

The overall impact of AIDS on the incidence of anal cancer is unclear as population studies have reached conflicting results. Some reports appear to show an increased risk of anal cancer in men with AIDS.

Table 12–2. ANAL CARCINOMA STAGING SYSTEMS

Primary Tumor (T)

TX	Primary tumor cannot be assessed
Tis	No evidence of primary tumor
T0	Carcinoma in situ
T1	Tumor 2 cm or less in greatest dimension
T2	Tumor more than 2 cm but not more than 5 cm in greatest dimension
T3	Tumor more than 5 cm in greatest dimension
T4	Tumor of any size invades adjacent organ(s), eg, vagina, urethra, bladder (involvement of sphincter muscle[s] alone is not classified as T4)

Lymph Node (N)

NX	Regional lymph nodes cannot be assessed
N0	No regional lymph node metastasis
N1	Metastasis in perirectal lymph node(s)
N2	Metastasis in unilateral internal iliac and/or inguinal lymph node(s)
N3	Metastasis in perirectal and inguinal lymph nodes and/or bilateral internal iliac and/or inguinal lymph nodes

Distant Metastasis (M)

MX	Presence of distant metastasis cannot be assessed
M0	No distant metastasis
M1	Distant metastasis

Stage Grouping

Stage 0	Tis	N0	M0
Stage 1	T1	N0	M0
Stage 2	T2	N0	M0
	T3	N0	M0
Stage 3A	T1	N1	M0
	T2	N1	M0
	T3	N1	M0
	T4	N0	M0
Stage 3B	T4	N1	M0
	Any T	N2	M0
	Any T	N3	M0
Stage 4	Any T	Any N	M1

American Joint Committee on Cancer, 1997.

Selik and Rabkin estimated that the relative risk of death with anal cancer in HIV-infected persons aged 25 to 44 years was 60.7 for men but only 1.6 for women.[37] Though based on only 39 cases of anal cancer in men with AIDS, Melbye and colleagues reported that the relative risk of developing anal cancer after the diagnosis of AIDS was 63.4 compared with the general population.[38] Moreover, in New York City, there was a 10-fold increase in anal cancer among men aged 20 to 49 from 1979 to 1985, possibly representing an early effect of the AIDS epidemic.[39] In Denmark, the incidence of anal cancer since 1957 has increased by 1.5 times in men and tripled in women; however, much of this increase occurred in the pre-AIDs era and may have been due to the increase in HPV infections.[24] The most compelling evidence that AIDS has had little impact on anal cancer comes from case-control studies of single men living in San Francisco where the incidence of anal cancer was not significantly different before the appearance of AIDS in 1980 and after the AIDS epidemic was established in the late 1980s. In contrast, the number of cases of Kaposi's sarcoma and non-Hodgkins lymphoma have increased significantly over the same time period.[40–42] When cancer and AIDS registries across the United States and Puerto Rico are linked, there is a trend toward increasing risk of anal cancer with the acquisition of AIDS that does not reach statistical significance.[43] Without controlling for receptive anal intercourse and prior HPV infection, it is very difficult to discern the true effect of HIV on anal cancer.

HIV appears to have had an impact on anal HPV infection and progressive anal dysplasia. Several studies have consistently shown that patients with HIV are at increased risk for developing anal HPV infection independent of the practice of anal receptive intercourse.[26,44–46] Progressive immunodeficiency associated with AIDS further increases the risk of persistent anal HPV infection. Sun and colleagues followed a cohort of HIV-positive and HIV-negative women recruited from sexually transmitted disease clinics in New York City.[47] HIV-positive women were more likely to develop HPV infection and more likely to have persistent HPV infection. Furthermore, persistent HPV infection was inversely correlated with the circulating CD4 count.

HIV disease may predispose to infection with more than one type of HPV, which is associated with an increased risk of abnormal anal cytology.[48,49] Critchlow and colleagues followed a cohort of homosexual men in a community-based clinic and found that HIV-positive men having less than 500 circulating CD4 cells/μL were 7.5 times more likely to develop high-grade AIN than HIV-negative men.[26] Despite this evidence, very little is known about the subsequent development of invasive anal cancer in patients with high-grade dysplasia, possibly due to the lack of reproducible, objective criteria in defining AIN.[50]

Conceivably, a greater number of HIV-infected patients with high-grade dysplasia will progress to invasive anal cancer as treatment for HIV-induced immunosuppression improves and immediate survival is prolonged. In support for this hypothesis, solid tumor transplant recipients have been shown to be at increased risk of developing anal cancer following chronic, iatrogenic immunosuppression.[51] Recipients of renal allografts may have a 100-fold risk of anogenital cancer, and this risk has been associated with persistent HPV infection.[52,53] A lesser rate of anal cancers has been reported thus far after heart transplantation, possibly because the follow-up period remains brief.[51,54] Chronic immunosuppression with steroids for the treatment of autoimmune diseases may also predispose patients to invasive anal cancer.[55–57]

Finally, several case-control studies have also found a statistically significant risk of anal cancers in smokers, and current smokers are at higher risk than past smokers.[18,30,31,58,59] Odds ratios for anal cancer in current male and female smokers are among the highest for any smoking-related malignancy. The etiology of this relationship is unknown.

THERAPY

Until recently, an abdominoperineal resection (APR) represented the treatment of choice for tumors arising in the anal canal. This radical operation requires the removal of the anorectum and the need for a permanent colostomy. The overall probability of 5-year survival following an APR ranges from 40 to 70 percent with an associated mortality of approximately 3 percent.[8,11–13,60–62] Over the past 30 years, the treatment of anal cancer has shifted to a nonsurgical paradigm.

Combined Modality Therapy

Extending prior observations by others who had demonstrated a radiation potentiating effect by the concomitant administration of fluoropyrimidines in a variety of gastrointestinal malignancies,[63–68] investigators at Wayne State administered preoperative 5-fluorouracil (5-FU) and mitomycin combined with intermediate-dose radiation therapy (30 Gy) to patients with anal canal cancers as a means of decreasing the surgical failure rate.[69] The surprising finding of complete pathologic responses in the first three patients on treatment resulted in a strategy directed at sphincter preservation. Patients were initially treated with chemoradiation therapy and subjected to subsequent APR only if residual tumor remained at the time of a postradiation biopsy.[70] The Wayne State investigators found that a majority of patients treated with combined modality therapy could be cured without an APR. This finding was subsequently confirmed by multiple investigators[70-94] (Table 12–3).

Typically, patients are treated with radiation fields initially encompassing the pelvis from the S1-S2 level, the inguinal lymph nodes, and the anus (Figure 12–9). After 30 to 36 Gy, the treatment fields are reduced to the low pelvis encompassing the anal tumor. With this technique, the total dose to the primary dose is escalated to 45 to 50 Gy. During the 5- to 6-week course of irradiation and chemotherapy, there is frequently marked regression of the tumor as well as a brisk perineal skin reaction. Figures 12–10 to 12–12 show the response of an anal cancer and surrounding normal tissues to combined modality therapy. Figure 12–13 shows fibrosis and retraction of the perianal and anal region several years following therapy of a similarly advanced tumor.

A combined modality approach has been used successfully in HIV-positive patients with similarly good response rates, though toxicity appears to be more common, particularly as radiation doses are increased above 30 Gy.[95,96]

Radiation Therapy Revisited

Many investigators questioned the additive benefit of chemotherapy to radiation in the treatment of anal cancer. The use of radiation therapy alone, either by external beam or brachytherapy (ie, direct intratumoral implantation of radioactive seeds), as primary treatment for anal canal cancer has been associated with local control and overall survival rates in approximately 70 to 90 percent of selected patients[14,87,91,97-104] (Table 12–4). However, the local control and survival rates for patients with large tumors or nodal involvement were less than 50 percent in some series.[14,91,105]

The optimal dose of radiation therapy in the treatment of anal cancer has been the subject of considerable debate. Retrospective studies have shown that the dose of radiation is a significant prognostic indicator with improved disease-free survival in patients receiving at least 54 Gy of external beam radiation.[91,106] Late toxicity from radiation therapy such as anal ulcers, stenosis, and necrosis can lead to colostomies in 6 to 12 percent of patients who are free of disease.[14,87,107] Allal and colleagues reviewed their experience with 144 patients with anal cancer and demonstrated that late complications were dose dependent. After 5 years, 10 percent of patients required an APR for late complications, and the rate of serious complications was 23 percent for patients who had at least 39 Gy to the pelvis before a boost of radiation to the tumor and 7 percent for patients who had less than 39 Gy of external beam radiation.[108] An attempt to reduce this toxicity by divid-

			Complete	Local	Colostomy-free	Disease-free	Overall
Source	No. of Patients	Follow-up (yrs)	Response (%)	Failure (%)	Survival (%)	Survival (%)	Survival (%)
Leichman (1985)[70]	45	4	84	16	NA	84	NA
Sischy (1989)[73]	79	3	90	27	NA	61	73
Tanum (1991)[121]	94	5	84	NA	NA	72	72
Doci (1992)[71]	56	4	87	37	NA	77	81
Allal (1993)[104]	68	5	NA	44	66	61	65
Martenson (1995)[75]	50	7	74	46	NA	53	58
John (1996)[76]	46	1.7	81	NA	70	NA	89
Doci (1996)*[72]	35	3	94	14	86	94	NA
Peiffert (1997)*[119]	30	1	96	NA	NA	NA	NA
Gerard (1998)*[130]	95	5	NA	20	71	90	84

Table 12–3. SELECTED SERIES OF COMBINED MODALITY THERAPY IN ANAL CANCER

Local failure = persistent and recurrent tumor; NA = not available. *Administered a cisplatin-containing regimen.

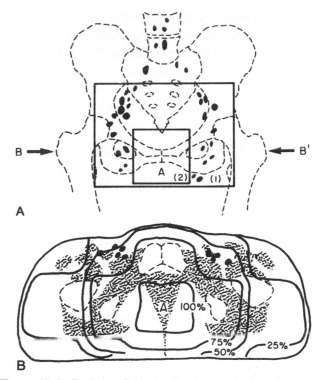

Figure 12–9. Radiation fields for the treatment of anal cancer. Reprinted with permission from Cummings BJ. Anal cancer. In: Perez CA, Brady LW, eds. Principles and practice of radiation oncology, 3rd ed. Philadelphia: Lippincott-Raven, 1997.

ing a total radiation dose of 59 Gy into a split-dose schedule (2-week delay after 36 Gy) proved unsuccessful, resulting in diminished tumor control but similar toxicity.[76]

Through a series of randomized studies, investigators in Europe and the United States have successfully addressed some of the questions surrounding the additive benefit of chemotherapy to radiation in the treatment of anal cancer.

Phase III Trials in Anal Cancer

There are currently a number of phase III trials ongoing for the treatment of anal cancer (Table 12–5). The Anal Cancer Trial Working Party of the United Kingdom Coordination Committee on Cancer Research (UKCCCR)[109] randomized 585 patients to receive either radiotherapy administered as 45 Gy of external beam with either a 15 Gy external beam boost or a 25 Gy brachytherapy boost, or radiotherapy with concurrent 5-fluorouracil (5-FU) and mitomycin. Similar response rates were noted in both groups, with a trend toward a more favorable response in the combined

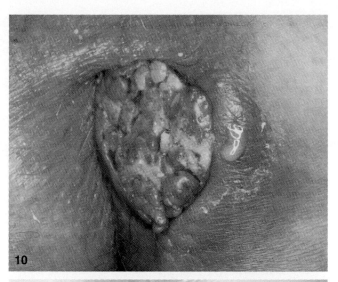

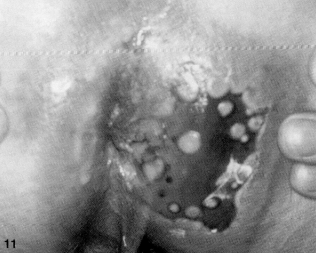

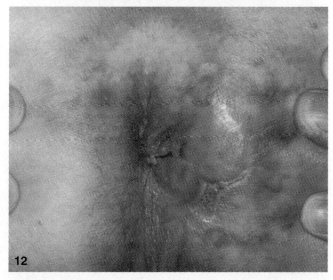

Figure 12–10 to 12–12. Treatment of anal cancer with combined modality therapy. This series of photographs demonstrates a squamous cell carcinoma of the anus prior to combined modality treatment (10), during treatment with perianal erythema and moist desquamation (11), and immediate post-treatment with healing of perianal tissue (12).

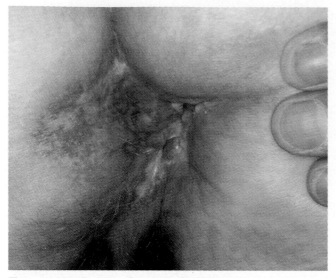

Figure 12–13. Radiation fibrosis. Radiation fibrosis can occur several years after treatment and its occurrence is related to dose of radiation. Severe fibrosis may have to be treated surgically with a colostomy.

modality therapy (CMT) arm. However, there was a significant improvement in local control for patients treated with CMT (61% vs 39%, $p = .0001$). Deaths from anal cancer were also reduced in the CMT arm (28% vs 39%, $p = .02$), but overall survival was not statistically significant. Of note, the CMT group experienced significantly more acute morbidity, including six deaths, but late morbidity was the same.

The European Organization for the Research and Treatment of Cancer (EORTC)[7] randomized 110 patients with T3-4, N0-3 or T1-2, N1-3 anal cancer

to receive either radiotherapy (45 Gy with a 15 or 30 Gy boost) with concurrent chemotherapy (5-FU and mitomycin) or radiotherapy alone. The CMT group experienced a higher pathologic complete remission rate (80% vs 54%), an 18 percent higher 5-year locoregional control rate ($p = .02$), a 32 percent higher colostomy-free rate ($p = .002$), a higher event-free survival rate, and a higher progression-free survival rate. Overall survival, however, was not significantly different. As opposed to the UKCCCR trial, acute and late side effects were not significantly different between the groups, and one death occurred in the CMT group. Multivariate analysis established that the presence of either skin ulceration or nodal involvement was a poor prognostic factor and that women had better local control and survival than men. These two trials have established that the addition of chemotherapy to radiation therapy improves local control and disease-free survival but not overall survival.

Role of Mitomycin

Assessing the contribution of mitomycin in a curative combined modality regimen was thought important since the drug is not a radiation sensitizer, has only modest antitumor activity against squamous cell cancers like those from the anus, and has been associated with chronic toxicity to the kidneys,[110–112]

Source	No. of Patients	Follow-up (yrs)	Therapy	Complete Response (%)	Local Control (%)	Colostomy-free Survival (%)	Overall Survival (%)
Puthawala 1982[97]	40	3	40–50 Gy XRT + BRT 35–40 Gy	NA	70*	NA	65*
Cantril 1983[99]	35	5	45–69 Gy XRT	91	80*	NA	79
Papillon 1983[100]	97	3	42 Gy XRT + 20 Gy BRT	NA	NA	55*	83*
Eschwege 1985[105]	61	5	30–65 Gy + 20 Gy BRT	67	80.3*	NA	79*
Doggett 1988[101]	35	5	45–75 Gy XRT	77	97	NA	92
Kin 1988[131]	32	5	36–50 Gy XRT + 15–28 Gy BRT		75	NA	49*
Schlienger 1989[132]	193	5	40–45 Gy XRT ± 20–25 Gy BRT	66	72*	55*	85 T1,2 59 T3,4
Cummings 1991[87]	57	5	45–55 Gy XRT ± BRT	56	53	NA	61
Dubois 1991[102]	61	5	30 65 Gy ± BRT	NA	80	NA	89
Martenson 1993[103]	18	7	55–67 Gy XRT	NA	90	NA	86
Allal 1993[104]	57	5	50–60 Gy XRT + 20–25 Gy BRT	NA	74	70	66

Table 12–4. SELECTED SERIES OF RADIATION THERAPY ALONE

*Crude statistics; XRT = external beam radiation; BRT = brachytherapy; local control includes patients who required surgery.

Table 12–5. PHASE III TRIALS IN ANAL CANCER

	Local Control at 3 Years (%)		Overall Survival at 3 Years (%)	
	Radiation Alone	Combined Modality	Radiation Alone	Combined Modality
EORTC[7]	39	58	65	72
UKCCR[109]	39	61	58	65

	Colostomy-free Survival at 4 Years (%)		Disease-free Survival at 4 Years (%)	
	RT + 5-FU	RT + 5-FU + Mito	RT + 5-FU	RT + 5FU + Mito
RTOG/ECOG[6]	59	71	51	73

RT = radiation therapy; 5-FU = 5-fluorouracil; Mito = mitomycin.

lungs,[113,114] and probably bone marrow.[115,116] The RTOG/ECOG[6] randomized 310 patients with anal cancer of any tumor or nodal stage to CMT with or without mitomycin. The addition of mitomycin resulted in a statistically significant improvement in colostomy-free survival at 4 years (71% vs 59%, p = .014), and disease-free survival at 4 years (73% vs 51%, p = .003). Overall survival and negative biopsy rate post-therapy did not differ significantly in the two arms. Grade IV toxicity (23% vs 7%) and fatal neutropenic sepsis (4 patients vs 1 patient, $p \leq$ .001) were significantly more common in the mitomycin arm. Of note, colostomy-free survival was 42 and 37 percent for node-positive patients in the 5-FU and 5-FU with mitomycin arms, respectively. Furthermore, the addition of mitomycin on the treatment plan for T3/4 tumors did not impact significantly on subset analysis.

Role of Local Excision

Whether local excision can ever be applied to the management of patients with squamous cell cancer of the anus remains an unresolved question. Early series reported that the probability of 5-year survival in patients with anal margin cancers less than 2 cm is greater than 80 percent.[11,12,61] It is difficult to draw conclusions from these early reports as some patients may have had cancers of the perianal skin and some patients received APRs for local tumor control. There is a lack of data demonstrating the natural history of high-grade AIN, incidentally noted squamous cell cancers after excision of high-grade AIN, and T1 tumors following local excision.

Two recent series have begun to shed light on these questions. Brown and colleagues have reported their experience with 46 patients who underwent local excision for high-grade AIN.[117] More than 40 percent of patients had positive surgical margins and over 50 percent of these patients had recurrent lesions after 1 year. For patients who had complete microscopic excision, 13 percent developed recurrent AIN. In addition, the morbidity of local excision was not trivial as 11 percent developed complications of anal stenosis and/or fecal incontinence. Hu and colleagues at Memorial Sloan Kettering Cancer Center reported their experience with local excision and CMT in a selected group of 25 patients.[118] For the entire group, 5-year, disease-free survival was 78 percent and overall survival was 86 percent. Of note, 30 Gy of radiation appeared to be an adequate dose.

These series demonstrate that AIN is a multifocal process due to HPV infection and complete local excision is often inadequate or not possible. By extension, the same concerns apply to small or incidentally found squamous cell carcinomas of the anus. Even when local excision is combined with chemoradiation, there appears to be a 20 percent risk of therapeutic failure. Therefore, local excision as sole therapy for anal cancer should not be considered adequate. More studies are needed to help define the best therapeutic options for patients with small (or incidentally found) tumors.

Platinum-Based Regimens

Presently, interest has arisen at replacing mitomycin with cisplatin. The platinum compounds, not available at the time the combined modality strategy evolved for anal canal cancers, are generally considered to be more effective than mitomycin in the treatment of squamous cell carcinomas. The combination of cisplatin and 5-FU given concurrently with radiation therapy in patients with anal cancer showed that only 14 percent of patients required a colostomy after 37 months and that 94 percent were alive.[72] This encouraging outcome has been confirmed in another series involving 30 patients.[119] An ongoing study in the United States is comparing cisplatin and 5-FU to mitomycin and 5-FU and also is examining the optimal dose of radiation.

Locally Recurrent Disease

Although some patients may be salvaged with surgery, locally recurrent anal cancer can be a difficult clinical problem associated with profound morbidity and suffering. Figures 12–14 and 12–15 show a photograph and CT scan of a patient with an anal cancer with massive recurrence filling the perineum and posterior pelvis. For patients with persistent disease after primary CMT, surgical removal either by local excision or APR remains the treatment of choice. A recent retrospective review of 21 patients who underwent APR after locoregional recurrence revealed a 58 percent 3-year survival rate.[120] In the UKCCCR trial, 29 patients with a less than 50 percent response were treated with an APR, 24 patients (83%) were rendered disease free, and 10 of the 24 patients (42%) eventually developed locoregional recurrence.

The RTOG/ECOG treated patients with persistent disease after primary chemoradiotherapy with salvage 5-FU, cisplatin, and radiation therapy (9 Gy boost). Of 22 patients, 12 (55%) were rendered disease free after salvage therapy. Of the 12 successfully salvaged patients, 4 had subsequent APR and are free of disease, 4 died (3 with recurrent disease), and 4 remain disease free. Of the 10 patients who had unsuccessful salvage therapy, 9 underwent APR. After 4 years, 3 remain alive without disease and 7 have died, including 6 with recurrent disease.

Metastatic Disease

In the EORTC and UKCCCR trial, 17 and 10 percent, respectively, of patients in the combined modality arms developed distant metastases. When reported, the liver is the most frequent site of distant metastases.[10,104,121] Reports of treatment for metastatic disease are rare and include partial responses with cisplatin, 5-FU, and methyl-CCNU.[122–124] There is little published experience with newer agents such as taxanes and irinotecan in this disease. Since cervical cancer and anal cancer are both HPV-related malignancies, it may be possible to extrapolate from the experience of chemotherapy in advanced cervical cancer. In cervical cancer, the two most active agents in the advanced setting are cisplatin and paclitaxel.[125–127] Two recent phase II studies of cisplatin and paclitaxel demonstrated an objective response rate of 47 and 46 percent, respectively, and have led

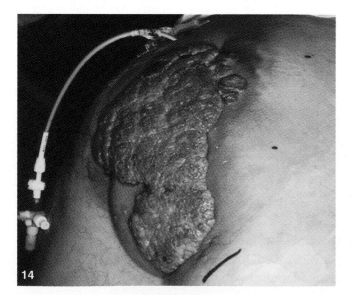

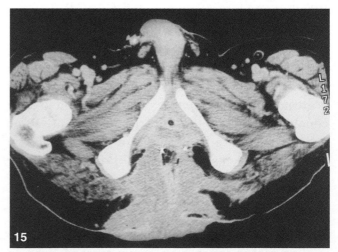

Figures 12–14 and 12–15. Recurrent anal cancer.

to a phase III effort by the Gynecologic Oncology Group comparing cisplatin versus the combination of cisplatin and paclitaxel.[128,129]

REFERENCES

1. Landis SH, Murray T, Bolden S, et al. Cancer statistics, 1999. CA Cancer J Clin 1999;49:8–31.

2. Kline RJ, Spencer RJ, Harrison EG. Carcinoma associated with fistulo-in-ano. Arch Surg 1964;89:989–94.

3. Buckwalter JA, Jurayj MN. Relationship of chronic anorectal disease to carcinoma. Arch Surg 1957;75: 352–61.

4. Klotz RG Jr, Pamukcoglu T, Souilliard DH. Transitional cloacogenic carcinoma of the anal canal. Clinicopathologic study of three hundred seventy-three cases. Cancer 1967;20:1727–45.

5. Myerson RJ, Karnell LH, Menck HR. The National Cancer Data Base report on carcinoma of the anus. Cancer 1997;80:805–15.

6. Flam M, John M, Pajak TF, et al. Role of mitomycin in combination with fluorouracil and radiotherapy, and of salvage chemoradiation in the definitive nonsurgical treatment of epidermoid carcinoma of the anal canal: results of a phase III randomized intergroup study. J Clin Oncol 1996;14:2527–39.

7. Bartelink H, Roelofsen F, Eschwege F, et al. Concomitant radiotherapy and chemotherapy is superior to radiotherapy alone in the treatment of locally advanced anal cancer: results of a phase III randomized trial of the European Organization for Research and Treatment of Cancer Radiotherapy and Gastrointestinal Cooperative Groups. J Clin Oncol 1997;15:2040–9.

8. Beahrs OH, Wilson SM. Carcinoma of the anus. Ann Surg 1976;184:422–8.

9. Frost DB, Richards PC, D. Montague ED, et al. Epidermoid cancer of the anorectum. Cancer 1984;53: 1285–93.

10. Greenall MJ, Quan SH, Stearns MW, et al. Epidermoid cancer of the anal margin. Pathologic features, treatment, and clinical results. Am J Surg 1985;149: 95–101.

11. Pintor MP, Northover JM, Nicholls RJ. Squamous cell carcinoma of the anus at one hospital from 1948 to 1984. Br J Surg 1989;76:806–10.

12. Schraut WH, Wang CH, Dawson PJ, et al. Depth of invasion, location, and size of cancer of the anus dictate operative treatment. Cancer 1983;51:1291–6.

13. Boman BM, Moertel CG, O'Connell MJ, et al. Carcinoma of the anal canal. A clinical and pathologic study of 188 cases. Cancer 1984;54:114–25.

14. Touboul E, Schlienger M, Buffat L, et al. Epidermoid carcinoma of the anal canal. Cancer 1994;73:1569–79.

15. Preston DM, Fowler EF, Lennard-Jones JE, et al. Carci-

noma of the anus in Crohn's disease. Br J Surg 1983; 70:346–7.

16. Slater G, Greenstein A, Aufses AH Jr. Anal carcinoma in patients with Crohn's disease. Ann Surg 1984;199: 348–50.

17. Daly JJ, Madrazo A. Anal Crohn's disease with carcinoma in situ. Dig Dis Sci 1980;25:464–6.

18. Holly EA, Whittemore AS, Aston DA, et al. Anal cancer incidence: genital warts, anal fissure or fistula, hemorrhoids, and smoking. J Natl Cancer Inst 1989; 81:1726–31.

19. Frisch M, Olsen JH, Bautz A, et al. Benign anal lesions and the risk of anal cancer. N Engl J Med 1994;331:300–2.

20. Daling JR, Weiss NS, Klopfenstein LL, et al. Correlates of homosexual behavior and the incidence of anal cancer. JAMA 1982;247:1988–90.

21. Peters RK, Mack TM. Patterns of anal carcinoma by gender and marital status in Los Angeles County. Br J Cancer 1983;48:629–36.

22. Daling JR, Weiss NS, Hislop TG, et al. Sexual practices, sexually transmitted diseases, and the incidence of anal cancer. N Engl J Med 1987;317:973–7.

23. Melbye M, Rabkin C, Frisch M, et al. Changing patterns of anal cancer incidence in the United States, 1940–1989. Am J Epidemiol 1994;139:772–80.

24. Frisch M, Melbye M, Mller H. Trends in incidence of anal cancer in Denmark. BMJ 1993;306:419–22.

25. Rabkin CS, Yellin F. Cancer incidence in a population with high prevalence of HIV-1 infection [meeting abstract]. Proc Annu Meet Am Assoc Cancer Res 1994;35:A1497.

26. Critchlow CW, Surawicz CM, Holmes KK, et al. Prospective study of high grade anal squamous intraepithelial neoplasia in a cohort of homosexual men: influence of HIV infection, immunosuppression and human papillomavirus infection. AIDS 1995;9:1255–62.

27. Frisch M, Glimelius B, van den Brule AJ, et al. Sexually transmitted infection as a cause of anal cancer. N Engl J Med 1997;337:1350–8.

28. Peters RK, Mack TM, Bernstein L. Parallels in the epidemiology of selected anogenital carcinomas. J Natl Cancer Inst 1984;72:609–15.

29. Melbye M, Sprogel P. Aetiological parallel between anal cancer and cervical cancer. Lancet 1991;338:657–9.

30. Frisch M, Olsen JH, Melbye M. Malignancies that occur before and after anal cancer: clues to their etiology. Am J Epidemiol 1994;140:12–9.

31. Rabkin CS, Biggar RJ, Melbye M, et al. Second primary cancers following anal and cervical carcinoma: evidence of shared etiologic factors. Am J Epidemiol 1992;136:54–8.

32. Tilston P. Anal human papillomavirus and anal cancer. J Clin Pathol 1997;50:625–34.

33. Fenger C. Anal neoplasia and its precursors: facts and controversies. Semin Diagn Pathol 1991;8:190–201.

34. Duggan MA, Boras VF, Inoue M, et al. Human papillomavirus DNA determination of anal condylomata, dysplasias, and squamous carcinomas with in situ hybridization. Am J Clin Pathol 92:16–21.

35. Palefsky J. Human papillomavirus infection among HIV-infected individuals. Implications for development of malignant tumors. Hematol Oncol Clin North Am 1991;5:357–70.

36. Williams GR, Lu QL, Love SB, et al. Properties of HPV-positive and HPV-negative anal carcinomas. J Pathol 1996;180:378–82.

37. Selik RM, Rabkin CS. Cancer death rates associated with human inmmunodeficiency virus infection in the United States. J Natl Cancer Inst 1998;90:1300–2.

38. Melbye M, Cote TR, Kessler L, et al. High incidence of anal cancer among AIDS patients. The AIDS/Cancer Working Group. Lancet 1994;343:636–9.

39. Biggar RJ, Burnett W, Mikl J, et al. Cancer among New York men at risk of acquired immunodeficiency syndrome. Int J Cancer 1989;43:979–85.

40. Rabkin CS, Yellin F. Cancer incidence in a population with a high prevalence of infection with human immunodeficiency virus type 1. J Natl Cancer Inst 1994;86:1711–16.

41. Biggar RJ, Horm J, Goedert JJ, et al. Cancer in a group at risk of acquired immunodeficiency syndrome (AIDS) through 1984. Am J Epidemiol 1987;126:578–86.

42. Harnly ME, Swan SII, Holly EΛ, et al. Temporal trends in the incidence of non-Hodgkin's lymphoma and selected malignancies in a population with a high incidence of acquired immunodeficiency syndrome (AIDS). Am J Epidemiol 1988;128:261–7.

43. Goedert JJ, Cote TR, Virgo P, et al. Spectrum of AIDS-associated malignant disorders. Lancet 1998;351:1833–9.

44. Caussy D, Goedert JJ, Palefsky J, et al. Interaction of human immunodeficiency and papilloma viruses: association with anal epithelial abnormality in homosexual men. Int J Cancer 1990;46:214–9.

45. Kiviat N, Rompalo A, Bowden R, et al. Anal human papillomavirus infection among human immunodeficiency virus-seropositive and -seronegative men. J Infect Dis 1990;162:358–61.

46. Williams AB, Darragh TM, Vranizan K, et al. Anal and cervical human papillomavirus infection and risk of anal and cervical epithelial abnormalities in human immunodeficiency virus-infected women. Obstet Gynecol 1994;83:205–11.

47. Sun XW, Kuhn L, Ellerbrock TV, et al. Human papillomavirus infection in women infected with the human immunodeficiency virus. N Engl J Med 1997;337:1343–9.

48. Palefsky JM, Gonzales J, Greenblatt RM, et al. Anal intraepithelial neoplasia and anal papillomavirus infection among homosexual males with group Iv HIV disease. JAMA 1990;263:2911–6.

49. Unger ER, Vernon SD, Lee DR, et al. Human papillomavirus type in anal epithelial lesions is influenced by human immunodeficiency virus. Arch Pathol Lab Med 1997;121:820–4.

50. Carter PS, Sheffield JP, Shepherd N, et al. Interobserver variation in the reporting of the histopathological grading of anal intraepithelial neoplasia. J Clin Pathol 1994;47:1032–4.

51. Penn I. Tumors after renal and cardiac transplantation. Hematol Oncol Clin North Am 1993;7:431–45.

52. Penn I. Cancers of the anogenital region in renal transplant recipients. Analysis of 65 cases. Cancer 1986;58:611–6.

53. Arends MJ, Benton EC, McLaren KM, et al. Renal allograft recipients with high susceptibility to cutaneous malignancy have an increased prevalence of human papillomavirus DNA in skin tumours and a greater risk of anogenital malignancy. Br J Cancer 1997;75:722–8.

54. Couetil JP, McGoldrick JP, Wallwork J, et al. Malignant tumors after heart transplantation. J Heart Transplant 1990;9:622–6.

55. Sillman F, Stanek A, Sedlis A, et al. The relationship between human papillomavirus and lower genital intraepithelial neoplasia in immunosuppressed women. Am J Obstet Gynecol 1984;150:300–8.

56. Sillman FH, Sedlis A. Anogenital papillomavirus infection and neoplasia in immunodeficient women: an update. Dermatol Clin 1991;9:353–69.

57. Sillman FH, Fruchter RG, Chen YS, et al. Vaginal intraepithelial neoplasia: risk factors for persistence, recurrence, and invasion and its management. Am J Obstet Gynecol 1997;176:93–9.

58. Holmes F, Borek D, Owen-Kummer M, et al. Anal cancer in women. Gastroenterology 1988;95:107–11.

59. Daling JR, Sherman KJ, Hislop TG, et al. Cigarette smoking and the risk of anogenital cancer. Am J Epidemiol 1992;135:180–9.

60. Singh R, Nime F, Mittelman A. Malignant epithelial tumors of the anal canal. Cancer 1981;48:411–15.

61. Greenall MJ, Quan SH, Urmacher C, et al. Treatment of epidermoid carcinoma of the anal canal. Surg Gynecol Obstet 1985;161:509–17.

62. Dougherty BG, Evans HL. Carcinoma of the anal canal: a study of 79 cases. Am J Clin Pathol 1985;83:159–64.

63. Foye LVJ, Willett FM, Hall B, et al. Potentiation of radiation effects with 5-fluorouracil. Cancer Chemother Rep 1960;6:12–5.

64. Allaire FJ, Thieme ET, Korst DR. Cancer chemotherapy with 5-fluorouracil alone and in combination with x-ray therapy. Cancer Chemother Rep 1961;14:59–75.

65. Frank W, Newcomer KL, Cirksena WJ, et al. Further

observations on concomitant use of x-rays and 5-flu-orouracil in neoplasms of humans. Cancer Chemother Rep 1962;22:55–8.

66. Childs DS, Moertel CG, Holbrook MA, et al. Treatment of unresectable adenocarcinomas of the stomach with a combination of 5-fluorouracil and radiation. Am J Roentgenol Radium Ther Nucl Med 1968;102:541–4.

67. Moertel CG, Childs DS, Reitemeier RJ, et al. Combined 5-fluorouracil and supervoltage radiation therapy of locally unresectable gastrointestinal cancer. Lancet 1969;2:865–67.

68. Henderson IW, Lipowska B, Lougheed MN. Clinical evaluation of combined radiation and chemotherapy in gastrointestinal malignancies. Am J Roentgenol Radium Ther Nucl Med 1968;102:545–51.

69. Nigro ND, Vaitkevicius VK, Considine B Jr. Combined therapy for cancer of the anal canal: a preliminary report. Dis Colon Rectum 1974;17:354–6.

70. Leichman L, Nigro N, Vaitkevicius VK, et al. Cancer of the anal canal. Model for preoperative adjuvant combined modality therapy. Am J Med 1985;78:211–5.

71. Doci R, Zucali R, Bombelli L, et al. Combined chemoradiation therapy for anal cancer. A report of 56 cases. Ann Surg 1992;215:150–6.

72. Doci R, Zucali R, La Monica G, et al. Primary chemoradiation therapy with fluorouracil and cisplatin for cancer of the anus: results in 35 consecutive patients. J Clin Oncol 1996;14:3121–5.

73. Sischy B, Doggett RL, Krall JM, et al. Definitive irradiation and chemotherapy for radiosensitization in management of anal carcinoma: interim report on Radiation Therapy Oncology Group Study No. 8314. J Natl Cancer Inst 1989;81:850–6.

74. Martenson JA, Lipsitz SR, Wagner H Jr, et al. Initial results of a phase II trial of high dose radiation therapy, 5-fluorouracil, and cisplatin for patients with anal cancer (E4292): an Eastern Cooperative Oncology Group study. Int J Radiat Oncol Biol Phys 1996;35:745–9.

75. Martenson JA, Lipsitz SR, Lefkopoulou M, et al. Results of combined modality therapy for patients with anal cancer (E7283). An Eastern Cooperative Oncology Group study. Cancer 1995;76:1731–6.

76. John M, Pajak T, Flam M, et al. Dose escalation in chemoradiation for anal cancer: preliminary results of RTOG 92-08. Cancer J Sci Am 1996;2:205–11.

77. Miller EJ, Quan SH, Thaler HT. Treatment of squamous cell carcinoma of the anal canal. Cancer 1991;67:2038–41.

78. Enker WE, Heilwell M, Janov AJ, et al. Improved survival in epidermoid carcinoma of the anus in association with preoperative multidisciplinary therapy. Arch Surg 1986;121:1386–90.

79. Michaelson RA, Magill GB, Quan SH, et al. Preopera-

tive chemotherapy and radiation therapy in the management of anal epidermoid carcinoma. Cancer 1983;51:390–5.

80. Nigro ND. Multidisciplinary management of cancer of the anus. World J Surg 1987;11:446–51.

81. Nigro ND. An evaluation of combined therapy for squamous cell cancer of the anal canal. Dis Colon Rectum 1984;27:763–6.

82. Nigro ND, Seydel HG, Considine B, et al. Combined preoperative radiation and chemotherapy for squamous cell carcinoma of the anal canal. Cancer 1983;51:1826–9.

83. Sischy B. The use of radiation therapy combined with chemotherapy in the management of squamous cell carcinoma of the anus and marginally resectable adenocarcinoma of the rectum. Int J Radiat Oncol Biol Phys 1985;11:1587–93.

84. Sischy B, Remington JH, Hinson EJ, et al. Definitive treatment of anal canal carcinoma by means of radiation therapy and chemotherapy. Dis Colon Rectum 1982;25:685–8.

85. John MJ, Flam M, Lovalvo L, et al. Feasibility of non-surgical definitive management of anal canal carcinoma. Int J Radiat Oncol Biol Phys 1987;13:299–303.

86. Flam MS, John M, Lovalvo LJ, et al. Definitive nonsurgical therapy of epithelial malignancies of the anal canal. A report of 12 cases. Cancer 1983;51:1378–87.

87. Cummings BJ, Keane TJ, O'Sullivan B, et al. Epidermoid anal cancer: treatment by radiation alone or by radiation and 5-fluorouracil with and without mitomycin C. Int J Radiat Oncol Biol Phys 1991;21:1115–25.

88. Cummings B, Keane T, Thomas G, et al. Results and toxicity of the treatment of anal canal carcinoma by radiation therapy or radiation therapy and chemotherapy. Cancer 1984;54:2062–8.

89. Fung CY, Willett CG, Efird JT, et al. Chemoradiotherapy for anal carcinoma: what is the optimal radiation dose? Radiat Oncol Investig 1994;2:152–6.

90. Johnson D, Lipsett J, Leong L, et al. Carcinoma of the anus treated with primary radiation therapy and chemotherapy. Surg Gynecol Obstet 1993;177:329–34.

91. Hughes LL, Rich TA, Delclos L, et al. Radiotherapy for anal cancer: experience from 1979–1987. Int J Radiat Oncol Biol Phys 1989;17:1153–60.

92. Meeker WR, Jr., Sickle-Santanello BJ, Philpott G, et al. Combined chemotherapy, radiation, and surgery for epithelial cancer of the anal canal. Cancer 1986;57:525–9.

93. John M, Flam M, Palma N. Ten year results of chemoradiation for anal cancer: focus on late morbidity. Int J Radiat Oncol Biol Phys 1995;34:65–9.

94. Nigh SS, Smalley SR, Elman AJ, et al. Conservative

therapy for anal carcinoma: an analysis of prognostic factors. Int J Radiat Oncol Biol Phys 1991;21 (Suppl 1):224.

95. Peddada AV, Smith DE, Rao AR, et al. Chemotherapy and low-dose radiotherapy in the treatment of HIV-infected patients with carcinoma of the anal canal. Int J Radiat Oncol Biol Phy 1997;37:1101–5.

96. Chadha M, Rosenblatt EA, Malamud S, et al. Squamous-cell carcinoma of the anus in HIV-positive patients. Dis Colon Rectum 1994;37:861–5.

97. Puthawala AA, Syed AM, Gates TC, et al. Definitive treatment of extensive anorectal carcinoma by external and interstitial irradiation. Cancer 1982;50: 1746–50.

98. Cummings BJ, Thomas GM, Keane TJ, et al. Primary radiation therapy in the treatment of anal canal carcinoma. Dis Colon Rectum 1982;25:778–82.

99. Cantril ST, Green JP, Schall GL, et al. Primary radiation therapy in the treatment of anal carcinoma. Int J Radiat Oncol Biol Phys 1983;9:1271–8.

100. Papillon J, Mayer M, Montbarbon JF, et al. A new approach to the management of epidermoid carcinoma of the anal canal. Cancer 1983;51:1830–7.

101. Doggett SW, Green JP, Cantril ST. Efficacy of radiation therapy alone for limited squamous cell carcinoma of the anal canal. Int J Radiat Oncol Biol Phys 1988; 15:1069–72.

102. Dubois JB, Garrigues JM, Pujol H. Cancer of the anal canal: report on the experience of 61 patients. Int J Radiat Oncol Biol Phys 1991;20:575–80.

103. Martenson JA, Jr., Gunderson LL. External radiation therapy without chemotherapy in the management of anal cancer. Cancer 1993;71:1736–40.

104. Allal A, Kurtz JM, Pipard G, et al. Chemoradiotherapy versus radiotherapy alone for anal cancer: a retrospective comparison. Int J Radiat Oncol Biol Phys 1993;27:59–66.

105. Eschwege F, Lasser P, Chavy A, et al. Squamous cell carcinoma of the anal canal: treatment by external beam irradiation. Radiother Oncol 1985;3:145–50.

106. Constantinou EC, Daly W, Fung CY, et al. Time-dose considerations in the treatment of anal cancer. Int J Radiat Oncol Biol Phys 1997;39:651–7.

107. Wagner JP, Mahe MA, Romestaing P, et al. Radiation therapy in the conservative treatment of carcinoma of the anal canal. Int J Radiat Oncol Biol Phys 1994; 29:17–23.

108. Allal AS, Mermillod B, Roth AD, et al. Impact of clinical and therapeutic factors on major late complications after radiotherapy with or without concomitant chemotherapy for anal carcinoma. Int J Radiat Oncol Biol Phys 1997;39:1099–105.

109. United Kingdom Coordination Committee on Cancer Research. Epidermoid anal cancer: results from the UKCCCR randomised trial of radiotherapy alone versus radiotherapy, 5-fluorouracil, and mitomycin. UKCCCR Anal Cancer Trial Working Party. UK Co-ordinating Committee on Cancer Research. Lancet 1996;348:1049–54.

110. Sheldon R, Slaughter D. A syndrome of microangiopathic hemolytic anemia, renal impairment, and pulmonary edema in chemotherapy-treated patients with adenocarcinoma. Cancer 1986;58:1428–36.

111. Verwey J, de Vries J, Pinedo HM. Mitomycin C-induced renal toxicity, a dose-dependent side effect? Eur J Cancer Clin Oncol 1987;23:195–9.

112. Lesesne JB, Rothschild N, Erickson B, et al. Cancer-associated hemolytic-uremic syndrome: analysis of 85 cases from a national registry. J Clin Oncol 1989;7:781–9.

113. Chang AY, Kuebler JP, Pandya KJ, et al. Pulmonary toxicity induced by mitomycin C is highly responsive to glucocorticoids. Cancer 1986;57:2285–90.

114. Verweij J, van Zanten T, Souren T, et al. Prospective study on the dose relationship of mitomycin C-induced interstitial pneumonitis. Cancer 1987;60:756–61.

115. Kantarjian HM, Keating MJ, Walters RS, et al. Therapy-related leukemia and myelodysplastic syndrome: clinical, cytogenetic, and prognostic features. J Clin Oncol 1986;4:1748 57.

116. Pedersen-Bjergaard J, Philip P, Larsen SO, et al. Therapy-related myelodysplasia and acute myeloid leukemia. Cytogenetic characteristics of 115 consecutive cases and risk in seven cohorts of patients treated intensively for malignant diseases in the Copenhagen series. Leukemia 1993;7:1975–86.

117. Brown SR, Skinner P, Tidy J, et al. Outcome after surgical resection for high-grade anal intraepithelial neoplasia (Bowen's disease). Br J Surg 1999;86:1063–6.

118. Hu K, Minsky BD, Cohen AM, et al. 30 Gy may be an adequate dose in patients with anal cancer treated with excisional biopsy followed by combined-modality therapy. J Surg Oncol 1999;70:71–7.

119. Peiffert D, Seitz JF, Rougier P, et al. Preliminary results of a phase II study of high-dose radiation therapy and neoadjuvant plus concomitant 5-fluorouracil with CDDP chemotherapy for patients with anal canal cancer: a French cooperative study. Ann Oncol 1997;8:575–81.

120. Pocard M, Tiret E, Nugent K, et al. Results of salvage abdominoperineal resection for anal cancer after radiotherapy. Dis Colon Rectum 1998;41:1488–93.

121. Tanum G, Tveit K, Karlsen KO, et al. Chemotherapy and radiation therapy for anal carcinoma. Survival and late morbidity. Cancer 1991;67:2462–6.

122. Zimm S, Wampler GL. Response of metastatic cloacogenic carcinoma to treatment with semustine. Cancer 1981;48:2575–6.

123. Khater R, Frenay M, Bourry J, et al. Cisplatin plus 5-fluorouracil in the treatment of metastatic anal squa-

mous cell carcinoma: a report of two cases [letter]. Cancer Treat Rep 1986;70:1345–6.

124. Ajani JA, Carrasco CH, Jackson DE, et al. Combination of cisplatin plus fluoropyrimidine chemotherapy effective against liver metastases from carcinoma of the anal canal. Am J Med 1989;87:221–4.

125. Bonomi P, Blessing JA, Stehman FB, et al. Randomized trial of three cisplatin dose schedules in squamous-cell carcinoma of the cervix: a Gynecologic Oncology Group study. J Clin Oncol 1985;3:1079–85.

126. Alberts DS, Kronmal R, Baker LH, et al. Phase II randomized trial of cisplatin chemotherapy regimens in the treatment of recurrent or metastatic squamous cell cancer of the cervix: a Southwest Oncology Group Study. J Clin Oncol 1987;5:1791–5.

127. McGuire WP, Blessing JA, Moore D, et al. Paclitaxel has moderate activity in squamous cervix cancer. A Gynecologic Oncology Group study. J Clin Oncol 1996;14:792–5.

128. Papadimitriou CA, Sarris K, Moulopoulos LA, et al. Phase II trial of paclitaxel and cisplatin in metastatic and recurrent carcinoma of the uterine cervix. J Clin Oncol 1999;17:761–6.

129. Rose PG, Blessing JA, Gershenson DM, et al. Paclitaxel and cisplatin as first-line therapy in recurrent or advanced squamous cell carcinoma of the cervix: a Gynecologic Oncology Group study. J Clin Oncol 1999;17:2676–80.

130. Gerard JP, Ayzac L, Hun D, et al. Treatment of anal canal carcinoma with high dose radiation therapy and concomitant fluorouracil-cisplatinum. Long-term results in 95 patients. Radiother Oncol 1998; 46:249–56.

131. Ng Ying Kin NY, Pigneux J, Auvray H, et al. Our experience of conservative treatment of anal canal carcinoma combining external irradiation and interstitial implant: 32 cases treated between 1973 and 1982. Int J Radiat Oncol Biol Phys 1988;14:253–9.

132. Schlienger M, Krzisch C, Pene F, et al. Epidermoid carcinoma of the anal canal treatment results and prognostic variables in a series of 242 cases. Int J Radiat Oncol Biol Phys 1989;17:1141–51.

13

Palliative Care for Patients with Lower Gastrointestinal Malignancies

ANTHONY L. BACK, MD

ROGER J. WALTZMAN, MD

Palliative care is comprehensive, interdisciplinary care, focusing primarily on promoting quality of life for patients living with a terminal illness and for their families.[1] Although cancer care in the U.S. has placed its primary focus on working toward a cure, the importance of end-of-life care has been recognized as a meaningful outcome of quality cancer care by the Institute of Medicine and the National Comprehensive Cancer Network.[2] Palliative care aims to help patients and their families live as well as possible in the face of life-threatening illness and requires attention to communication issues, symptom control, psychological issues, and end-of-life care. In the past, cancer care has often been conceptualized as a period of anticancer therapy, followed by an abrupt switch in goals to palliative therapy. But newer models of cancer care suggest that palliative therapy ought to begin when cancer is diagnosed and, as a patient approaches death, the emphasis should change gradually from anticancer therapy to palliative therapy[3] (Figure 13–1).

Which clinician should be responsible for palliative care? Even though palliative care teams are being developed at many cancer centers, the basic aspects of palliative care are an integral part of an oncology practice. Medical oncologists, surgical oncologists, and radiation oncologists are involved with people with cancer in a way that gives them unique opportunities to make life-enhancing interventions. The American Society of Clinical Oncology has recognized the need for oncologists to develop competence in end-of-life care by developing a specialized curriculum.

Despite improvements in cancer treatment, colorectal cancer is a leading cause of cancer morbidity and mortality. In the U.S. and Europe, about 300,000

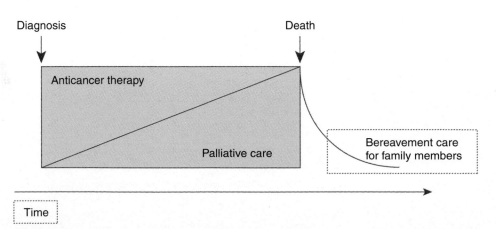

Figure 13–1. The balance of anticancer therapy and palliative care as a patient reaches the end of life.

new cases of colorectal cancer are diagnosed each year and about 200,000 people die of colorectal cancer.[4] Although hospices are involved with many patients dying of colorectal cancer, the potential impact of hospice care is limited by late referrals. Currently in the U.S. most hospice referrals are made within 3 weeks of death. Also in the U.S., reimbursement for hospice is structured so that some patients must choose between hospice and anticancer therapy. Many patients could benefit from palliative care delivered earlier in the course of their illness.

In this chapter, we have chosen to summarize key issues in palliative care of importance to clinicians involved in colorectal cancer care. More extensive discussions are available elsewhere, notably in the *Oxford Textbook of Palliative Medicine* and *Principles and Practice of Supportive Oncology*.[5,6] Within palliative care, cancer has been generally treated as a single diagnosis, with little attention paid to the different demands of different tumor types. Yet oncologists know that the supportive care needs of patients with different tumor types are quite different. This is common clinical knowledge but there are few data to back it up. So while we will highlight palliative issues commonly encountered in dealing with patients with colorectal cancer, many of our choices are based more on clinical experience than empirical data. By pointing out where data are lacking, we hope to stimulate interest and research in this area.

COMMUNICATION ISSUES

Giving Bad News

One of the first tasks facing physicians caring for patients with colorectal cancer is that they must give patients bad news. Giving bad news is a skill that can be learned and retained by physicians who have received specific communication skills training. Physicians who have taken communication skills training rate their own skills as improved and perform better with standardized patients. Unfortunately, few physicians have received this sort of training, and most oncologists have learned to do this by watching role models during their training. Communications training is available through organizations such as the American Academy for the

Physician and Patient and the Bayer Institute for Healthcare Communications.

Studies of patients with cancer indicate significant diversity in how they wish to be told bad news.[7] Patients differ on who should give the news, whether they want to be alone or with a companion, and whether they want detailed information or the big picture. Physicians should thus not count on using a stock routine successfully when giving bad news to different patients and families.

A thoughtful protocol for giving bad news was described by Robert Buckman. This protocol involves six steps (Table 13–1).[8] A helpful feature of the protocol is its emphasis on having physicians find out what a patient already knows before going on to give the bad news; this allows the physician to gauge something of the patient's educational level, affective state, and comprehension of the medical issue. A physician with this knowledge in hand can then match the patient's preferences and informational needs more closely. The protocol has been used at national workshops but has not been studied empirically.

Discussing Benefits and Burdens of Anticancer Treatment

The next most common issue in physician-patient communication about cancer involves benefits and burdens of anticancer treatment. Studies have shown that patients commonly leave consultations with

---

Table 13–1. GIVING BAD NEWS

A six-step protocol for giving bad news.

1. **Prepare**—Choose an appropriate physical location where all participants can be comfortably seated and verify the important information before sitting down.

2. **Find out how much the patient knows**—Getting both patient and physician on the same page at the outset can allow the physician to provide context for the information and get insight into the patient's emotional state.

3. **Find out how much the patient wants to know**—Asking what level of detail to cover can help the physician tailor the information and give the patient some control over the flow of information.

4. **Share the information**—Avoid medical jargon; give information in pieces and check for understanding after each piece.

5. **Respond to the patient's feelings**—This may need to be done after each piece of information and allowing the patient to react as the information unfolds can help prevent the patient from being overwhelmed.

6. **Make concrete follow-up plans for the next step**.

incorrect impressions about anticancer therapy.[9] Oncologists tend to quote statistics, which assumes a level of education not shared by some patients. In addition, statistics can be used selectively, sometimes unwittingly. For instance, the benefit of adjuvant chemotherapy after resection of a stage III colon cancer can be stated as a relative reduction in recurrence by 35 percent or as an absolute reduction in recurrence of 5 percent.[4] Educational interventions have been described for a small number of cancer treatment decisions. These interventions tend to rely on written material; presentation of material in lay language; time for patient comprehension, thought, and decision making; and nonjudgmental language.

In discussing benefits and burdens of anticancer treatment, patients also rely heavily on trust in their physician or oncologist. The importance of patient trust has been identified most clearly in studies of patients entering Phase I studies. In the Phase I situation, trust in the physician is an important factor— second only to the possibility of personal benefit from experimental therapy.[10] Yet physicians tend to be influenced by their own background and tend to believe more strongly in the benefits of medical intervention than laypersons.

Discussing Prognosis

Patients commonly ask physicians for their prognosis, a survival estimate. Even though this information is extremely important for patients, physicians are notoriously poor at predicting survival. For instance, if a patient with colorectal cancer has finished primary therapy, there is no empirical method that gives physicians probability of patient survival. Physicians commonly quote findings from clinical trials, but the patients who participate in clinical trials tend to be a selected subset of all patients, and in particular these patients tend to be younger and not to have comorbid medical conditions.

Even when patients are near death, physicians are commonly inaccurate in predicting survival time.[11] Interestingly, physician error in predicting survival occurs mostly in the optimistic direction. In one study of hospice patients in which physicians were prospectively asked to predict survival time, only 20 percent of predictions were accurate. Both increased time since the last contact with the patient and increasing duration of the patient-physician relationship correlated with overoptimistic predictions.[11]

These rosy predictions influence patient decision making near death. Patients who overestimate their remaining survival tend to opt for more life-sustaining therapy—specifically, they are more likely to want to have mechanical ventilation or CPR. In the SUPPORT study, which included patients with metastatic colorectal cancer admitted to intensive care units as well as patients with other conditions expected to have < 6 months survival, many patients wildly overestimated their survival. The patients who overestimated their survival were the ones most likely to continue wanting mechanical ventilation and CPR, and, consequently, they were more likely to die after having had mechanical ventilation or CPR.[12]

Understanding Patient Concerns

Cancer involving the colon or rectum can cause loss of bodily function, damage to body image, and a heightened sense of mortality. For example, a patient with rectal cancer who has undergone abdominoperineal resection must now live with an anus in the abdominal wall, and a colostomy bag that may leak, smell, and make embarrassing noises. The patient may certainly find life with a colostomy preferable to dying from unresected rectal cancer, but this new life requires a large readjustment. Several studies show that this readjustment depends in large part on the confidence and flexibility that the patient can bring to this new situation and also by the degree to which people feel that the cancer-related changes make them feel different from others.[13]

One indicator of adjustment to life with cancer is sexual functioning. Sexual functioning after cancer surgery involves physiologic and psychological issues. In male patients after surgery for rectal cancer that may disrupt pelvic sympathetic and parasympathetic nerves, ejaculatory dysfunction occurs in 30 to 50 percent and erectile dysfunction in 50 to 75 percent.[14] Women patients have not been studied as extensively, although one study describes decreased vaginal lubrication and frequency of orgasm after abdominoperineal resection for rectal cancer.[15] Furthermore, psychological issues of shame and stigma may affect patients whether or not physiologic changes can be easily identified. In one study involving patients with colorectal cancer, 27 percent of patients felt that they had permanently become less attractive to their sexual partners, and about the same proportion felt that their libido had decreased.[15] Together, these physiologic and psychological changes can result in fear, grief, and depression.

Patients tend to withhold the full nature and extent of their problems in order to protect health care professionals, family members, and caregivers. Cancer care settings implicitly teach patients what is required to be "a good patient," and patients follow these unspoken guidelines in the hope that being a good patient may increase their chances of receiving benefit from the treatment. When anticancer treatment is discontinued, many patients will no longer have regular appointments with their primary oncologist or clinic staff, resulting in the loss of supportive relationships dating back for years in some cases. This can result in feelings of abandonment, and patients may continue to opt for anticancer therapy in order to preserve the relationship.

Thus, physicians should not assume that a patient who does not volunteer concerns is actually free of concerns. In a study in which research nurses interviewed patients dying of colorectal cancer, patient concerns were frequently undetected by physicians.[16] The nurses received communications skills training and used a semi-structured instrument to elicit concerns. The most common physical complaints were appetite loss, nausea/vomiting, pain, breathlessness, and fever. These patients' physicians correctly identified these concerns 0 to 42 percent of the time. The physicians recognized less than half of the cases of affective disorder. The authors concluded that physicians often underestimate physical symptoms and fail to recognize anxiety and depression.

Talking with Family Members

Cancer affects the entire family (here family is meant to include both biologic relatives and emotional intimates). Family members may have differing perspectives, their own emotional needs, and their own coping mechanisms. Collusion is a particular problem. Family members may collude with patients to deny the seriousness of the illness. This may be evident in denial or overoptimism, but the classic manifestation is to ask the physician to pro-

tect the patient from the truth. Physicians and other medical caregivers should promote open approaches to discussing the cancer. A helpful step is to clarify the reasons for the family member's desire to protect the patient, as collusion is often done at significant emotional cost.[17] Family conferences can be useful at key decision-making points (Table 13–2).

Advance-Care Plans

Advance-care planning can be an important part of cancer care, especially at the end of life, if it stimulates conversation between patient, family caregiver, and physician. Advance-care planning includes conversations about patient wishes and values, as well as written documents called advance directives or living wills. Ideally, patient, family, and physician could discuss the patient's current medical situation and possible future outcomes of illness, and reach some consensus on future treatments such as mechanical

---

Table 13–2. CONDUCTING A FAMILY CONFERENCE

1. **Prepare:**
   a. Invite the key people—Patient (usually), surrogate decision maker (if applicable) or durable power of attorney for health care, important family members or friends, other health care providers. If key people are excluded, they may undo any decisions that are made, but if the conference includes too many people it will be unwieldy.
   b. Find a quiet room where all participants can be seated.
   c. Verify important medical information ahead of time.
   d. Formulate concrete goals for the conference.

2. **Conduct the meeting:**
   a. Introductions—Have participants introduce themselves.
   b. Establish goals for the conference; explicitly state any decisions that need to be made and the time frame available for making the decisions.
   c. Establish ground rules that each person will have a chance to express opinions and views.
   d. Review medical information.
   e. Ask patient to comment (for instance, "How do you view the pros and cons of treatment x?")
   f. Ask family or friends to express their views or concerns.
   g. Allow time for questions and discussion.
   h. If no decision is reached, ask if they would like to think it over for a period of time if this is medically possible; consider a follow-up conference the next day or at some appropriate time later.

3. **Summarize the discussion:**
   a. State your understanding of the decision reached (or not reached).
   b. Identify a family spokesperson, if the family requires, to simplify further communication.
   c. Document the conference and decision reached in the chart.

ventilation. This would enable future decision making to occur in the context of known patient wishes, physician judgments about what procedures would be medically reasonable, and family concerns. For example, a patient with metastatic colon cancer and liver metastases could specify that she would want to try some palliative chemotherapy but could also place a high priority on dying at home with a husband who agrees to be a full-time caregiver when needed.

However, few Americans have advance directives or living wills, and even when they exist, studies indicate that these documents are ignored by medical staff. Several barriers prevent advance-care planning from being more effective. First, neither physicians nor patients tend to raise the issue early in the course of illness. The possibility of future treatment failure is uncomfortable for both parties, and few physicians have been trained in the required communication skills. Second, the advance directives rarely address cancer-specific problems. Most living wills address situations of irreversible coma, for instance, because of rare but well-publicized cases of young adults in persistent vegetative states; unfortunately, these situations are usually irrelevant to patients with colon cancer. Third, the advance directives are sometimes not known to medical staff. In the SUPPORT study, which included patients with metastatic colon cancer and liver metastases who were admitted to intensive care units, physicians rarely knew patient preferences for CPR and were often unaware that a patient had filled out an advance directive.[18]

Advance directives might be more useful to patients with colorectal cancer and physicians if they addressed the problems a cancer patient is likely to encounter. Berry and Singer have developed a cancer-specific advance directive that discusses a variety of issues specifically related to advanced cancer[19]; the will is available on the World Wide Web at www.utoronto.ca/jcb. This living will was developed through a process of literature review, key informant interviews, and focus groups and has undergone testing with patients that showed that most patients preferred this living will to a generic living will. The subject areas it asks patients about are CPR, mechanical ventilation, radiation therapy, chemotherapy, surgery, blood product transfusion, antibiotics, and tube feeding. However, even a cancer-specific living will is at best a very general guide for future decision making. It is important for patients to identify a surrogate, or proxy, decision maker who can represent the patient's wishes if the patient becomes incapacitated.

Two interventions not specifically addressed in the Singer living will are important for physicians to discuss because of the empirical data describing patient outcomes: intensive unit care and CPR for patients with metastatic cancer. The prognosis is poor for cancer patients admitted to an intensive care unit (ICU) for reasons other than recovery from planned surgery. In one study, approximately 75 percent of cancer patients admitted to an ICU who survived to hospital discharge lived less than 3 months. In the most comprehensive mortality prediction model that has been developed to date specifically for cancer patients admitted to an ICU, Groeger identified three cancer-specific variables as significant: allogeneic bone marrow transplantation, disease progression, and poor performance status (all correlate with increased mortality).[20] The other 13 variables include laboratory values (such as PaO_2/FiO_2) and clinical variables (such as days of hospitalization before ICU admission). This model may prove more useful for patients with cancer but was developed in four tertiary cancer centers and has not been validated in other settings.

Patients with metastatic cancer who undergo in-hospital cardiopulmonary resuscitation are unlikely to survive to discharge. A review of studies, summarized by Faber-Langendoen, revealed that 0 percent of patients with metastatic cancer survived to hospital discharge after in-hospital CPR,[21] even though some patients initially responded. A meta-analysis of CPR-survival studies identified metastatic cancer as highly associated with failure to survive to discharge. Thus, physicians should counsel patients with advanced metastatic colorectal cancer that ICU transfers and CPR at the time of death are unlikely to meaningfully prolong life.

Referring Patients to Hospice

In most areas of the U.S., hospice is a system of home care delivered by a multidisciplinary team aiming to address physical, psychological, social, and spiritual issues as the patient approaches death. Most insurers follow the Medicare standard of patient eligibility at

6 months estimated survival. Yet most patients are referred much closer to death—often days before death. Some patients resist referral because they feel this represents loss of hope and loss of continuity with their cancer care team, whom they often know extremely well. But the most important barrier to hospice utilization is failure of physician referral. The reasons are assumed to be that physicians resist referral because they fail to recognize that the patient is near death or because their medical systems do not facilitate ways to maintain continuity of care after hospice referral. Hospices are an underutilized resource for end-of-life care for patients with cancer.

PSYCHOLOGICAL ISSUES

Distress

Distress is a common psychosocial aspect of cancer experience. An expert panel for the National Comprehensive Cancer Network developed the following definition: Distress is an unpleasant emotional experience of a psychological (cognitive, behavioral, emotional), social, and/or spiritual nature that interferes with the ability to cope effectively with cancer and its treatment.[22] Distress extends along a continuum, ranging from common normal feelings of vulnerability, sadness, and fear to problems that can become disabling, such as depression, anxiety, panic, social isolation, and spiritual crisis. Distress can be a normal response to cancer, along with sadness, worry, and fear, but distress levels can rise to encompass depression requiring intervention. Because oncologists often miss distress,[23] a screening tool, which is graphically represented as a thermometer, and an interview guide (Table 13–3) have been developed to facilitate inquiry into psychosocial problems. These tools are useful as guides even though the outcomes of their use are not yet documented.

Anxiety

There is little literature specifically documenting anxiety disorders in patients with colorectal cancer. However, anxiety is one of the most common reasons for psychosocial consultation. Patients with anxiety find their minds filled with recurring, intru-

sive thoughts and images of cancer. Their thinking tends to focus on catastrophic events and often casts the patient as a helpless victim in an uncontrollable situation. These thoughts can be accompanied by autonomic arousal such as tachycardia, sweating, and a sinking sensation in the stomach. Medical procedures, including blood draws and CT scans, are common triggers for anxiety. Oncologists and primary care providers can make the diagnosis of anxiety and prescribe pharmacologic management with benzodiazepines, and also consider referral to other psychosocial clinicians for psychotherapy, behavioral techniques, support groups, or more complex pharmacologic management.

Table 13–3. DISTRESS MANAGEMENT
During the past week, how distressed have you been?
Extreme distress = 10
No distress = 0
Check the causes of your distress
Practical problems
housing
insurance
work/school
transportation
child care
Family problems
dealing with partner
dealing with children
Emotional problems
worry
sadness
depression
nervousness
Spiritual/religious concerns
relating to God
loss of faith
other problems
Physical problems
pain
nausea
fatigue
sleep
getting around
bathing/dressing
breathing
mouth sores
indigestion
constipation/diarrhea
bowel changes
changes in urination
fevers
skin dry/itchy
nose dry/congested
tingling in hands/feet
feeling swollen
sexual

From NCCN.[22]

Depression

There are no data specifically addressing the prevalence of depression in patients with colorectal cancer, although studies of patients with advanced cancer (all diagnoses included) found from one-quarter to one-half of patients were depressed.[24] In patients with cancer, the diagnosis of depression depends on psychological symptoms of dysphoric mood, feelings of helplessness and hopelessness, loss of self-esteem, and feelings of worthlessness or guilt. In one study, the screening question "Are you depressed?" was found to be useful.[25] Somatic symptoms such as weight loss or anorexia are often not useful clues to depression in these patients because of the possibility that the symptoms are caused by treatment side effects or disease progression. In patients who are terminally ill, a major difficulty is sorting out depression from sadness and grief. Block suggests that grief characteristically comes in waves, that grieving patients retain a capacity for pleasure, and that their feelings relate to specific losses.[26] Depressed patients have unremitting gloom, enjoy nothing, and tend to generalize distress to all facets of their life. For oncologists and primary care providers, the important tasks are to recognize depression, initiate treatment with pharmacologic medications[27] such as serotonin reuptake inhibitors or, for patients with advanced cancer, psychostimulants such as Ritalin, and consider referral to a psychosocial clinician for psychotherapy.

Fear and Grief

For patients who are near dying, two major issues are fear and grief. Fear arises from the patient's reaction to imminent death. Grief is the reaction to the ongoing and future losses entailed by dying.[13] Oncologists and primary-care physicians are often in a unique position to help people through turning points in their lives such as cancer, cancer treatment, and approaching death. Even though fear and grief may not be a primary focus for most oncologists, a small degree of attention to this area can be surprisingly rewarding. It is extremely useful to ask about fears, as this can help patients articulate feelings they did not themselves know about. Since fear tends to aggravate itself, simply naming and acknowledging fears is important. A plan for medical care can then take into account the patient's fears and address the fears explicitly. Physicians should not assume they know what a particular patient fears. Similarly, for an oncologist to simply acknowledge a patient's grief can be extremely therapeutic. More extensive approaches to dealing with grief and loss are available.[5]

SYMPTOM CONTROL

Pain Management

The principles of dependence, tolerance, and addiction should be well understood when prescribing the often-needed opioid therapy for analgesia of cancer pain. Dependence is a normal physiologic response to chronic use of opioid therapy and will cause withdrawal symptoms if opioids are abruptly discontinued. Physical dependence does not preclude withdrawal of medications but does warrant a tapering of drug when withdrawal is indicated. Tolerance is a normal physiologic response to chronic opioid therapy in which increasing doses of drug may be needed to produce the same effect. Increases in dosage usually indicate progressive disease. Psychological dependence or addiction is an abnormal behavioral response that involves a compulsion to take the opioid drug on a continuous or periodic basis to experience its psychic effects. It may be associated with destructive behaviors and with forsaking other interests or needs in order to obtain access to the opioid.

In general, the WHO analgesic ladder can be followed for the treatment of pain. Mild pain is treated with non-opioids such as nonsteroidal anti-inflammatory drugs (NSAIDs) and acetaminophen. Moderate and severe pain are treated with opioid analgesics. The so-called weak opioids, codeine and hydrocodone, may be limited by their composition with acetaminophen or aspirin. Total daily dose of acetaminophen should not exceed 4 g; fatalities have been reported at 7.5 g/day. Since acetaminophen is 95 percent excreted by the liver, caution should be taken when prescribing the drug for patients with liver metastases and potentially compromised organ function. The strong opioids include morphine, oxycodone, hydromorphone, fentanyl, and methadone. Adjuvant analgesics usually include tricyclic antidepressants such as amitriptyline, desipramine, or nortriptyline and anticonvulsant agents such as gabapentin and valproic acid for the treatment of neuropathic pain. Steroids such as dexamethasone and prednisone may also be used, especially to treat pain associated with new-onset nerve compression. Mexilitine, the anti-arrhythmic, can be used for refractory neuropathic pain.

The importance of the use of non-opioid analgesics should be underscored as the NSAIDs in particular are very effective therapies for the treatment of metastatic bone pain. They are also an effective class of drugs to use for night sweats, skin pain (allodynia), and diaphoresis associated with intravenous (IV) morphine. Side effects include the commonly seen gastrointestinal effects of dyspepsia and peptic ulcer disease and less commonly headache, confusion, anxiety, fluid retention, elevated liver function tests, and urticaria. One of the most useful of the NSAIDs is choline magnesium trisalicylate because of its minimal gastrointestinal intolerance. It can be dosed from 500 to 2,000 mg PO bid. The widely used and efficacious ibuprofen can be administered at 400 to 800 mg PO to a maximum of 3,200 mg/day.

The use of strong opioids is frequently appropriate in patients with metastatic disease and chronic pain. Dosing should be around the clock, rather than prn, in order to gain adequate control over chronic pain and limit its associated complications, including inactivity, fatigue, anorexia, insomnia, and others. Morphine sulfate is the gold standard, based as much on its frequency of use in studies and greater level of clinical experience and comfort as on its reasonable cost. General recommendations are to begin at 15 to 30 mg PO q4h with breakthrough dosing qh. Immediate release preparations are available in a variety of forms, including capsules, oral and IV solutions, sublingual, suppositories, and tablets. Long-acting morphine may be given every 8 to 12 hours but must not be chewed or crushed as this will render it short-acting. Equianalgesic scales are available to convert dosing of either weak to strong opioids or from one opioid

to another. Due to differences in cross-tolerance between opioids, when calculating a conversion from one opioid drug to another, a reduction of 25 to 50 percent of the total daily dose should be made in order to avoid the onset of undesirable side effects related to overmedication. Rescue doses should always be made available when this type of drug conversion occurs (Table 13–4).

Always begin a bowel regimen of a stool softener and a laxative when starting chronic opioid therapy. Tolerance to the constipating side effect of opioids rarely develops. By contrast, fortunately, tolerance to nausea usually develops within approximately 3 days but should be treated with routine antiemetics in the interim. Sedation from opioid therapy, if it occurs, will likely resolve in a similar period of time.

Anorexia

One of the most disturbing symptoms for the family, although usually not for the patient, is loss of appetite. It should be distinguished from early satiety, a sense of feeling full after minimal oral intake, which may develop as a consequence of ascites or hepatomegaly. Early satiety is best treated by encouraging small and frequent meals. Some causes of anorexia, such as poorly fitting dentures or loss of taste for particular foods, can be easily corrected. In general, treatment of anorexia often begins with explaining to the family the frequency of this symptom in advanced cancer and listening to their fears and concerns. It is important to both discourage the sense of trying to force feedings when not desired and to encourage offering small amounts of the patient's favorite foods. Physicians should acknowledge that time spent with the patient is valuable and that it need not be associated with typical social customs involving food. Medical therapies for the treatment of anorexia include megestrol acetate 180 to 800 mg PO qd, prednisone 15 to 30 mg PO qam, and dronabinol 2.5 to 20 mg PO bid. Dietary supplementation may be assisted with the use of high-calorie nutritional drinks, such as Ensure. The use of nasogastric, gastrostomy, or jejunostomy feeding, however, is unlikely to reverse anorexia and resultant cachexia. Although tube feeds may be appropriate for patients with mechanical difficulties who otherwise require and desire nutrition, hyperalimentation is rarely an appropriate or comfortable

Table 13–4. PAIN MANAGEMENT

Key principles for using opioids

1. Use long-acting opioids as the mainstay of treatment and provide breakthrough doses of short-acting opioids.

2. Treat side effects promptly so that patients do not decrease opioids and compromise pain relief.

3. Use an equianalgesic table if switching opioids and adjust the new dose downwards by 25% to allow for cross-tolerance.

PO/PR (mg)	Analgesic	SC/IV/IM (mg)
100	codeine	60
15	hydrocodone	—
4	hydromorphone	1.5
15	morphine	5
10	oxycodone	—

4. Be careful to distinguish inadequate pain control from addiction, a psychological syndrome of use despite harm that rarely develops as a consequence of cancer pain treatment.

component of a patient's end-of-life care. It should be noted that there is no scientific evidence that tube feeding avoids risks of aspiration. Spoon feeding, although more labor intensive, at least provides the patient with an opportunity for oral gratification and the family with a means to provide comfort and enjoyment for the patient.

Ascites

The development of ascites may be associated with the presence of metastatic carcinoma on the serosal surface of the bowel, thereby increasing oncotic pressure, leading to third-spacing of fluids. Ascites may also occur secondary to hepatic infiltration of tumor, hepatomegaly, and passive congestion of venous flow to the liver. Complete portal venous thrombus (Budd-Chiari syndrome) may lead to the rapid development of ascites. Considerable ascites often cause symptoms that include abdominal pain or distension, impaired intestinal motility, early satiety, dyspepsia, nausea and vomiting, peripheral edema, and dyspnea.

The treatment of malignant ascites can be challenging. Although paracentesis is a relatively simple bedside procedure and may be guided by ultrasound placement of the catheter if the presence of ascites is in doubt or loculated ascites is suspected, its duration of palliation is often measured in days. It should be reserved for instances in which symptoms are signif-

icant: dyspnea, inability to lie supine, or abdominal pain. Long-term shunting of malignant ascites with a peritoneovenous catheter is feasible but is associated with infectious and thrombotic risks as well as the development of disseminated intravascular coagulation (DIC); generally, shunts function for only a few weeks or months. Medical therapy is centered on diuretics, including spironolactone and furosemide. The suggested doses are spironolactone 200 mg PO plus furosemide 40 mg PO qd, although they may be increased to spironolactone 200 mg PO bid plus furosemide 120 mg PO qd. Furosemide should be given on an empty stomach and with the patient lying recumbent for 2 hours after administration. The onset of action of spironolactone is longer, approximately 5 to 7 days. Since it is a potassium-sparing diuretic, supplemental potassium should not routinely be given. It is important to keep in mind that analgesics are also needed to treat the pain associated with ascites. Opioids will exacerbate bowel stasis, which may already be compromised by disease. Stool softeners and laxatives should always be started concomitantly with opioid analgesia, unless the particular clinical situation dictates otherwise.

Constipation

Constipation may occur as a side effect of diminished activity, opioid analgesia, and in conjunction with a partial bowel obstruction. The most common cause of intestinal obstruction is stool. A colonic fecal impaction with significant constipation may lead to watery diarrhea, as stool is passed through a narrow lumen around an impaction. Once constipation develops, it is critical to determine that a colonic impaction is not present and that a complete bowel obstruction does not exist. If there has been no bowel movement in 2 to 3 days, a digital rectal examination should be performed before oral laxatives are administered as the peristaltic action against a fixed obstruction may cause a bowel perforation. When obstipation is suspected and manual disimpaction is not successful, oil retention or soap suds enemas may be effective. A high colonic, a good therapy for impacted stool, consists of 2 liters of body-temperature warmed saline infused into the rectum from ceiling height over 30 minutes using gravity to infuse the solution. When possible, the patient should be encouraged to ambulate and be adequately hydrated, preferably with fruit juices. Commodes and hand rails by toilet seats allow patients to use their abdominal muscles when trying to move their bowels and may be much more effective than a bedpan.

Prevention is the best defense against constipation. All patients on opioids must be on laxatives. Prevention of constipation may be effected by judicious use of laxatives and stool softeners when opioid analgesia is started. Since opioids induce constipation by enhancing intestinal ring contractions, the most effective therapy is a stimulant laxative that relaxes ring contractions. It is generally important to combine a stool softener with a stimulant laxative; rectal suppositories, enemas, and digital evacuation may also be necessary. Frequent recommendations include Senekot plus a stool softener (Senekot-S), once-daily dosing with no maximum dose. Lactulose and sorbitol 30 to 60 mL PO qd may also be used, with no maximum dose, at 2-hour intervals until bowel movement. Since these compounds are osmotic laxatives, the patient must be well hydrated. Milk of magnesia 30 mL combined with cascara 5 mL or prune juice 30 mL is also an effective combination. However, it should be expected that up to one-third of patients will require rectal measures, such as suppositories, enemas, and manual removals, in addition to oral medications.

Intestinal Obstruction

Bowel obstruction may be caused by a variety of factors, including cancerous tumor growth; benign adhesions or hernia from a prior surgical procedure; postradiation bowel changes, relevant more so for patients with a history of rectal cancer; immobility; and medications. Intraluminal tumor blockage may lead to intestinal obstruction and watery diarrhea. If the patient's life expectancy is greater than 2 months, functional status is good, and a reversible cause is anticipated, then nasogastric suction followed by a diverting surgical procedure should be considered. Surgical management is generally inappropriate in cases of peritoneal carcinomatosis, rapidly reaccumulating ascites, or when a prior laparotomy would preclude a successful diversion procedure. Prolonged nasogastric suction is not ideal for symptom relief as it is itself uncomfort-

able. The treatment of intestinal obstruction is focused on the treatment of pain, the obstruction itself, and associated symptoms of nausea, vomiting, anxiety, and colicky pain. Pain should be treated with morphine or dilaudid PR or IV. In order to administer medication per rectum, the rectum should be completely cleaned of stool. Treatment of the obstruction and its associated symptoms of nausea and vomiting usually requires multiple medications with different modes of action. If the patient has mild or no colic and is able to pass flatus, a prokinetic drug such as metoclopramide is acceptable. Prokinetic drugs, however, are contraindicated for those with severe colic or who are not passing flatus. Instead, an antispasmodic and antisecretory drug should be used. Several commonly used combinations include metoclopramide 20 mg, decadron 8 mg, haloperidol 1 mg in suppository form or metoclopramide 3 mg/hr, decadron 1.5 mg/hr, and haloperidol 0.25 mg/hr administered intravenously. A subcutaneous preparation includes decadron 1.5 mg/hr, haloperidol 0.25 mg/hr, and midazolam (versed) 0.125 mg/hr. The use of steroids in bowel obstruction is controversial but may be effective for reducing local edema and improving patency of the bowel lumen.

When a complete obstruction exists, somatostatin can be considered at a dose of 100 µg subcutaneously (SQ) tid or 10 µg/hr to a maximum of 600 µg/24 hr as an antisecretory agent. 5-HT3-receptor antagonists may be useful as increased intraluminal pressure results in the release of serotonin from the enterochromaffin cells in the bowel wall. For the treatment of colicky pain, dicyclomine hydrochloride 20 to 40 mg PO qid is recommended. Rectal manipulation with digital examination followed by a soap suds, milk, or molasses enema may be used. Oral laxatives such as lactulose should be used with extreme caution and only if no nausea or vomiting exists. If the symptoms of intestinal obstruction improve, the patient may be weaned off medications. Laxatives, however, should be increased. On occasion, patients may experience spontaneous remission of intestinal obstruction. When malignant intestinal obstruction is refractory to symptomatic therapy in a dying patient, terminal sedation may be appropriate.

Dehydration

In the last days and hours of life, dehydration is common but not painful, as evidenced by observations of thousands. The symptoms of mouth dryness can easily be treated with adequate mouth care, including artificial saliva, ice chips, and a wet sponge applied to the lips. Intravenous fluids may be appropriate to counteract symptoms of discomfort brought on by dehydration, such as confusion and disorientation related to alterations in serum sodium or calcium. However, intravenous hydration does not treat symptoms of thirst, and when patients refuse oral food and drink because of anorexia-cachexia, they will likely gain no improvement in symptom control from the addition of intravenous fluids or nutrition. A time-limited trial of 2 to 3 days may be appropriate to determine if symptoms improve with IV or SQ hydration, but prolonged periods of IV rehydration in the moribund patient ultimately leads to worsening edema, anasarca, and increased respiratory secretions.

Diarrhea

There are many potential causes of diarrhea, including laxative overuse, fecal impaction, and partial bowel obstruction, as well as treatment-related causes. Diarrhea may occur as a side effect of chemotherapy and/or radiotherapy. Both 5-fluorouracil and irinotecan, the most commonly used drugs for the treatment of metastatic colorectal cancer, have diarrhea as one of their dose-limiting toxicities. It is critical to treat these symptoms immediately as they can be life threatening when severe. Loperamide 4 mg PO followed by 2 mg PO should be judiciously used after each loose stool to a maximum dosage of 32 mg/day, although it is rare for use to exceed 16 mg/day. Diphenoxylate 2 tablets or 10 mL PO qid may also be used. Paregoric (camphorated tincture of opium) is frequently effective when the former agents are not. It is administered in liquid form 4 to 8 mL PO after each loose stool to a maximum of 32 mL/day. Codeine 30 to 60 mg PO may be given bid or qid but may be associated with nausea.

Severe refractory diarrhea, as can be associated with carcinoid syndrome, may require treatment with somatostatin 100 to 600 µg/day, given in two to four divided doses IV/SQ over 24 hours or as a continuous infusion at 4 to 24 µg/hr IV/SQ. Diarrhea secondary to radiation therapy may respond to sucralfate 1 g PO qid.

Mucositis

Apart from diarrhea and myelosuppression, mucositis is the next most common symptom suffered by patients receiving treatment for colorectal cancer. It may be treated with a variety of medications, including analgesics, antifungals, and antivirals. The mainstay of therapy is a mouthwash providing analgesia. Diphenhydramine and viscous lidocaine usually serve as the analgesic and may be combined with oral fluconazole 100 mg/10 mL, prednisone 15 mg/5 mL, and tetracycline 125 mg/5 mL. Generally, equal proportions of these compounds are mixed into a mouthwash, then taken 15 to 30 mL PO qid swish and swallow. For the particular treatment of oropharyngeal thrush, the following regimens are effective for the treatment of oropharyngeal thrush: fluconazole 200 mg PO qd × 1 week, followed by 100 mg PO qd × 1 week; nystatin 100,000 units/mL, 5 to 10 mL PO qid swish and swallow; clotrimazole troche qid. If pain does not resolve despite these treatments, then herpetic infection should be suspected. Famcyclovir 500 mg PO tid × 5 to 7 days and acyclovir 200 mg 5 ×/day × 1 week are the recommended treatments. Sucralfate liquid 5 mL PO qid swish and swallow may be useful for generalized oral discomfort. If significant oropharyngeal bleeding is associated with the mucositis, aminocaproic acid 3.75 g (15 mL) PO qid with viscous lidocaine swish and swallow may be effective.

Nausea and Vomiting

The etiology of nausea and vomiting may direct the clinician to the most effective therapy for its treatment. There are four general etiologies: cerebral cortex, chemoreceptor trigger zone, constipation, and vestibular alteration. Etiologies stemming from the cerebral cortex include meningeal carcinomatosis, metastatic intraparenchymal disease, and meningitis. Treatment is with dexamethasone 4 mg PO qid and lorazepam 0.5 to 1 mg PO q4h. The chemoreceptor trigger zone is likely to be an etiology given the multiplicity of syndromes that involve this pathway, including chemotherapy, dehydration, hepatic capsule distension, hypercalcemia, medication-related or radiation-induced renal failure, and syndrome of inappropriate antidiuretic hormone (SIADH). Treatment for this etiology of nausea and vomiting should include dopaminergic agents such as prochlorperazine 15 mg PO or 25 mg PR qid, haloperidol 1 mg PO or PR bid-tid, metoclopramide 10 to 20 mg PO or PR qid, steroidal agents such as dexamethasone 2 mg PO or PR qid, benzodiazepines such as lorazepam 0.5 mg PO or PR qid, and 5-HT3 antagonists such as ondansetron 8 mg PO tid, granisetron 1 mg PO qd, or dolasetron 100 mg qd. Mechanical causes of nausea and vomiting are usually related to constipation as a result of medications or obstruction secondary to tumor. Treatment is directed at correcting the constipation, providing antiemetic therapy with dopaminergic antagonists such as prochlorperazine, steroids such as dexamethasone, and promotility agents such as metoclopramide. Vestibular alteration is usually related to bone metastases at the skull base or tumors at the base of the skull. Therapy may include the previously mentioned agents as well as meclizine 25 mg PO bid.

Pruritus

Pruritus occurring in metastatic colorectal cancer is usually a result of hepatic insufficiency and impaired bile adsorption. Cholestyramine 1 to 2 packets/day is frequently helpful, as can be 5-HT3 antagonists. Correcting skin dryness may be beneficial. Keep nails clipped closely and discourage scratching. Use ointments or creams as soap substitutes. Avoid overheating or hot baths.

Delirium

Hepatic insufficiency is generally the etiology of delirium in patients with advanced colorectal cancer. Protective measures should be taken to shield the patient from harm. Encourage the family to focus on the lucid intervals and be certain to treat the patient with the same degree of respect. Avoid restraints and bedrails and always provide accompaniment for the patient when walking. Reduce unnecessary medications and

use low doses of haloperidol 1.5 to 5 mg PO, maintaining qd or bid dosing once the symptom is well controlled. Terminal agitation may occur rather than progressive somnolence. It should be treated with an increased dose of haloperidol of 10 to 30 mg/24 hours with the addition of a benzodiazepine.

Fatigue

When possible, attempt to identify an etiology of fatigue. On occasion, laboratory abnormalities may be corrected and fatigue will improve. The sedation caused by opioids will diminish as tolerance develops; alternatively, opioid-induced sedation may be effectively relieved by altering opioid agents while still maintaining adequate analgesia. Psychostimulants such as methyphenidate may relieve opioid-induced sedation without compromising adequate analgesia. If anorexia is a significant contributor to the sensation of fatigue, then an appetite stimulant such as megestrol acetate may be helpful. Megestrol acetate has been shown to be an effective agent for the treatment of fatigue even when a catabolic state cannot be reversed. It should be noted, however, that aggressive nutrition has not been noted to improve significantly the sensation of fatigue in cancer patients. Erythropoietin has been demonstrated to improve fatigue related to chemotherapy-induced anemia in patients with cancer. The usual starting dose of erythropoietin for this indication is 10,000U SQ tiw, with dose escalation if no response is observed.

More comprehensive guides to symptom management are available.[5,6,28]

CONCLUSION

Palliative care is comprehensive, interdisciplinary care, focusing primarily on promoting quality of life for patients and their families. In the past, hospice and palliative care were considered only when anticancer therapy had been exhausted. However, many patients with colorectal cancer could benefit from palliative care delivered earlier in the course of their illness. Key elements of palliative care include communication skills, management of psychological issues, and symptom control. Other important aspects of palliative care, such as spiritual or existential issues, are addressed in more comprehensive references.

ACKOWLEDGMENT

The principal investigator and first author of this chapter is an employee of the U.S. government whose work is in the public domain. The views of the contributors do not necessarily reflect the view or policies of the U.S. government.

REFERENCES

1. Billings JA. What is palliative care? J Palliat Med 1998; 1:73–81.
2. Hewitt M, Simone JV. Ensuring quality cancer care. Washington, DC: National Academy Press; 1999.
3. Field MJ, Cassel CK. Approaching death. Improving care at the end of life. Washington, DC: National Academy Press; 1997.
4. Midgley R, Kerr D. Colorectal cancer. Lancet 1999; 353:391–9.
5. Doyle D, Hanks GWC, MacDonald N. Oxford textbook of palliative medicine. New York: Oxford University Press; 1998.
6. Berger A, Portenoy RK, Weissman D. Principles and practice of supportive oncology. Philadelphia: Lippincott-Raven; 1998.
7. Butow PN, Kazemi JN, Beeney LJ, et al. When the diagnosis is cancer: patient communication experiences and preferences. Cancer 1996;77:2630–7.
8. Buckman R. How to break bad news: a guide for health care professionals. Baltimore: Johns Hopkins University Press, 1992.
9. Richards MA, Ramirez AJ, Degner LF, et al. Offering choice of treatment to patients with cancers. A review based on a symposium held at the 10th annual conference of The British Psychosocial Oncology Group, December 1993. Eur J Cancer 1995;1:112–6.
10. Daugherty C, Ratain MJ, Grochowski E, et al. Perceptions of cancer patients and their physicians involved in phase I trials [published erratum appears in J Clin Oncol 1995;13:2476]. J Clin Oncol 1995;13: 1062–72.
11. Christakis NA, Lamont EB. Extent and determinants of error in doctors' prognoses in terminally ill patients: prospective cohort study. BMJ 2000;320:469–73.
12. Weeks JC, Cook EF, O'Day SJ, et al. Relationship between cancer patients' predictions of prognosis and their treatment preferences. JAMA 1998; 279:1709–14.
13. Parkes CM, Markus A. Coping with loss: helping patients and their families. London: BMJ Books; 1998.
14. Bernhard J, Hurny C. Gastrointestinal Cancer. In: Holland J, editor. Psychooncology. New York: Oxford; 1998. p. 324–39.
15. Schag CA, Ganz PA, Wing DS. Quality of life in adult survivors of lung, colon, and prostate cancers. Qual Life Res 1994;2:127–41.
16. Maguire P, Walsh S, Jeacock J, Kingston R. Physical and psychological needs of patients dying from colorectal cancer. Palliat Med 1999;13:45–50.
17. Faulkner A, Maguire P. Talking to cancer patients and their relatives. New York: Oxford University Press; 1994.
18. Teno JM, Licks S, Lynn J, et al. Do advance directives provide instructions that direct care? SUPPORT Investigators. Study to Understand Prognoses and Preferences for Outcomes and Risks of Treatment. J Am Geriatr Soc 1997;45:508–12.
19. Berry SR, Singer PA. The cancer specific advance directive. Cancer 1998;82:1570–7.
20. Groeger JS, Lemeshow S, Price K, et al. Multicenter outcome study of cancer patients admitted to the intensive care unit: a probability of mortality model. J Clin Oncol 1998;16:761–70.
21. Faber-Langendoen K. Resuscitation of patients with metastatic cancer. Is transient benefit still futile? Arch Intern Med 1991;151:235–9.
22. NCCN practice guidelines for the management of psychosocial distress. National Comprehensive Cancer Network. Oncology (Huntingt) 1999;13:113–47.
23. Ford S, Fallowfield L, Lewis S. Can oncologists detect distress in their out-patients and how satisfied are they with their performance during bad news consultations? Br J Cancer 1994;70:767–70.
24. Sellick SM, Crooks DL. Depression and cancer: an appraisal of the literature for prevalence, detection, and practice guideline development for psychological interventions. Psychooncology 1999;8:315–33.
25. Chochinov HM, Wilson KG, Enns M, Lander S. "Are you depressed?" Screening for depression in the terminally ill. Am J Psychiatry 1997;154:674–6.
26. Block SD. Assessing and managing depression in the terminally ill patient. ACP-ASIM End-of-Life Care Consensus Panel. American College of Physicians-American Society of Internal Medicine. Ann Intern Med 2000;132:209–18.
27. Petitto JM, Evans DL. Treatment of depression in individuals with cancer: implications of antidepressant pharmacotherapy. Semin Clin Neuropsychiatry 1998;3:131–6.
28. Twycross RG. Symptom management in advanced cancer. Abingdon: Radcliff Medical Press; 1997.

Index